2017
Nelson's Pediatric Antimicrobial Therapy

23rd Edition

John S. Bradley, MD
Editor in Chief

John D. Nelson, MD
Emeritus

Elizabeth D. Barnett, MD
Joseph B. Cantey, MD
David W. Kimberlin, MD
Paul E. Palumbo, MD
Jason Sauberan, PharmD
William J. Steinbach, MD
Contributing Editors

American Academy of Pediatrics

DEDICATED TO THE HEALTH OF ALL CHILDREN®

American Academy of Pediatrics Publishing Staff

Mark Grimes, *Director, Department of Publishing*
Peter Lynch, *Manager, Digital Strategy and Product Development*
Barrett Winston, *Senior Editor, Professional and Clinical Publishing*
Shannan Martin, *Production Manager, Consumer Publications*
Jason Crase, *Manager, Editorial Services*
Mary Lou White, *Director, Department of Marketing and Sales*
Linda Smessaert, MSIMC, *Marketing Manager, Professional Publications*

Published by the American Academy of Pediatrics
141 Northwest Point Blvd, Elk Grove Village, IL 60007-1019
847/434-4000
Facsimile: 847/434-8000
www.aap.org

The recommendations in this publication do not indicate an exclusive course of treatment or serve as a standard of medical care. Variations, taking into account individual circumstances, may be appropriate.
Statements and opinions expressed are those of the authors and not necessarily those of the American Academy of Pediatrics.
Web sites are mentioned for informational purposes only and do not imply an endorsement by the American Academy of Pediatrics. Web site addresses are as current as possible but may change at any time.
Brand names are furnished for identifying purposes only. No endorsement of the manufacturers or products listed is implied.
This publication has been developed by the American Academy of Pediatrics. The authors, editors, and contributors are expert authorities in the field of pediatrics. No commercial involvement of any kind has been solicited or accepted in the development of the content of this publication.
Every effort has been made to ensure that the drug selection and dosages set forth in this text are in accordance with current recommendations and practice at the time of publication. It is the responsibility of the health care professional to check the package insert of each drug for any change in indications or dosage and for added warnings and precautions.
Special discounts are available for bulk purchases of this publication. E-mail our Special Sales Department at aapsales@aap.org for more information.
Please see our Web site for content-related notices and updates: www.aap.org/nelsonsabx.

Printed in the United States of America.
9-378/1216   1 2 3 4 5 6 7 8 9 10
MA0809
ISSN: 2164-9278 (print)
ISSN: 2164-9286 (electronic)
ISBN: 978-1-61002-074-9
eBook: 978-1-61002-075-6

Editor in Chief

John S. Bradley, MD
Professor of Pediatrics
Chief, Division of Infectious Diseases,
    Department of Pediatrics
University of California, San Diego,
    School of Medicine
Director, Division of Infectious Diseases,
    Rady Children's Hospital San Diego
San Diego, CA

Emeritus

John D. Nelson, MD
Professor Emeritus of Pediatrics
The University of Texas
Southwestern Medical Center at Dallas
Southwestern Medical School
Dallas, TX

Contributing Editors

Elizabeth D. Barnett, MD
Professor of Pediatrics
Boston University School of Medicine
Director, International Clinic and Refugee
    Health Assessment Program,
    Boston Medical Center
GeoSentinel Surveillance Network,
    Boston Medical Center
Boston, MA

Joseph B. Cantey, MD
Assistant Professor of Pediatrics
Divisions of Pediatric Infectious Diseases and
    Neonatology/Perinatal Medicine
Texas A&M Health Science Center
Baylor/Scott and White Health
Dallas, TX

David W. Kimberlin, MD
Professor of Pediatrics
Codirector, Division of Pediatric
    Infectious Diseases
Sergio Stagno Endowed Chair in
    Pediatric Infectious Diseases
University of Alabama at Birmingham
Birmingham, AL

Paul E. Palumbo, MD
Professor of Pediatrics and Medicine
Geisel School of Medicine at Dartmouth
Director, International Pediatric HIV Program
Dartmouth-Hitchcock Medical Center
Lebanon, NH

Jason Sauberan, PharmD
Assistant Clinical Professor
University of California, San Diego,
    Skaggs School of Pharmacy and
    Pharmaceutical Sciences
Rady Children's Hospital San Diego
San Diego, CA

William J. Steinbach, MD
Professor of Pediatrics
Professor in Molecular Genetics
    and Microbiology
Chief, Division of Pediatric Infectious Diseases
Director, International Pediatric Fungal
    Network
Duke University School of Medicine
Durham, NC

Contents

Introduction

Welcome to the 23rd edition of *Nelson's Pediatric Antimicrobial Therapy*, now 42 years since the first edition was created by John Nelson and shipped from his garage from his home in Dallas, TX. He had decided to put down his thoughts in a small pocketbook to help clinicians select the most appropriate therapy for children with infections! The book has grown extensively since the first edition, and the printed version does not so easily fit in one's pocket. We continue our close and productive collaboration with the American Academy of Pediatrics (AAP) to address the important infectious diseases in childhood and the antimicrobials available to treat them. We hope to provide clinicians with accurate, relevant, practical, and easily accessed information as they care for children. We are very pleased that many providers appreciate the references that we share in the print and app versions so they can get the important facts that go into our recommendations for therapy. The references are designed to share important studies and reviews so clinicians may take our suggestions and use them to help treat children with unusual infections or unusual presentations of common infections.

Jason Sauberan continues to carefully update the antimicrobial drugs and dosages for all children, an increasing challenge (Chapter 11), with particular attention to children with obesity (Chapter 12) and neonates (Chapter 5), which he writes with JB Cantey (under the watchful eye of Pablo Sanchez) and John van den Anker, a neonatologist/pharmacologist from Children's National Medical Center, Washington, DC, who has again generously agreed to review our neonatal antibiotic chapter. Neonatal pharmacology of antimicrobials continues to be an area of intense study. We help with the writing of the AAP *Red Book* (an official policy of the AAP, approved by its Board of Directors). Although the *Nelson's* book is not official policy, the doses and drugs recommended should be very similar between the two.

All of our editors have substantial clinical weeks "on service," which clearly shows in the insights provided by the antimicrobial recommendations, particularly for difficult infections. They are some of the best clinicians in the field of pediatric infectious diseases, all having academic interests in performing investigations to find out which newer as well as older agents work best to treat infections. They take the time, working with the AAP, to provide advice and insight into their particular areas of interest, knowledge, and experience. The "Comments" columns in this book's tables are designed to provide a personal discussion on some interesting or controversial areas that may be very important for managing children.

The advice, experience, and knowledge of published/unpublished data are provided with a grading of our recommendations: our assessment of how strongly we feel about a recommendation and the strength of the evidence to support our recommendation (noted on the next page).

Strength of Recommendation	Description
A	Strongly recommended
B	Recommended as a good choice
C	One option for therapy that is adequate, perhaps among many other adequate therapies

Level of Evidence	Description
I	Based on well-designed, prospective, randomized, and controlled studies in an appropriate population of children
II	Based on data derived from prospectively collected, small comparative trials, or noncomparative prospective trials, or reasonable retrospective data from clinical trials in children, or data from other populations (eg, adults)
III	Based on case reports, case series, consensus statements, or expert opinion for situations in which sound data do not exist

As we state each year, many of the recommendations by the editors for specific situations have not been systematically evaluated in controlled, prospective, comparative clinical trials. Many of the recommendations may be supported by published data, but the data may never have been presented to or reviewed by the US Food and Drug Administration (FDA) and, therefore, are not in the package label. We in pediatrics find ourselves in this situation frequently. Many of us are working closely with the FDA to try to narrow the gap in our knowledge of antimicrobial agents between adults and children; the FDA is providing an exceptional effort to shed light on the doses that are safe and effective for neonates, infants, and children.

We are all deeply grateful for the hard work and tireless efforts of our AAP colleagues. Alain Park, our senior product development editor for many years, has decided to take his interest in teaching to the next level, and we will miss his kind and steady input for future directions of our book. However, we have just met Barrett Winston, who, along with Peter Lynch (who has been working on developing *Nelson's* online), will together be our primary AAP contacts for the specifics of development and production of the book. Barrett has considerable experience in medical publications, and we believe her input, along with Peter's, will be critical to ensuring the success and accuracy of our book. We continue to appreciate the teamwork of all those at AAP who make sure this book gets to all the clinicians who may benefit. Thanks to Mark Grimes, Director, Department of Publishing, and our steadfast friends and supporters in the AAP departments of Publishing and Marketing and Sales—Jeff Mahony, Director, Division of

Professional and Consumer Publishing; Linda Smessaert, Marketing Manager, Professional Publications; and the entire staff—who make certain that important clinical recommendations are provided to clinicians as effectively and effortlessly as possible.

Please let us know if there are new chapters or sections you wish for us to develop—and whether you find certain sections particularly helpful, so we don't change or delete them! Please send your suggestions to nelsonabx@aap.org. We will be putting in a new short chapter on all the new antibiotics for multidrug-resistant gram-negative pathogens in the next edition!

John S. Bradley, MD

John D. Nelson, MD

Notable Changes to *2017 Nelson's Pediatric Antimicrobial Therapy*, 23rd Edition

Antifungals

- Isavuconazole US Food and Drug Administration (FDA) approval and dosing in adults provided

- New Infectious Diseases Society of America (IDSA) guidelines for candidiasis incorporated

- New IDSA guidelines for aspergillosis incorporated

Parasites

- Mebendazole included again after it was not available at the time the 2016 edition published

- The emphasis on use of miltefosine (available from the Centers for Disease Control and Prevention) for the treatment of free-living amoebae

HIV

- Updated HIV treatment and postexposure prophylaxis recommendations

Ceftaroline

- New FDA-approved option for intravenous (IV) therapy for invasive methicillin-resistant *Staphylococcus aureus* (MRSA) infections in children down to 3 months of age: ceftaroline is a fifth-generation cephalosporin (with excellent activity against *S aureus* and most other gram-positive pathogens, including MRSA, as well as methicillin-resistant coagulase-negative *S aureus*). We now have another option beyond vancomycin and clindamycin. Best studied in complicated skin infections and pneumonia.

Ceftazidime/Avibactam

- New IV therapy option for children with meropenem/imipenem-resistant gram-negative bacilli (eg, *Escherichia coli, Klebsiella*) that is approved for adults and under study in children: ceftazidime/avibactam. It is available in most hospital pharmacies for patients with resistant organisms. Our use will be mostly in children with urologic anomalies and recurrent urinary tract infection.

Pneumonia

- The Pediatric Infectious Diseases Society/IDSA community-acquired pneumonia (CAP) guidelines from 2011 recommending plain old ampicillin IV for empiric therapy in immunized children has held up to post-implementation review in new publications—a big score for decreasing unnecessary routine exposure of children to ceftriaxone. Amoxicillin can be used for CAP if hospitalization is not required.

Fluoroquinolones

- No reports of any tendon/joint toxicity of fluoroquinolones (ciprofloxacin, levofloxacin, moxifloxacin) in children when you need to use them: pathogens resistant to everything else; or an option for oral therapy when the only alternative is IV therapy. Overuse in adults has led to new warnings in the package label; an update of our American Academy of Pediatrics statement addressing fluoroquinolone use in children is due to be published by the end of 2016.

Traveler's Diarrhea

- For those who prescribe antibiotics for children who travel to foreign countries to prevent traveler's diarrhea: new data in adults suggest that if you are taking antibiotics, you are more likely to get colonized with the local resistant organisms and bring them home, even if you are not acutely infected. Another reason to take precautions and watch what you eat and drink, rather than just taking antibiotics.

Sexually Transmitted Infections

- For those who care for adolescents with sexually transmitted infections: resistance in gonorrhea to multiple antibiotics is still increasing, and current recommendations are to treat with *both* ceftriaxone AND azithromycin or doxycycline.

1. Choosing Among Antibiotics Within a Class: Beta-lactams, Macrolides, Aminoglycosides, and Fluoroquinolones

New drugs should be compared with others in the same class regarding (1) antimicrobial spectrum; (2) degree of antibiotic exposure (a function of the pharmacokinetics of the nonprotein-bound drug at the site of infection and the pharmacodynamic properties of the drug); (3) demonstrated efficacy in adequate and well-controlled clinical trials; (4) tolerance, toxicity, and side effects; and (5) cost. If there is no substantial benefit for efficacy or safety for one antimicrobial over another for the isolated or presumed bacterial pathogen(s), one should opt for using an older, more extensively used (with presumably better-defined efficacy and safety), and less expensive drug with the narrowest spectrum of activity.

Beta-lactams

Oral Cephalosporins (cephalexin, cefadroxil, cefaclor, cefprozil, cefuroxime, cefixime, cefdinir, cefpodoxime, cefditoren [tablet only], and ceftibuten). As a class, the oral cephalosporins have the advantages over oral penicillins of somewhat greater spectrum of activity, greater safety, and greater palatability of the suspension formulations (penicillins have a bitter taste). The serum half-lives of cefpodoxime, ceftibuten, and cefixime are greater than 2 hours. This pharmacokinetic feature accounts for the fact that they may be given in 1 or 2 doses per day for certain indications, particularly otitis media, where the middle ear fluid half-life is likely to be much longer than the serum half-life. For more resistant pathogens, twice daily is preferred (see Chapter 3). The spectrum of activity increases for gram-negative organisms as one goes from the first-generation cephalosporins (cephalexin and cefadroxil), to the second generation (cefaclor, cefprozil, and cefuroxime) that demonstrates activity against *Haemophilus influenzae* (including beta-lactamase–producing strains), to the third-generation agents (cefdinir, cefixime, cefpodoxime, and ceftibuten) that have enhanced coverage of many enteric gram-negative bacilli (*Escherichia coli, Klebsiella* spp). However, ceftibuten and cefixime, in particular, have a disadvantage of less activity against *Streptococcus pneumoniae* than the others, particularly against penicillin (beta-lactam) non-susceptible strains. None of the currently available oral cephalosporins have activity against *Pseudomonas* or methicillin-resistant *Staphylococcus aureus* (MRSA). The palatability of generic versions of these products may not have the same pleasant characteristics as the original products.

Parenteral Cephalosporins. First-generation cephalosporins, such as cefazolin, are used mainly for treatment of gram-positive infections caused by *S aureus* (excluding MRSA) and group A streptococcus and for surgical prophylaxis; the gram-negative spectrum is limited but more extensive than ampicillin. Cefazolin is well tolerated on intramuscular or intravenous (IV) injection.

A second-generation cephalosporin (cefuroxime) and the cephamycins (cefoxitin and cefotetan) provide increased activity against many gram-negative organisms, particularly *Haemophilus* and *E coli*. Cefoxitin has, in addition, activity against approximately 80% of strains of *Bacteroides fragilis* and can be considered for use in place of the more active agents, like metronidazole or carbapenems, when that organism is implicated in nonserious disease.

Third-generation cephalosporins (cefotaxime, ceftriaxone, and ceftazidime) all have enhanced potency against many enteric gram-negative bacilli. As with all cephalosporins, they are inactive against enterococci and *Listeria;* only ceftazidime has significant activity against *Pseudomonas.* Cefotaxime and ceftriaxone have been used very successfully to treat meningitis caused by pneumococcus (mostly penicillin-susceptible strains), *H influenzae* type b, meningococcus, and susceptible strains of *E coli* meningitis in a small number of young infants. These drugs have the greatest usefulness for treating gram-negative bacillary infections due to their safety, compared with other classes of antibiotics. Because ceftriaxone is excreted to a large extent via the liver, it can be used with little dosage adjustment in patients with renal failure. Furthermore, it has a serum half-life of 4 to 7 hours and can be given once a day for all infections, including meningitis, that are caused by susceptible organisms.

Cefepime, a fourth-generation cephalosporin approved for use in children in 1999, exhibits (1) enhanced antipseudomonal activity over ceftazidime; (2) the gram-positive activity of second-generation cephalosporins; (3) better activity against gram-negative enteric bacilli; and (4) stability against the inducible ampC beta-lactamases of *Enterobacter, Serratia,* and some strains of *Proteus* and *Citrobacter* that can hydrolyze third-generation cephalosporins. It can be used as single-drug antibiotic therapy against these pathogens, rather than paired with an aminoglycoside to prevent the emergence of ampC resistance.

Ceftaroline is a fifth-generation cephalosporin, the first of the cephalosporins with activity against MRSA. Ceftaroline was approved by the US Food and Drug Administration (FDA) in December 2010 for adults and approved for children in June 2016 for treatment of complicated skin infections (including MRSA) and community-acquired pneumonia. The pharmacokinetics of ceftaroline have been evaluated in all pediatric age groups, including neonates; clinical studies for pediatric community-acquired pneumonia and complicated skin infection have now been published.[1-3] Global studies in neonatal sepsis are in progress. Based on these published data and review by the FDA, for infants and children 2 months and older, ceftaroline should be effective and safer than vancomycin for treatment of MRSA infections. Just as beta-lactams are preferred over vancomycin for methicillin-susceptible *S aureus* infections, ceftaroline should be considered preferred treatment over vancomycin for MRSA infection. Neither renal function nor drug levels need to be followed with ceftaroline therapy. We will follow safety and efficacy closely.

Penicillinase-Resistant Penicillins (dicloxacillin [capsules only]; nafcillin and oxacillin [parenteral only]). "Penicillinase" refers specifically to the beta-lactamase produced by *S aureus* in this case and not those produced by gram-negative bacteria. These antibiotics are active against penicillin-resistant *S aureus* but not against MRSA. Nafcillin differs pharmacologically from the others in being excreted primarily by the liver rather than by the kidneys, which may explain the relative lack of nephrotoxicity compared with methicillin, which is no longer available in the United States. Nafcillin pharmacokinetics are erratic in persons with liver disease, and it often burns with IV infusion.

Antipseudomonal Beta-lactams (ticarcillin/clavulanate, piperacillin, piperacillin/ tazobactam, ceftolozane/tazobactam, aztreonam, ceftazidime, cefepime, meropenem, and imipenem). Timentin (ticarcillin/clavulanate), Zosyn (piperacillin/tazobactam), and Zerbaxa (ceftolozane/tazobactam) represent combinations of 2 beta-lactam drugs. One beta-lactam drug in the combination, known as a "beta-lactamase inhibitor" (clavulanic acid or tazobactam in these combinations), binds irreversibly to and neutralizes specific beta-lactamase enzymes produced by the organism, allowing the second beta-lactam drug (ticarcillin, piperacillin, or ceftolozane) to act as the active antibiotic to bind effectively to the intracellular target site (transpeptidase), resulting in death of the organism. Thus, the combination only adds to the spectrum of the original antibiotic when the mechanism of resistance is a beta-lactamase enzyme and only when the beta-lactamase inhibitor is capable of binding to and inhibiting that particular organism's beta-lactamase enzyme(s). The combinations extend the spectrum of activity of the primary antibiotic to include many beta-lactamase–positive bacteria, including some strains of enteric gram-negative bacilli (*E coli, Klebsiella,* and *Enterobacter*), *S aureus,* and *B fragilis.* Ticarcillin/ clavulanate, piperacillin/tazobactam, and ceftolozane/tazobactam have no significant activity against *Pseudomonas* beyond that of ticarcillin, piperacillin, or ceftolozane because their beta-lactamase inhibitors do not effectively inhibit all of the many relevant beta-lactamases of *Pseudomonas.*

Pseudomonas has an intrinsic capacity to develop resistance following exposure to any beta-lactam, based on the activity of several inducible chromosomal beta-lactamases, upregulated efflux pumps, and changes in the permeability of the cell wall. Because development of resistance during therapy is not uncommon (particularly beta-lactamase–mediated resistance against ticarcillin, piperacillin, or ceftazidime), an aminoglycoside such as tobramycin is often used in combination, in hopes that the tobramycin will kill strains developing resistance to the beta-lactams. Cefepime, meropenem, and imipenem are relatively stable to the beta-lactamases induced while on therapy and can be used as single-agent therapy for most *Pseudomonas* infections, but resistance may still develop to these agents based on other mechanisms of resistance. For *Pseudomonas* infections in compromised hosts or in life-threatening infections, these drugs, too, should be used in combination with an aminoglycoside or a second active agent.

Aminopenicillins (amoxicillin and amoxicillin/clavulanate [oral formulations only, in the United States], ampicillin [oral and parenteral], and ampicillin/sulbactam [parenteral only]). Amoxicillin is very well absorbed, good tasting, and associated with very few side effects. Augmentin is a combination of amoxicillin and clavulanate (see Antipseudomonal Beta-lactams for more information on beta-lactam/beta-lactamase inhibitor combinations) that is available in several fixed proportions that permit amoxicillin to remain active against many beta-lactamase–producing bacteria, including *H influenzae* and *S aureus* (but not MRSA). Amoxicillin/clavulanate has undergone many changes in formulation since its introduction. The ratio of amoxicillin to clavulanate was originally 4:1, based on susceptibility data of pneumococcus and *Haemophilus* during the 1970s. With the emergence of penicillin-resistant pneumococcus, recommendations for increasing the dosage of amoxicillin, particularly for upper respiratory tract infections, were made. However, if one increases the dosage of clavulanate even slightly, the incidence of diarrhea increases dramatically. If one keeps the dosage of clavulanate constant while increasing the dosage of amoxicillin, one can treat the relatively resistant pneumococci while not increasing gastrointestinal side effects of the combination. The original 4:1 ratio is present in suspensions containing 125-mg and 250-mg amoxicillin/ 5 mL and the 125-mg and 250-mg chewable tablets. A higher 7:1 ratio is present in the suspensions containing 200-mg and 400-mg amoxicillin/5 mL and in the 200-mg and 400-mg chewable tablets. A still higher ratio of 14:1 is present in the suspension formulation Augmentin ES-600 that contains 600-mg amoxicillin/5 mL; this preparation is designed to deliver 90 mg/kg/day of amoxicillin, divided twice daily, for the treatment of ear (and sinus) infections. The high serum and middle ear fluid concentrations achieved with 45 mg/kg/dose, combined with the long middle ear fluid half-life (4–6 hours) of amoxicillin, allow for a therapeutic antibiotic exposure to pathogens in the middle ear with a twice-daily regimen. However, the prolonged half-life in the middle ear fluid is not necessarily found in other infection sites (eg, skin, lung tissue, joint tissue), for which dosing of amoxicillin and Augmentin should continue to be 3 times daily for most susceptible pathogens.

For older children who can swallow tablets, the amoxicillin to clavulanate ratios are as follows: 500-mg tablet (4:1); 875-mg tablet (7:1); 1,000-mg tablet (16:1).

Sulbactam, another beta-lactamase inhibitor like clavulanate, is combined with ampicillin in the parenteral formulation Unasyn. The cautions regarding spectrum of activity for Timentin and Zosyn with respect to the limitations of the beta-lactamase inhibitor in increasing the spectrum of activity (see Antipseudomonal Beta-lactams) also apply to Unasyn.

Carbapenems. Meropenem, imipenem, doripenem, and ertapenem are carbapenems with a broader spectrum of activity than any other class of beta-lactam currently available. Meropenem, imipenem, and ertapenem are approved by the FDA for use in children, while doripenem is under investigation in children. At present, we recommend them for treatment of infections caused by bacteria resistant to standard therapy or for mixed infections involving aerobes and anaerobes. Imipenem has greater central nervous system irritability compared with other carbapenems, leading to an increased risk of seizures in children with meningitis. Meropenem was not associated with an increased rate of seizures, compared with cefotaxime in children with meningitis. Imipenem and meropenem are active against virtually all coliform bacilli, including cefotaxime-resistant (extended spectrum beta-lactamase–producing or ampC-producing) strains, against *Pseudomonas aeruginosa* (including most ceftazidime-resistant strains), and against anaerobes, including *B fragilis*. While ertapenem lacks the excellent activity against *P aeruginosa* of the other carbapenems, it has the advantage of a prolonged serum half-life, which allows for once-daily dosing in adults and children aged 13 years and older and twice-daily dosing in younger children. Newly emergent strains of *Klebsiella pneumoniae* contain *K pneumoniae* carbapenemases that degrade and inactivate all the carbapenems. These strains, as well as strains carrying the less common New Delhi metallo-beta-lactamase (also active against carbapenems), have begun to spread to many parts of the world, reinforcing the need to keep track of your local antibiotic susceptibility patterns.

Macrolides

Erythromycin is the prototype of macrolide antibiotics. Almost 30 macrolides have been produced, but only 3 are FDA approved for children in the United States: erythromycin, azithromycin (also called an azalide), and clarithromycin, while a fourth, telithromycin (also called a ketolide), is approved for adults and only available in tablet form. As a class, these drugs achieve greater concentrations intracellularly than in serum, particularly with azithromycin and clarithromycin. As a result, measuring serum concentrations is usually not clinically useful. Gastrointestinal intolerance to erythromycin is caused by the breakdown products of the macrolide ring structure. This is much less of a problem with azithromycin and clarithromycin. Azithromycin, clarithromycin, and telithromycin extend the activity of erythromycin to include *Haemophilus;* azithromycin and clarithromycin also have substantial activity against certain mycobacteria. Azithromycin is also active in vitro and effective against many enteric gram-negative pathogens, including *Salmonella* and *Shigella*. Solithromycin, a fluoroketolide with enhanced activity against gram-positive organisms, including MRSA, is currently in pediatric clinical trials.

Aminoglycosides

Although 5 aminoglycoside antibiotics are available in the United States, only 3 are widely used for systemic therapy of aerobic gram-negative infections and for synergy in the treatment of certain gram-positive and gram-negative infections: gentamicin, tobramycin, and amikacin. Streptomycin and kanamycin have more limited utility due to increased toxicity compared with the other agents. Resistance in gram-negative bacilli to aminoglycosides is caused by bacterial enzymes that adenylate, acetylate, or phosphorylate the aminoglycoside, resulting in inactivity. The specific activities of each enzyme against each agent in each pathogen are highly variable. As a result, antibiotic susceptibility tests must be done for each aminoglycoside drug separately. There are small differences in toxicities to the kidneys and eighth cranial nerve hearing/vestibular function, although it is uncertain whether these small differences are clinically significant. For all children receiving a full treatment course, it is advisable to monitor peak and trough serum concentrations early in the course of therapy, as the degree of drug exposure correlates with toxicity and elevated trough concentrations may predict impending drug accumulation. With amikacin, desired peak concentrations are 20 to 35 µg/mL and trough drug concentrations are less than 10 µg/mL; for gentamicin and tobramycin, depending on the frequency of dosing, peak concentrations should be 5 to 10 µg/mL and trough concentrations less than 2 µg/mL. Children with cystic fibrosis require greater dosages to achieve equivalent therapeutic serum concentrations due to enhanced clearance. Inhaled tobramycin has been very successful in children with cystic fibrosis as an adjunctive therapy of gram-negative bacillary infections. The role of inhaled aminoglycosides in other gram-negative pneumonias (eg, ventilator-associated pneumonia) has not yet been defined.

Once-Daily Dosing of Aminoglycosides. Once-daily dosing of 5 to 7.5 mg/kg gentamicin or tobramycin has been studied in adults and in some neonates and children; peak serum concentrations are greater than those achieved with dosing 3 times daily. Aminoglycosides demonstrate concentration-dependent killing of pathogens, suggesting a potential benefit to higher serum concentrations achieved with once-daily dosing. Regimens giving the daily dosage as a single infusion, rather than as traditionally split doses every 8 hours, are effective and safe for normal adult hosts and immune-compromised hosts with fever and neutropenia and may be less toxic. Experience with once-daily dosing in children is increasing, with similar results as noted for adults. Once-daily dosing should be considered as effective as multiple, smaller doses per day and may be safer for children.

Fluoroquinolones

More than 30 years ago, fluoroquinolone (FQ) toxicity to cartilage in weight-bearing joints in experimental juvenile animals was documented to be dose and duration of therapy dependent. Pediatric studies were, therefore, not initially undertaken with ciprofloxacin or other FQs. However, with increasing antibiotic resistance in pediatric pathogens and an accumulating database in pediatrics suggesting that joint toxicity may be uncommon, the FDA allowed prospective studies to proceed in 1998. As of July 2016, no cases of documented FQ-attributable joint toxicity have occurred in children with FQs that are approved for use in the United States. Limited published data are available from prospective, blinded studies to accurately assess this risk. A prospective, randomized, double-blind study of moxifloxacin for intraabdominal infection, with 1-year follow-up specifically designed to assess tendon/joint toxicity, demonstrated no concern for toxicity. Unblinded studies with levofloxacin for respiratory tract infections and unpublished randomized studies comparing ciprofloxacin versus other agents for complicated urinary tract infection suggest the possibility of an uncommon, reversible, FQ-attributable arthralgia, but these data should be interpreted with caution. The use of FQs in situations of antibiotic resistance where no other active agent is available is reasonable, weighing the benefits of treatment against the low risk of toxicity of this class of antibiotics. The use of an oral FQ in situations in which the only alternative is parenteral therapy is also justified.[4]

Ciprofloxacin usually has very good gram-negative activity (with great regional variation in susceptibility) against enteric bacilli (*E coli, Klebsiella, Enterobacter, Salmonella,* and *Shigella*) and against *P aeruginosa*. However, it lacks substantial gram-positive coverage and should not be used to treat streptococcal, staphylococcal, or pneumococcal infections. Newer-generation FQs are more active against these pathogens; levofloxacin has documented efficacy and safety in pediatric clinical trials for respiratory tract infections, acute otitis media, and community-acquired pneumonia. Children with any question of joint/tendon/bone toxicity in the levofloxacin studies were followed up to 5 years after treatment, with no difference in outcomes in these randomized studies, compared with the standard FDA-approved antibiotics used as comparators in these studies.[5] None of the newer-generation FQs are more active against gram-negative pathogens than ciprofloxacin. Quinolone antibiotics are bitter tasting. Ciprofloxacin and levofloxacin are currently available in a suspension form; ciprofloxacin is FDA approved in pediatrics for complicated urinary tract infections and inhalation anthrax, while levofloxacin is approved for inhalation anthrax only, as the sponsor chose not to apply for approval for pediatric respiratory tract infections. For reasons of safety and to prevent the emergence of widespread resistance, FQs should still not be used for primary therapy of pediatric infections and should be limited to situations in which safe and effective oral therapy with other classes of antibiotics does not exist.

2. Choosing Among Antifungal Agents: Polyenes, Azoles, and Echinocandins

Separating antifungal agents by class, much like navigating the myriad of antibacterial agents, allows one to best understand the underlying mechanisms of action and then appropriately choose which agent would be optimal for empirical therapy or a targeted approach. There are certain helpful generalizations that should be considered, eg, echinocandins are fungicidal against yeast and fungistatic against molds, while azoles are the opposite. Coupled with these concepts is the need for continued surveillance for fungal resistance patterns. While some fungal species are inherently or very often resistant to specific agents or even classes, there are also an increasing number of fungal isolates that are developing resistance due to environmental pressure or chronic use in individual patients. In 2017, there are 14 individual antifungal agents approved by the US Food and Drug Administration (FDA) for systemic use, and for each agent there are often several formulations (each with unique pharmacokinetics that one has to understand to optimize the agent, particularly in patients who are critically ill). Therefore, it is more important than ever to establish a firm foundation in understanding how these antifungal agents work and where they work best.

Polyenes

Amphotericin B (AmB) is a polyene antifungal antibiotic that has been available since 1958 (discovered in the soil in Venezuela) for the treatment of invasive fungal infections. Its name originates from the drug's amphoteric property of reacting as an acid as well as a base. Nystatin is another polyene antifungal, but, due to systemic toxicity, it is only used in topical preparations. It was named after the research laboratory where it was discovered, the New York State Health Department Laboratory. AmB remains the most broad-spectrum antifungal available for clinical use. This lipophilic drug binds to ergosterol, the major sterol in the fungal cell membrane, and creates transmembrane pores that compromise the integrity of the cell membrane and create a rapid fungicidal effect through osmotic lysis. Toxicity is likely due to the cross-reactivity with the human cholesterol bi-lipid membrane, which resembles ergosterol. The toxicity of the conventional formulation, AmB deoxycholate (AmB-D)—the parent molecule coupled with an ionic detergent for clinical use—can be substantial from the standpoints of systemic reactions (fever, rigors) and acute and chronic renal toxicity. Premedication with acetaminophen, diphenhydramine, and meperidine is often required to prevent systemic reactions during infusion. Renal dysfunction manifests primarily as decreased glomerular filtration with a rising serum creatinine concentration, but substantial tubular nephropathy is associated with potassium and magnesium wasting, requiring supplemental potassium for many neonates and children, regardless of clinical symptoms associated with infusion. Fluid loading with saline pre– and post–AmB-D infusion seems to mitigate renal toxicity.

Three lipid preparations approved in the mid-1990s decrease toxicity with no apparent decrease in clinical efficacy. Decisions on which lipid AmB preparation to use should, therefore, largely focus on side effects and costs. Two clinically useful lipid formulations exist: one in which ribbonlike lipid complexes of AmB are created (amphotericin B lipid complex [ABLC], Abelcet, and one in which AmB is incorporated into true liposomes (liposomal amphotericin B [L-AmB]), AmBisome. The standard dosage used of these preparations is 5 mg/kg/day, in contrast to the 1 mg/kg/day of AmB-D. In most studies, the side effects of L-AmB were somewhat less than those of ABLC, but both have significantly fewer side effects than AmB-D. The advantage of the lipid preparations is the ability to safely deliver a greater overall dose of the parent AmB drug. The cost of conventional AmB-D is substantially less than either lipid formulation. A colloidal dispersion of AmB in cholesteryl sulfate, Amphotec, which is no longer available in the United States, with decreased nephrotoxicity, but infusion-related side effects are closer to AmB-D than to the lipid formulations and preclude recommendation for its use. The decreased nephrotoxicity of the 3 lipid preparations is thought to be due to the preferential binding of its AmB to high-density lipoproteins, compared with AmB-D binding to low-density lipoproteins. Despite in vitro concentration-dependent killing, a clinical trial comparing L-AmB at doses of 3 mg/kg/day versus 10 mg/kg/day found no efficacy benefit for the higher dose and only greater toxicity.[1] Therefore, it is generally not recommended to use any AmB preparations at very high dosages (>5 mg/kg/day), as it will likely only incur greater toxicity with no real therapeutic advantage. There are reports of using higher dosing in very difficult infections where AmB is the first-line therapy (eg, mucormycosis), and while experts remain divided on this practice, it is clear that at least 5 mg/kg/day of a lipid AmB formulation should be used. AmB has a long terminal half-life and, coupled with the concentration-dependent killing, the agent is best used as single daily doses. These pharmacokinetics explain the use in some studies of once-weekly AmB for antifungal prophylaxis. If the overall AmB exposure needs to be decreased due to toxicity, it is best to increase the dosing interval (eg, 3 times weekly) but retain the full mg/kg dose for optimal pharmacokinetics.

AmB-D has been used for nonsystemic purposes, such as in bladder washes, intraventricular instillation, intrapleural instillation, and other modalities, but there are no firm data supporting those clinical indications, and it is likely that the local toxicities outweigh the theoretic benefits. One exception is aerosolized AmB for antifungal prophylaxis (not treatment) in lung transplant recipients due to the different pathophysiology of invasive aspergillosis (often originating at the bronchial anastomotic site, more so than parenchymal disease) in that specific patient population. Due to the lipid chemistry, the L-AmB does not interact well with renal tubules and L-AmB is recovered from the urine at lower levels than AmB-D, so there is a theoretic concern with using a lipid formulation, as opposed to AmB-D, when treating isolated urinary fungal disease. This theoretic concern is likely outweighed by the real concern of toxicity with AmB-D. Most experts believe AmB-D should be reserved for use in resource-limited settings in which no alternative agents (eg, lipid formulations) are available. An exception might be in neonates, where limited retrospective data suggest that the AmB-D formulation had better efficacy.[2] Importantly, there are several pathogens that are inherently or functionally resistant to AmB, including *Candida lusitaniae*, *Trichosporon* spp, *Aspergillus terreus*, *Fusarium* spp, and *Pseudallescheria boydii* (*Scedosporium apiospermum*) or *Scedosporium prolificans*.

Azoles

This class of systemic agents was first approved in 1981 and is divided into imidazoles (ketoconazole), triazoles (fluconazole, itraconazole), and second-generation triazoles (voriconazole, posaconazole, and isavuconazole) based on the number of nitrogen atoms in the azole ring. All of the azoles work by inhibition of ergosterol synthesis (fungal cytochrome P450 [CYP] sterol 14-demethylation) that is required for fungal cell membrane integrity. While the polyenes are rapidly fungicidal, the azoles are fungistatic against yeasts and fungicidal against molds. However, it is important to note that ketoconazole and fluconazole have no mold activity. The only systemic imidazole is ketoconazole, which is primarily active against *Candida* spp and is available in an oral formulation. Three azoles (itraconazole, voriconazole, posaconazole) need therapeutic drug monitoring with trough levels within the first 4 to 7 days (when patient is at pharmacokinetic steady state); it is unclear at present if isavuconazole will require drug-level monitoring. It is less clear if therapeutic drug monitoring is required during primary azole prophylaxis, although low levels have been associated with a higher probability of breakthrough infection.

Fluconazole is active against a broader range of fungi than ketoconazole and includes clinically relevant activity against *Cryptococcus, Coccidioides,* and *Histoplasma.* Like most other azoles, fluconazole requires a double loading dose on the first day, which has been nicely studied in neonates[3] and is likely also beneficial, but not definitively studied yet, in all children. Fluconazole achieves relatively high concentrations in urine and cerebrospinal fluid (CSF) compared with AmB due to its low lipophilicity, with urinary concentrations often so high that treatment against even "resistant" pathogens that are isolated only in the urine is possible. Fluconazole remains one of the most active, and so far one of the safest, systemic antifungal agents for the treatment of most *Candida* infections. *Candida albicans* remains generally sensitive to fluconazole, although some resistance is present in many non-*albicans Candida* spp as well as in *C albicans* in children repeatedly exposed to fluconazole. For instance, *Candida krusei* is considered inherently resistant to fluconazole, and *Candida glabrata* demonstrates dose-dependent resistance to fluconazole (and usually voriconazole). Fluconazole is available in parenteral and oral (with >90% bioavailability) formulations and toxicity is unusual and primarily hepatic.

Itraconazole is active against an even broader range of fungi and, unlike fluconazole, includes molds such as *Aspergillus.* It is currently available as a capsule or oral solution (the intravenous [IV] form was discontinued); the oral solution provides higher, more consistent serum concentrations than capsules and should be used preferentially. Absorption using itraconazole oral solution is improved on an empty stomach (unlike the capsule form, which is best administered under fed conditions and with a cola beverage to increase absorption), and monitoring itraconazole serum concentrations, like most azole antifungals, is a key principal in management (generally, itraconazole trough levels should be >0.5–1 μg/mL; trough levels >5 μg/mL may be associated with increased toxicity). In adult patients, itraconazole is recommended to be loaded at 200 mg twice daily for 2 days, followed by 200 mg daily starting on the third day. Loading dose studies have not been performed in children. Dosing itraconazole in children requires twice-daily dosing throughout treatment. Limited pharmacokinetic data are available in children; itraconazole has not been approved by the FDA for pediatric indications. Itraconazole is indicated in adults for therapy of mild/moderate disease with blastomycosis, histoplasmosis, and others. Although it possesses antifungal activity, itraconazole is not indicated as primary therapy against invasive aspergillosis, as voriconazole is a far superior option. Itraconazole is not active against *Zygomycetes* (eg, mucormycosis). Toxicity in adults is primarily hepatic.

Voriconazole was approved in 2002 and is only FDA approved for children 12 years and older, although there are now substantial pharmacokinetic data and experience for children aged 2 to 12 years.[4] Voriconazole is a fluconazole derivative, so think of it as having the greater tissue and CSF penetration of fluconazole but the added antifungal spectrum to include molds. While the bioavailability of voriconazole in adults is approximately 96%, multiple studies have shown that it is only approximately 60% in children, requiring clinicians to carefully monitor voriconazole trough concentrations in patients taking the oral formulation, further complicated by great inter-patient variability in clearance. Voriconazole serum concentrations are tricky to interpret, but monitoring concentrations is essential to using this drug, like all azole antifungals, and especially important in circumstances of suspected treatment failure or possible toxicity. Most experts suggest voriconazole trough concentrations of 2 µg/mL (at a minimum, 1 µg/mL) or greater, which would generally exceed the pathogen's minimum inhibitory concentration, but, generally, toxicity will not be seen until concentrations of approximately 6 µg/mL or greater. One important point is the acquisition of an accurate trough concentration, one obtained just before the next dose is due and not obtained through a catheter infusing the drug. These simple trough parameters will make interpretation possible. The fundamental voriconazole pharmacokinetics are different in adults versus children; in adults, voriconazole is metabolized in a nonlinear fashion, whereas in children, the drug is metabolized in a linear fashion. This explains the increased pediatric starting dosing for voriconazole at 9 mg/kg/dose versus loading with 6 mg/kg/dose in adult patients. Younger children, especially, require even higher dosages of voriconazole and also have a larger therapeutic window for dosing. However, many studies have shown an inconsistent relationship between dosing and levels, highlighting the need for close monitoring after the initial dosing scheme and then dose adjustment as needed in the individual patient. Given the poor clinical and microbiological response of *Aspergillus* infections to AmB, voriconazole is now the treatment of choice for invasive aspergillosis and many other mold infections (eg, pseudallescheriasis, fusariosis). Importantly, infections with *Zygomycetes* (eg, mucormycosis) are resistant to voriconazole. Voriconazole retains activity against most *Candida* spp, including some that are fluconazole resistant, but it is unlikely to replace fluconazole for treatment of fluconazole-susceptible *Candida* infections. Importantly, there are increasing reports of *C glabrata* resistance to voriconazole. Voriconazole produces some unique transient visual field abnormalities in about 10% of adults and children. There are an increasing number of reports, seen in as high as 20% of patients, of a photosensitive sunburn-like erythema that is not aided by sunscreen (only sun avoidance). In some rare long-term (mean of 3 years of therapy) cases, this voriconazole phototoxicity has developed into cutaneous squamous cell carcinoma. Discontinuing voriconazole is recommended in patients experiencing chronic phototoxicity. The rash is the most common indication for switching from voriconazole to posaconazole/isavuconazole if a triazole antifungal is required. Hepatotoxicity is uncommon, occurring only in 2% to 5% of patients. Voriconazole is CYP metabolized (CYP2C19), and allelic polymorphisms in the population have shown that some Asian patients will achieve higher toxic serum concentrations than other patients. Voriconazole also interacts with many similarly P450 metabolized drugs to produce some profound changes in serum concentrations of many concurrently administered drugs.

Posaconazole, an itraconazole derivative, was FDA approved in 2006 as an oral suspension for children 13 years and older. An extended-release tablet formulation was approved in November 2013, also for 13 years and older, and an IV formulation was approved in March 2014 for patients 18 years and older. Effective absorption of the oral suspension strongly requires taking the medication with food, ideally a high-fat meal; taking posaconazole on an empty stomach will result in approximately one-fourth of the absorption as in the fed state. The tablet formulation has better absorption due to its delayed release in the small intestine, but absorption will still be slightly increased with food. If the patient can take the (relatively large) tablets, the extended-release tablet is the preferred form due to the ability to easily obtain higher and more consistent drug levels. Due to the low pH (<5) of IV posaconazole, a central venous catheter is required for administration. The IV formulation contains only slightly lower amounts of the cyclodextrin vehicle than voriconazole, so similar theoretic renal accumulation concerns exist. The exact pediatric dosing for posaconazole has not been completely determined and requires consultation with a pediatric infectious diseases expert. The pediatric oral suspension dose recommended by some experts for treating invasive disease is 18 mg/kg/day divided 3 times daily, but the true answer is likely higher and serum trough level monitoring is recommended. A study with a new pediatric formulation for suspension, essentially the tablet form that is able to be suspended, is underway. Importantly, the current tablet cannot be broken for use due to its chemical coating. Pediatric dosing with the current IV or extended-release tablet dosing is completely unknown, but adolescents can likely follow the adult dosing schemes. In adult patients, IV posaconazole is loaded at 300 mg twice daily on the first day, and then 300 mg once daily starting on the second day. Similarly, in adult patients, the extended-release tablet is dosed as 300 mg twice daily on the first day, and then 300 mg once daily starting on the second day. In adult patients, the maximum amount of posaconazole oral suspension given is 800 mg per day due to its excretion, and that has been given as 400 mg twice daily or 200 mg 4 times a day in severely ill patients due to findings of a marginal increase in exposure with more frequent dosing. Greater than 800 mg per day is not indicated in any patient. Like voriconazole and itraconazole, trough levels should be monitored, and most experts feel that posaconazole levels for treatment should be at least greater than 700 ng/mL (0.7 µg/mL). The in vitro activity of posaconazole against *Candida* spp is better than that of fluconazole and similar to voriconazole. Overall in vitro antifungal activity against *Aspergillus* is also equivalent to voriconazole, but, notably, it is the first triazole with substantial activity against some *Zygomycetes*, including *Rhizopus* spp and *Mucor* spp, as well as activity against *Coccidioides*, *Histoplasma*, and *Blastomyces* and the pathogens of phaeohyphomycosis. Posaconazole treatment of invasive aspergillosis in patients with chronic granulomatous disease appears to be superior to voriconazole in this specific patient population for an unknown reason. Posaconazole is eliminated by hepatic glucuronidation but does demonstrate inhibition of the CYP3A4 enzyme system, leading to many drug interactions with other P450 metabolized drugs. It is currently approved for prophylaxis of *Candida* and *Aspergillus* infections in high-risk adults and for treatment of *Candida* oropharyngeal disease or esophagitis in adults. Posaconazole, like itraconazole, has generally poor CSF penetration.

Isavuconazole is a new triazole that was FDA approved in March 2015 for treatment of invasive aspergillosis and invasive mucormycosis with oral (capsules only) and IV formulations. Isavuconazole has a similar antifungal spectrum as voriconazole and some activity against *Zygomycetes* (yet, potentially, not as potent against *Zygomycetes* as posaconazole). A phase 3 clinical trial in adult patients demonstrated non-inferiority versus voriconazole against invasive aspergillosis and other mold infections. Isavuconazole is actually dispensed as the prodrug isavuconazonium sulfate. Dosing in adults patients is loading with isavuconazole 200 mg (equivalent to 372-mg isavuconazonium sulfate) every 8 hours for 2 days (6 doses), followed by 200 mg once daily for maintenance dosing. The half-life is long (>5 days), there is 98% bioavailability in adults, and there is no reported food effect with oral isavuconazole. The IV formulation does not contain the vehicle cyclodextrin, unlike voriconazole, which could make it more attractive in patients with renal failure. Early experience suggests a much lower rate of photosensitivity and skin disorders as well as visual disturbances compared with voriconazole. No specific pediatric dosing data exist for isavuconazole yet.

Echinocandins

This class of systemic antifungal agents was first approved in 2001. The echinocandins inhibit cell wall formation (in contrast to acting on the cell membrane by the polyenes and azoles) by noncompetitively inhibiting beta-1,3-glucan synthase, an enzyme present in fungi but absent in mammalian cells. These agents are generally very safe, as there is no beta-1,3-glucan in humans. The echinocandins are not metabolized through the CYP system, so fewer drug interactions are problematic, compared with the azoles. There is no need to dose-adjust in renal failure, but one needs a lower dosage in the setting of very severe hepatic dysfunction. As a class, these antifungals generally have poor CSF penetration, although animal studies have shown adequate brain parenchyma levels, and do not penetrate the urine well. While the 3 clinically available echinocandins each individually have some unique and important dosing and pharmacokinetic parameters, especially in children, efficacy is generally equivalent. Opposite the azole class, the echinocandins are fungicidal against yeasts but fungistatic against molds. The fungicidal activity against yeasts has elevated the echinocandins to the preferred therapy against invasive candidiasis. Echinocandins are thought to be best utilized against invasive aspergillosis only as salvage therapy if a triazole fails or in a patient with suspected triazole resistance, but not as primary monotherapy against invasive aspergillosis or any other mold infection. Improved efficacy with combination therapy with the echinocandins and triazoles against *Aspergillus* infections is unclear, with disparate results in multiple smaller studies and a definitive clinical trial demonstrating minimal benefit over voriconazole monotherapy in only certain patient populations. Some experts have used combination therapy in invasive aspergillosis with a triazole plus echinocandin only during the initial phase of waiting for triazole drug levels to be appropriately high. There are reports of echinocandin resistance in *Candida* spp, as high as 12% in *C glabrata* in some studies, and the echinocandins as a class are often somewhat less active against *Candida parapsilosis* isolates (approximately 10%–15% respond poorly, but most are still susceptible).

Caspofungin received FDA approval for children aged 3 months to 17 years in 2008 for empiric therapy of presumed fungal infections in febrile, neutropenic children; treatment of candidemia as well as *Candida* esophagitis, peritonitis, and empyema; and salvage therapy of invasive aspergillosis. Due to its earlier approval, there are generally more reports with caspofungin than the other echinocandins. Caspofungin dosing in children is calculated according to body surface area, with a loading dose on the first day of 70 mg/m^2, followed by daily maintenance dosing of 50 mg/m^2, and not to exceed 70 mg regardless of the calculated dose. Significantly higher doses of caspofungin have been studied in adult patients without any clear added benefit in efficacy, but if the 50 mg/m^2 dose is tolerated and does not provide adequate clinical response, the daily dose can be increased to 70 mg/m^2. Dosing for caspofungin in neonates is 25 mg/m^2/day.

Micafungin was approved in adults in 2005 for treatment of candidemia, *Candida* esophagitis and peritonitis, and prophylaxis of *Candida* infections in stem cell transplant recipients, and in 2013 for pediatric patients aged 4 months and older. Micafungin has the most pediatric and neonatal data available of all 3 echinocandins, including more extensive pharmacokinetic studies surrounding dosing and several efficacy studies.[5-7] Micafungin dosing in children is age dependent, as clearance increases dramatically in the younger age groups (especially neonates), necessitating higher doses for younger children. Doses in children are generally thought to be 2 mg/kg/day, with higher doses likely needed for younger patients, and premature neonates dosed at 10 mg/kg/day. Adult micafungin dosing (100 or 150 mg once daily) is to be used in patients who weigh more than 40 kg. Unlike the other echinocandins, a loading dose is not required for micafungin.

Anidulafungin was approved for adults for candidemia and *Candida* esophagitis in 2006 and is not officially approved for pediatric patients. Like the other echinocandins, anidulafungin is not P450 metabolized and has not demonstrated significant drug interactions. Limited clinical efficacy data are available in children, with only some pediatric pharmacokinetic data suggesting weight-based dosing (3 mg/kg/day loading dose, followed by 1.5 mg/kg/day maintenance dosing).[8] The adult dose for invasive candidiasis is a loading dose of 200 mg on the first day, followed by 100 mg daily.

3. How Antibiotic Dosages Are Determined Using Susceptibility Data, Pharmacodynamics, and Treatment Outcomes

Factors Involved in Dosing Recommendations

Our view of how to use antimicrobials is continually changing. As the published literature and our experience with each drug increases, our recommendations evolve as we compare the efficacy, safety, and cost of each drug in the context of current and previous data from adults and children. Every new antibiotic must demonstrate some degree of efficacy and safety in adults before we attempt to treat children. Occasionally, due to unanticipated toxicities and unanticipated clinical failures at a specific dosage, we will modify our initial recommendations for this book.

Important considerations in any new recommendations we make include (1) the susceptibilities of pathogens to antibiotics, which are constantly changing, are different from region to region, and are often hospital- and unit-specific; (2) the antibiotic concentrations achieved at the site of infection over a 24-hour dosing interval; (3) the mechanism of how antibiotics kill bacteria; (4) how often the dose we select produces a clinical and microbiological cure; (5) how often we encounter toxicity; (6) how likely the antibiotic exposure will lead to antibiotic resistance in the treated child and in the population in general; and (7) effect on the child's microbiome.

Susceptibility

Susceptibility data for each bacterial pathogen against a wide range of antibiotics are available from the microbiology laboratory of virtually every hospital. This antibiogram can help guide you in antibiotic selection for empiric therapy. Many hospitals can separate the inpatient culture results from outpatient results, and many can give you the data by ward of the hospital (eg, pediatric ward vs neonatal intensive care unit vs adult intensive care unit). Susceptibility data are also available by region and by country from reference laboratories or public health laboratories. The recommendations made in *Nelson's Pediatric Antimicrobial Therapy* reflect overall susceptibility patterns present in the United States. Tables A and B in Chapter 7 provide some overall guidance on susceptibility of gram-positive and gram-negative pathogens, respectively. Wide variations may exist for certain pathogens in different regions of the United States and the world.

Drug Concentrations at the Site of Infection

With every antibiotic, we can measure the concentration of antibiotic present in the serum. We can also directly measure the concentrations in specific tissue sites, such as spinal fluid or middle ear fluid. Because free, nonprotein-bound antibiotic is required to inhibit and kill pathogens, it is also important to calculate the amount of free drug available at the site of infection. While traditional methods of measuring antibiotics focused on the peak concentrations in serum and how rapidly the drugs were excreted, complex models of drug distribution in plasma and tissue sites (eg, cerebrospinal fluid, urine, peritoneal fluid) and elimination from plasma and tissue compartments now exist. Antibiotic exposure to pathogens at the site of infection can be described mathematically in many ways: (1) the percentage of time in a 24-hour dosing interval that the antibiotic concentrations are above the minimum inhibitory concentration (MIC; the antibiotic concentration required for inhibition of growth of an organism) at the site of infection (%T>MIC); (2) the mathematically calculated area below the serum concentration-versus-time curve (area under the curve [AUC]); and (3) the maximal concentration of drug achieved at the tissue site (Cmax). For each of these 3 values, a ratio of that value to the MIC of the pathogen in question can be calculated and provides more useful information on specific drug activity against a specific pathogen than simply looking at the MIC. It allows us to compare the exposure of different antibiotics (that achieve quite different concentrations in tissues) to a pathogen (where the MIC for each drug may be different) and to assess the activity of a single antibiotic that may be used for empiric therapy against the many different pathogens (potentially with many MICs) that may be causing an infection at that tissue site.

Pharmacodynamics

Pharmacodynamic descriptions provide the clinician with information on *how* the bacterial pathogens are killed (see Suggested Reading). Beta-lactam antibiotics tend to eradicate bacteria following prolonged exposure of the antibiotic to the pathogen at the site of infection, usually expressed as the percent of time over a dosing interval that the antibiotic is present at the site of infection in concentrations greater than the MIC (%T>MIC). For example, amoxicillin needs to be present at the site of pneumococcal infection (eg, middle ear) at a concentration above the MIC for only 40% of a 24-hour dosing interval. Remarkably, neither higher concentrations of amoxicillin nor a more prolonged exposure will substantially increase the cure rate. On the other hand, gentamicin's activity against *Escherichia coli* is based primarily on the absolute concentration of free antibiotic at the site of infection, in the context of the MIC of the pathogen (Cmax:MIC). The more antibiotic you can deliver to the site of infection, the more rapidly you can sterilize the tissue; we are only limited by the toxicities of gentamicin. For fluoroquinolones like ciprofloxacin, the antibiotic exposure best linked to clinical and microbiologic success is, like aminoglycosides, concentration-dependent rather than time-dependent, as is present with penicillins. However, the best mathematical correlate to microbiologic (and clinical) outcomes is the AUC:MIC, rather than Cmax:MIC.

Assessment of Clinical and Microbiological Outcomes

In clinical trials of anti-infective agents, most adults and children will hopefully be cured, but a few will fail therapy. For those few, we may note inadequate drug exposure (eg, more rapid drug elimination in a particular patient; the inability of a particular antibiotic to be present at the site of infection in its active form, not bound to salts or proteins) or infection caused by a pathogen with a particularly high MIC. By analyzing the successes and the failures based on the appropriate exposure parameters outlined previously (%T>MIC, AUC:MIC, or Cmax:MIC), we can often observe a particular value of exposure, above which we observe a higher rate of cure and below which the cure rate drops quickly. Knowing this target value in adults (the "antibiotic exposure break point") allows us to calculate the dosage that will create treatment success in most children. We do not have failure rates in children sufficient to calculate a pediatric exposure break point. It is the adult *exposure value* that leads to success that we subsequently offer to you for children, as one likely to cure your patient. US Food and Drug Administration (FDA)-approved break points that are reported by microbiology laboratories (S, I, and R) are now determined by outcomes linked to drug pharmacokinetics and exposure, the MIC, and the pharmacodynamic parameter for that agent. Recommendations to the FDA for break points for the United States often come from "break point organizations," such as the US Committee on Anti-microbial Susceptibility Testing (www.uscast.org) or the Clinical Laboratory Standards Institute Subcommittee on Antimicrobial Susceptibility Testing.

Suggested Reading

Bradley JS, et al. *Pediatr Infect Dis J.* 2010;29(11):1043–1046 PMID: 20975453

Drusano GL. *Clin Infect Dis.* 2007;45(Suppl 1):S89–S95 PMID: 17582578

4. Community-Associated Methicillin-Resistant *Staphylococcus aureus*

Community-associated methicillin-resistant *Staphylococcus aureus* (CA-MRSA) is a community pathogen for children (that can also spread from child to child in hospitals) that first appeared in the United States in the mid-1990s and currently represents 30% to 80% of all community isolates in various regions of the United States (check your hospital microbiology laboratory for your local rate); it is increasingly present in many areas of the world, with some strain variation documented. This CA-MRSA, like the hospital-associated MRSA strain that has been prevalent for the past 40 years, is resistant to methicillin and to all other beta-lactam antibiotics, except for ceftaroline, a fifth-generation cephalosporin antibiotic newly US Food and Drug Administration (FDA) approved for pediatrics in June 2016 (see Chapter 2).

There are an undetermined number of pathogenicity factors that make CA-MRSA more aggressive than methicillin-susceptible *S aureus* (MSSA) strains that circulated 20 years ago. Community-associated MRSA seems to cause greater tissue necrosis, an increased host inflammatory response, an increased rate of complications, and an increased rate of recurrent infections compared with MSSA. Response to therapy with non–beta-lactam antibiotics (eg, vancomycin, clindamycin) seems to be inferior compared with the response of MSSA to oxacillin/nafcillin or cefazolin, but it is unknown whether poorer outcomes are due to a hardier, better-adapted, more aggressive CA-MRSA or whether these alternative agents are just not as effective against MRSA as beta-lactam agents are against MSSA. Studies in children using ceftaroline to treat skin infections (many caused by MRSA) were conducted using a non-inferiority clinical trial design, compared with vancomycin, with the finding that ceftaroline was equivalent to vancomycin. Guidelines for management of MRSA infections were published by the Infectious Diseases Society of America in 2011.[1]

Antimicrobials for CA-MRSA

Vancomycin (intravenous [IV]) has been the mainstay of parenteral therapy of MRSA infections for the past 4 decades and continues to have activity against more than 98% of strains isolated from children. A few cases of intermediate resistance and "heteroresistance" (transient moderately increased resistance based on thickened staphylococcal cell walls) have been reported, most commonly in adults who are receiving long-term therapy or who have received multiple exposures to vancomycin. Unfortunately, the response to therapy using standard vancomycin dosing of 40 mg/kg/day in the treatment of the new CA-MRSA strains has not been as predictably successful as in the past with MSSA. Increasingly, data in adults suggest that serum trough concentrations of vancomycin in treating serious CA-MRSA infections should be kept in the range of 15 to 20 µg/mL, which frequently causes toxicity in adults. For children, serum trough concentrations of 15 to 20 µg/mL can usually be achieved using the old pediatric "meningitis dosage" of vancomycin of 60 mg/kg/day and have also been associated with renal toxicity. Although no prospectively collected data are available, it appears that this dosage in children is reasonably effective and not associated with the degree of nephrotoxicity observed in adults. For vancomycin, the ratio of the area under the serum concentration curve to minimum inhibitory concentration (AUC:MIC) that appears to be the exposure that best predicts a successful outcome is about 400 or greater (see Chapter 3 for more on the AIC:MIC). This ratio is achievable for CA-MRSA strains with in vitro MIC values of 1 μg/mL or less but difficult to achieve for strains with 2 μg/mL or greater.[2] Strains with MIC values of 4 μg/mL or greater should generally be considered resistant to vancomycin. When using these higher "meningitis" treatment dosages, one needs to follow renal function carefully for the development of toxicity.

Clindamycin (oral [PO] or IV) is active against approximately 70% to 90% of strains of either MRSA or MSSA, with great geographic variability (again, check with your hospital laboratory). The dosage for moderate to severe infections is 30 to 40 mg/kg/day, in 3 divided doses, using the same mg/kg dose PO or IV. Clindamycin is not as bactericidal as vancomycin but achieves higher concentrations in abscesses (based on high intracellular concentrations in neutrophils). Some CA-MRSA strains are susceptible to clindamycin on initial testing but have inducible clindamycin resistance (methylase-mediated) that is usually assessed by the "D-test" and, more recently, in automated multi-well microtiter plates. Within each population of these CA-MRSA organisms, a rare organism (between 1 in 10^6 and 10^8 organisms) will have a mutation that allows for constant (rather than induced) resistance.[3] Although still somewhat controversial, clindamycin should be effective therapy for infections that have a relatively low organism load (cellulitis, small abscesses) and are unlikely to contain a significant population of these methylase-producing mutants that are truly resistant (in contrast to those non-methylase–producing organisms that are actually poorly induced by clindamycin). Infections with a high organism load (empyema) may have a greater risk of failure against strains positive on the D-test (as a large population is more likely to have a significant number of truly resistant organisms), and clindamycin should not be used as the preferred agent for these strains. Many laboratories no longer report D-test results but simply call the organism "resistant." This forces the clinician to use alternative therapy that may not be needed.

Clindamycin is used to treat most CA-MRSA infections that are not life-threatening, and, if the child responds, therapy can be switched from IV to PO (although the oral solution is not very well tolerated). *Clostridium difficile* enterocolitis is a concern as a clindamycin-associated complication; however, despite a great increase in the use of clindamycin in children during the past decade, there are no recent published data on a clinically significant increase in the rate of this complication in children.

Trimethoprim/sulfamethoxazole (TMP/SMX) (PO, IV), Bactrim/Septra, is active against CA-MRSA in vitro. New, prospective comparative data on treatment of skin or skin structure infections in adults and children document efficacy equivalent to clindamycin.[4] Given our current lack of prospective, comparative information in MRSA bacteremia, pneumonia, and osteomyelitis (in contrast to skin infections), TMP/SMX should not be used routinely to treat these more serious infections at this time.

Linezolid (PO, IV), Zyvox, active against virtually 100% of CA-MRSA strains, is another reasonable alternative but is considered bacteriostatic and has relatively frequent hematologic toxicity in adults (neutropenia, thrombocytopenia) and some infrequent neurologic toxicity (peripheral neuropathy, optic neuritis), particularly when used for courses of 2 weeks or longer (a complete blood cell count should be checked every week or 2 in children receiving prolonged linezolid therapy). The cost of linezolid is substantially more than clindamycin or vancomycin, although the drug is soon to go off patent.

Daptomycin (IV), FDA approved for adults for skin infections in 2003 and, subsequently, for bacteremia/endocarditis, is a new class of antibiotic, a lipopeptide, and is highly bactericidal. Daptomycin should be considered for treatment of skin infection and bacteremia in failures with other, better studied antibiotics. **Daptomycin should not be used to treat pneumonia,** as it is inactivated by pulmonary surfactant. Pediatric studies for skin infections have been completed, and those for bacteremia and osteomyelitis have just concluded, but data from the trials have not yet been analyzed or presented. Some newborn animal neurologic toxicity data suggest additional caution for the use of daptomycin in infants younger than 1 year, prompting a change in the package label. Sponsored pediatric clinical trial investigations in these younger infants are not proceeding at this time.

Tigecycline and fluoroquinolones, both of which may show in vitro activity, are not generally recommended for children if other agents are available and are tolerated due to potential toxicity issues for children with tetracyclines and fluoroquinolones and rapid emergence of resistance with fluoroquinolones.

Ceftaroline, a fifth-generation cephalosporin antibiotic, the first FDA-approved beta-lactam antibiotic to be active against MRSA, was finally FDA-approved *for children* in June 2016. The gram-negative coverage is similar to cefotaxime, with no activity against *Pseudomonas*. Published data are available for pediatric pharmacokinetics, as well as for prospective, randomized comparative treatment trials of skin and skin structure infections[5] and community-acquired pneumonia.[6,7] The efficacy and toxicity profile in adults is what one would expect from most cephalosporins. Based on these published data and review by the FDA, for infants and children 2 months and older, ceftaroline should be effective and safer than vancomycin for treatment of MRSA infections. Just as beta-lactams are preferred over vancomycin for MSSA infections, ceftaroline should be considered preferred treatment over vancomycin for MRSA infection. Neither renal function nor drug levels need to be followed with ceftaroline therapy. We will be closely following post-marketing experience in children, and recommendations may change if unexpected clinical data on lack of efficacy or unexpected toxicity should be presented.

Combination therapy for serious infections, with vancomycin and rifampin (for deep abscesses) or vancomycin and gentamicin (for bacteremia), is often used, but no prospective, controlled human clinical data exist on improved efficacy over single antibiotic therapy. Some experts use vancomycin and clindamycin in combination, particularly for children with a toxic-shock clinical presentation. Ceftaroline has also been used in combination therapy with other agents in adults, but no prospective, controlled clinical data exist to assess benefits.

4

Community-Associated Methicillin-Resistant *Staphylococcus aureus*

Investigational Agents Recently Approved for Adults to Be Studied in Children

Dalbavancin and Oritavancin. Both antibiotics are IV glycopeptides, structurally very similar to vancomycin but with enhanced in vitro activity against MRSA and a much longer serum half-life, allowing once-weekly dosing or even just a single dose to treat skin infections.

Telavancin. A glyco-lipopeptide with mechanisms of activity that include cell wall inhibition and cell membrane depolarization, telavancin is administered once daily.

Tedizolid. A second-generation oxazolidinone like linezolid, tedizolid is more potent in vitro against MRSA than linezolid, with somewhat decreased toxicity to bone marrow in adult clinical studies.

Recommendations for Empiric Therapy of Suspected MRSA Infections

Life-threatening and Serious Infections. If any CA-MRSA is present in your community, empiric therapy for presumed staphylococcal infections that are life-threatening or infections for which any risk of failure is unacceptable (eg, meningitis) should follow the recommendations for CA-MRSA and include *high-dose* vancomycin, clindamycin, or linezolid, in addition to nafcillin or oxacillin (beta-lactam antibiotics are considered better than vancomycin or clindamycin for MSSA). Ceftaroline is now another option, particularly for children with some degree of renal injury.

Moderate Infections. If you live in a location with greater than 10% methicillin resistance, consider using the CA-MRSA recommendations for hospitalized children with presumed staphylococcal infections of any severity, and start empiric therapy with clindamycin (usually active against >90% of CA-MRSA), ceftaroline, vancomycin, or linezolid IV.

In skin and skin structure abscesses, drainage of the abscess may be completely curative in some children, and antibiotics may not be necessary following incision and drainage.

Mild Infections. For nonserious, presumed staphylococcal infections in regions with significant CA-MRSA, empiric topical therapy with mupirocin (Bactroban) or retapamulin (Altabax) ointment, or oral therapy with TMP/SMX or clindamycin, are preferred. For older children, doxycycline and minocycline are also options based on data in adults.

Prevention of Recurrent Infections

For children with problematic, recurrent infections, no well-studied, prospectively collected data provide a solution. Bleach baths (one-half cup of bleach in a full bathtub[8]) seems to be able to transiently decrease the numbers of colonizing organisms but was not shown to decrease the number of infections in a prospective, controlled study of children with eczema. Similarly, a regimen to decolonize with twice-weekly bleach baths in an attempt to prevent recurrent infection did not lead to a statistically significant decrease.[9] Bathing with chlorhexidine (Hibiclens, a preoperative antibacterial skin disinfectant) daily or a few times each week should provide topical anti-MRSA activity for several hours following a bath, but no prospective data exist yet to document benefit. Nasal mupirocin ointment (Bactroban) designed to eradicate colonization may also be used. All of these measures have advantages and disadvantages and need to be used together with environmental measures (eg, washing towels frequently, using hand sanitizers, not sharing items of clothing). Helpful advice can be found on the Centers for Disease Control and Prevention Web site at www.cdc.gov/mrsa (accessed September 13, 2016).

Vaccines are being investigated but are not likely to be available for several years.

5. Antimicrobial Therapy for Newborns

NOTES

- Prospectively collected data in newborns continue to become available, thanks in large part to federal legislation (including the US Food and Drug Administration [FDA] Safety and Innovation Act of 2012 that mandates neonatal studies). In situations of inadequate data, suggested doses are based on efficacy, safety, and pharmacologic data from older children or adults. These may not account for the effect of developmental changes (effect of ontogeny) on drug metabolism that occur during early infancy and among premature and full-term newborns.[1] These values may vary widely, particularly for the unstable premature newborn. Oral convalescent therapy for neonatal infections has not been well studied but may be used cautiously in non–life-threatening infections in adherent families with ready access to medical care.[2]

- The recommended antibiotic dosages and intervals of administration are given in the tables at the end of this chapter.

- **Adverse drug reaction:** Neonates should not receive intravenous (IV) ceftriaxone while receiving IV calcium-containing products, including parenteral nutrition, by the same or different infusion lines, as fatal reactions with ceftriaxone-calcium precipitates in lungs and kidneys in neonates have occurred. There are no data on interactions between IV ceftriaxone and oral calcium-containing products or between intramuscular ceftriaxone and IV or oral calcium-containing products. Current information is available on the FDA Web site.[3] Cefotaxime is preferred over ceftriaxone for neonates.[4]

- **Abbreviations:** 3TC, lamivudine; ABLC, lipid complex amphotericin; ABR, auditory brainstem response; ALT, alanine transaminase; AmB, amphotericin B; AmB-D, AmB deoxycholate; amox/clav, amoxicillin/clavulanate; AOM, acute otitis media; AST, aspartate transaminase; AUC, area under the curve; bid, twice daily; CBC, complete blood cell count; CDC, Centers for Disease Control and Prevention; CLD, chronic lung disease; CMV, cytomegalovirus; CNS, central nervous system; CSF, cerebrospinal fluid; CT, computed tomography; div, divided; echo, echocardiogram; ECMO, extracorporeal membrane oxygenation; ESBL, extended spectrum beta-lactamase; FDA, US Food and Drug Administration; GA, gestational age; GBS, group B streptococcus; G-CSF, granulocyte colony stimulating factor; HIV, human immunodeficiency virus; HSV, herpes simplex virus; IAI, intra-abdominal infection; ID, infectious diseases; IM, intramuscular; IUGR, intrauterine growth restriction; IV, intravenous; IVIG, intravenous immune globulin; L-AmB, liposomal AmB; MIC, minimal inhibitory concentration; MRSA, methicillin-resistant *Staphylococcus aureus;* MSSA, methicillin-susceptible *S aureus;* NEC, necrotizing enterocolitis; NICU, neonatal intensive care unit; NVP, nevirapine; PCR, polymerase chain reaction; pip/tazo, piperacillin/tazobactam; PO, orally; RSV, respiratory syncytial virus; spp, species; ticar/clav, ticarcillin/clavulanate; tid, 3 times daily; TIG, tetanus immune globulin; TMP/SMX, trimethoprim/sulfamethoxazole; UCSF, University of California, San Francisco; UTI, urinary tract infection; VCUG, voiding cystourethrogram; VDRL, Venereal Disease Research Laboratories; ZDV, zidovudine.

A. RECOMMENDED THERAPY FOR SELECTED NEWBORN CONDITIONS

Condition	Therapy (evidence grade) See Tables 5B–D for neonatal dosages.	Comments
Conjunctivitis		
– Chlamydia[5–8]	Azithromycin 10 mg/kg/day PO for 1 day, then 5 mg/kg/day PO for 4 days (AII), or erythromycin ethylsuccinate PO for 10–14 days (AII)	Macrolides PO preferred to topical eye drops to prevent development of pneumonia; association of erythromycin and pyloric stenosis in young neonates.[9] Alternative: 3-day course of higher-dose azithromycin at 10 mg/kg/dose once daily, although safety not well defined in neonates (CIII). Oral sulfonamides may be used after the immediate neonatal period for infants who do not tolerate erythromycin.
– Gonococcal[10–14]	Ceftriaxone 25–50 mg/kg (max 125 mg) IV, IM once, AND azithromycin 10 mg/kg PO q24h for 5 days (AII)	Ceftriaxone no longer recommended as single agent therapy due to increasing cephalosporin resistance; therefore, addition of azithromycin recommended (no data in neonates; azithromycin dose is that recommended for pertussis). Cefotaxime is preferred for neonates with hyperbilirubinemia. Saline irrigation of eyes. Evaluate for chlamydial infection. All neonates born to mothers with untreated gonococcal infection (regardless of symptoms) require therapy. Cefixime and ciprofloxacin no longer recommended for empiric maternal therapy.
– Staphylococcus aureus[15–17]	Topical therapy sufficient for mild S aureus cases (AII), but oral or IV therapy may be considered for moderate to severe conjunctivitis. MSSA: oxacillin/nafcillin IV or cefazolin (for non-CNS infections) IM, IV for 7 days. MRSA: vancomycin IV or clindamycin IV, PO.	Neomycin or erythromycin (BIII) ophthalmic drops or ointment No prospective data for MRSA conjunctivitis (BIII) Cephalexin PO for mild-moderate disease caused by MSSA Increased S aureus resistance with ciprofloxacin/levofloxacin ophthalmic formulations (AII)
– Pseudomonas aeruginosa[18–20]	Ceftazidime IM, IV AND tobramycin IM, IV for 7–10 days (alternatives: meropenem, cefepime, pip/tazo) (BIII)	Aminoglycoside or polymyxin B–containing ophthalmic drops or ointment as adjunctive therapy

– Other gram-negative	Aminoglycoside or polymyxin B–containing ophthalmic drops or ointment if mild (AII). Systemic therapy if moderate to severe or unresponsive to topical therapy (AIII).	Duration of therapy dependent on clinical course and may be as short as 5 days if clinically resolved.

Cytomegalovirus

– Congenital[21–24]	For moderately to severely symptomatic neonates with congenital infection syndrome and multisystem disease: oral valganciclovir at 16 mg/kg/dose bid for 6 mo[24] (AI); IV ganciclovir 6 mg/kg/dose IV q12h can be used for some or all of the first 6 wk of therapy if oral therapy not advised (AII).	Benefit for hearing loss and neurodevelopmental outcomes (AI). Treatment recommended for neonates with moderate or severe symptomatic congenital CMV disease, with or without CNS involvement. Treatment is not routinely recommended for "mildly symptomatic" neonates congenitally infected with CMV (eg, only 1 or perhaps 2 manifestations of congenital CMV infection, which are mild in scope [eg, slight IUGR, mild hepatomegaly] or transient and mild in nature [eg, a single platelet count of 80,000 or an ALT of 130]), as the risks of treatment may not be balanced by benefits in mild disease that is often reversible without long-term sequelae.[25] This includes neonates who are asymptomatic except for sensorineural hearing loss. Treatment for asymptomatic neonates congenitally infected with CMV is not recommended. Neutropenia in 20% (oral valganciclovir) to 68% (IV ganciclovir) of neonates on long-term therapy (responds to G-CSF or temporary discontinuation of therapy). Treatment for congenital CMV should start within the first month of life. CMV-IVIG not recommended.
– Perinatally or postnatally acquired[23]	Ganciclovir 12 mg/kg/day IV div q12h for 14–21 days (AIII)	Antiviral treatment has not been studied in this population but can be considered in patients with acute, severe, visceral (end-organ) disease, such as pneumonia, hepatitis, encephalitis, necrotizing enterocolitis, or persistent thrombocytopenia. If such patients are treated with parenteral ganciclovir, a reasonable approach is to treat for 2 wk and then reassess responsiveness to therapy. If clinical data suggest benefit of treatment, an additional 1 wk of parenteral ganciclovir can be considered if symptoms and signs have not fully resolved. Observe for possible relapse after completion of therapy (AIII).

5

A. RECOMMENDED THERAPY FOR SELECTED NEWBORN CONDITIONS (continued)

Condition	Therapy (evidence grade) *See Tables 5B–D for neonatal dosages.*	Comments
Fungal infections (See also Chapter 8.)		
– Candidiasis[26–34]	**Treatment** AmB-D (1 mg/kg/day) is recommended therapy (AII). Fluconazole (12 mg/kg/day q24h, after a load of 25 mg/kg/day) is an alternative if patient has not been on fluconazole prophylaxis (AII).[26] For treatment of neonates and young infants (<120 days) on ECMO, fluconazole loading dose is 35 mg/kg on day 1, then 12 mg/kg q24h (BII). Lipid formulation AmB is an alternative but carries a theoretic risk of less urinary tract penetration compared with AmB-D (CIII). Duration of therapy for candidemia without obvious metastatic complications is for 2 wk after documented clearance and resolution of symptoms. **Prophylaxis** In nurseries with high rates of candidiasis (>10%),[35] IV or oral fluconazole prophylaxis (AI) (3–6 mg/kg twice weekly for 6 wk) in high-risk neonates (birth weight <1,000 g) is recommended. Oral nystatin, 100,000 units 3 times daily for 6 wk, is an alternative to fluconazole in neonates with birth weights <1,500 g if availability or resistance preclude fluconazole use (CII).	Evaluate for other sites of infection: CSF analysis, echo, abdominal ultrasound to include bladder; retinal eye examination. Length of therapy dependent on disease (BIII), usually 2 wk after all clearance. Antifungal susceptibility testing is suggested with persistent disease. *C krusei* inherently resistant to fluconazole; *C parapsilosis* may be less susceptible to echinocandins; increasing resistance of *C glabrata* to fluconazole and echinocandins. No proven benefit for combination antifungal therapy in candidiasis. Change from AmB or fluconazole to echinocandin if cultures persistently positive (BII). Although fluconazole prophylaxis has been shown to reduce colonization, it has not reduced mortality.[29] Lumbar puncture and dilated retinal examination recommended in neonates with cultures positive for *Candida* spp from blood (AIII). Same recommended for all infants with birth weight <1,500 g with candiduria with or without candidemia (AIII). CT or ultrasound imaging of genitourinary tract, liver, and spleen should be performed if blood culture results are persistently positive (AIII). Meningoencephalitis in the neonate occurs at a higher rate than in older children/adults. Central venous catheter removal strongly recommended. Infected CNS devices, including ventriculostomy drains and shunts, should be removed, if possible. See Skin and Soft Tissues later in this Table for management of congenital cutaneous candidiasis.

Neonates and children on ECMO: fluconazole 12 mg/kg on day 1, followed by 6 mg/kg/day (BII).

Echinocandins should be used with caution and generally limited to salvage therapy or situations in which resistance or toxicity preclude use of AmB-D or fluconazole (CIII).

Role of flucytosine in neonates with meningitis is questionable and not routinely recommended due to toxicity concerns. The addition of flucytosine (100 mg/kg/day div q6h) may be considered as salvage therapy in patients who have not had a clinical response to initial AmB therapy, but adverse effects are frequent (CIII).

A. RECOMMENDED THERAPY FOR SELECTED NEWBORN CONDITIONS (continued)

Condition	Therapy (evidence grade) See Tables 5B–D for neonatal dosages.	Comments
– Aspergillosis (usually cutaneous infection with systemic dissemination)[24,36-38]	Voriconazole initial dosing same as pediatric >2 y: 18 mg/kg/day IV div q12h for a loading dose on the first day, then 16 mg/kg/day IV div q12h as a maintenance dose. Continued dosing is guided by monitoring of trough serum concentrations (AII). When stable, may switch from voriconazole IV to voriconazole PO 18 mg/kg/day div bid (AII). Unlike in adults, PO bioavailability in children is only approximately 60%. Trough monitoring is crucial after switch.[23] Alternatives for primary therapy when voriconazole cannot be administered: L-AmB 5 mg/kg/day (AII). ABLC is another possible alternative. Echinocandin primary monotherapy should not be used for treating invasive aspergillosis (CII). AmB deoxycholate should be used only in resource-limited settings in which no alternative agent is available (AII).	Aggressive antifungal therapy, early debridement of skin lesions (AIII). Voriconazole is preferred primary antifungal therapy for all clinical forms of aspergillosis (AI). Early initiation of therapy in patients with strong suspicion of disease is important while a diagnostic evaluation is conducted. Therapeutic voriconazole trough serum concentrations of 2–5 mg/L are important for success. It is critical to monitor trough concentrations to guide therapy due to high inter-patient variability.[25] Low voriconazole concentrations are a leading cause of clinical failure. Neonatal and infant voriconazole dosing is not well defined, but doses required to achieve therapeutic troughs are generally higher than in children >2 y (AII). No experience with posaconazole or isavuconazole in neonates. Total treatment course is for a minimum of 6–12 wk, largely dependent on the degree and duration of immunosuppression and evidence of disease improvement. Salvage antifungal therapy options after failed primary therapy include a change of antifungal class (using L-AmB or an echinocandin), switching to posaconazole (trough concentrations >0.7 μg/mL), or using combination antifungal therapy. Combination therapy with voriconazole + an echinocandin may be considered in select patients.[26] In vitro data suggest some synergy with 2 (but not 3) drug combinations: an azole + an echinocandin is the most well studied. If combination therapy is employed, this is likely best done initially when voriconazole trough concentrations may not yet be therapeutic. Routine susceptibility testing is not recommended but is suggested for patients suspected of having an azole-resistant isolate or who are unresponsive to therapy.

Azole-resistant *Aspergillus fumigatus* is increasing. If local epidemiology suggests >10% azole resistance, empiric initial therapy should be voriconazole OR L-AmB, and subsequent therapy guided based on antifungal susceptibilities.[39]

Micafungin likely has equal efficacy to caspofungin against aspergillosis.[27]

Gastrointestinal infections

– NEC or peritonitis secondary to bowel rupture[40–45]	Ampicillin IV AND gentamicin IM, IV for ≥10 days (AII). Alternatives: pip/tazo AND gentamicin (AII); ceftazidime/cefotaxime AND gentamicin ± metronidazole (BIII); OR meropenem (BI). ADD fluconazole if known to have gastrointestinal colonization with *Candida* (BIII).	Surgical drainage (AII). Definitive antibiotic therapy based on culture results (aerobic, anaerobic, and fungal); meropenem or cefepime if ceftazidime-resistant gram-negative bacilli isolated. Vancomycin rather than ampicillin if MRSA prevalent. *Bacteroides* colonization may occur as early as the first week of life (AIII).[45] Duration of therapy dependent on clinical response and risk of persisting intra-abdominal abscess (AIII). Probiotics may prevent NEC in neonates born <1,500 g, but agent, dose, and safety not fully known.[42,45]
– *Salmonella*[46]	Ampicillin IM, IV (if susceptible) OR cefotaxime IM, IV for 7–10 days (AII)	Observe for focal complications (eg, meningitis, arthritis) (AIII).

Herpes simplex infection

– CNS and disseminated disease[47–49]	Acyclovir 60 mg/kg/day div q8h IV for 21 days (AII) (if eye disease present, ADD topical 1% trifluridine or 0.15% ganciclovir ophthalmic gel) (AII).	For CNS disease, perform CSF HSV PCR near end of 21 days of therapy and continue acyclovir until PCR negative. Serum AST/ALT may help identify early disseminated infection. Foscarnet for acyclovir-resistant disease. Acyclovir PO (300 mg/m²/dose tid) suppression for 6 mo recommended following parenteral therapy (AI).[51] Monitor for neutropenia during suppressive therapy. Different dosages than those listed in Table 5B have been modeled, but there are no safety or efficacy data in humans to support them.[51]

A. RECOMMENDED THERAPY FOR SELECTED NEWBORN CONDITIONS (continued)

Condition	Therapy (evidence grade) See Tables 5B–D for neonatal dosages.	Comments
– Skin, eye, or mouth disease[47-49]	Acyclovir 60 mg/kg/day div q8h IV for 14 days (AII) (if eye disease present, ADD topical 1% trifluridine or 0.15% ganciclovir ophthalmic gel) (AII). Obtain CSF PCR for HSV to assess for CNS infection.	Acyclovir PO (300 mg/m²/dose tid) suppression for 6 mo recommended following parenteral therapy (AI).[50] Monitor for neutropenia during suppressive therapy. Different dosages than those listed in Table 5B have been modeled, but there are no safety or efficacy data in humans to support them.[51]
Human immuno- deficiency virus infection[52,53]	There has been recent interest in using "treatment" antiretroviral regimens for high-risk, exposed neonates in an attempt to achieve a remission or possibly even a cure. This was initially stimulated by the experience of a baby from Mississippi: high-risk neonate treated within the first 2 days of life with subsequent infection documentation; off therapy at 18 mo of age without evidence of circulating virus until 4 y of age, at which point virus became detectable.[54] While a clinical trial is ongoing to study issues further, full treatment dosing of high-risk neonates is not currently recommended due to lack of safety and dosing data and lack of defined efficacy.	
	Peripartum presumptive preventive therapy for HIV-exposed newborns: ZDV for the first 6 wk of age (AI). Note: if the mother was treated with combination antiretroviral therapy during pregnancy with complete viral suppression, newborn prevention therapy for 4 wk can be considered. GA ≥35 wk: ZDV 8 mg/kg/day PO div bid OR 6 mg/kg/day IV div q8h for 6 wk. GA <35 wk but ≥30 wk: ZDV 4 mg/kg/day PO (OR 3 mg/kg/day IV) div q12h. Increase at 2 wk of age to 6 mg/kg/day PO (OR 4.6 mg/kg/day IV) div q12h. GA <30 wk: ZDV 4 mg/kg/day PO (OR 3 mg/kg/day IV) div q12h. Increase at 4 wk of age to 6 mg/kg/day PO (OR 4.6 mg/kg/day IV) div q12h.	For detailed information: https://aidsinfo.nih.gov/guidelines/html/1/adult-and-adolescent-treatment-guidelines/0 (accessed September 15, 2016). UCSF Clinician Consultation Center (888/448-8765) provides free clinical consultation. Start prevention therapy as soon after delivery as possible, but by 6–8 h of age for best effectiveness (AII). Monitor CBC at birth and 4 wk (AII). Some experts consider the use of ZDV in combination with other anti-retroviral drugs in certain situations (eg, mothers with minimal intervention before delivery, with high viral load, and/or with known resistant virus). Consultation with a pediatric HIV specialist is recommended (BIII). Perform HIV-1 DNA PCR or RNA assays at 14–21 days, 1–2 mo, and 4–6 mo (AI). Initiate prophylaxis for pneumocystis pneumonia at 6 wk of age if HIV infection not yet excluded (AII).

For newborns whose mothers received NO antenatal antiretroviral therapy, add 3 doses of NVP (first dose at 0–48 h; second dose 48 h later; third dose 96 h after second dose) to the 6 wk of ZDV treatment (AI).

NVP dose: birth weight 1.5–2 kg: 8 mg/dose PO; birth weight >2 kg: 12 mg/dose PO (AI).[55]

The preventive ZDV doses listed herein for neonates are also treatment doses for infants with diagnosed HIV infection. Note that antiretroviral treatment doses for neonates are established only for ZDV and 3TC (4 mg/kg/day div q12h). Treatment of HIV-infected neonates should be considered only with expert consultation.

Influenza A and B viruses[56–59]	Preterm, <38 wk postmenstrual age: 1 mg/kg/dose PO bid Preterm, 38–40 wk postmenstrual age: 1.5 mg/kg/dose PO bid Preterm, >40 wk postmenstrual age: 3 mg/kg/dose PO bid[57] Term, birth–8 mo: 3 mg/kg/dose PO bid[57,60]	Oseltamivir chemoprophylaxis not recommended for infants <3 mo unless the situation is judged critical because of limited safety and efficacy data in this age group.[61] This formulation of the drug is not yet approved in the United States, though. Studies of parenteral zanamivir have been completed in children.[61]
Omphalitis and funisitis		
– Empiric therapy for omphalitis and necrotizing funisitis direct therapy against coliform bacilli, S aureus (consider MRSA), and anaerobes[62–64]	Cefotaxime OR gentamicin, AND clindamycin for ≥10 days (AII)	Need to culture to direct therapy. Alternatives for coliform coverage if resistance likely: cefepime, meropenem. For suspect MRSA: ADD vancomycin. Alternatives for combined MSSA and anaerobic coverage: pip/tazo or ticar/clav. Appropriate wound management for infected cord and necrotic tissue (AIII).

5

Antimicrobial Therapy for Newborns

5

A. RECOMMENDED THERAPY FOR SELECTED NEWBORN CONDITIONS (continued)

Condition	Therapy (evidence grade) See Tables 5B–D for neonatal dosages.	Comments
– Group A or B strepto-cocci[65]	Penicillin G IV for ≥7–14 days (shorter course for superficial funisitis without invasive infection) (AII)	Group A streptococcus usually causes "wet cord" without pus and with minimal erythema; single dose of benzathine penicillin IM adequate. Consultation with pediatric ID specialist is recommended for necrotizing fasciitis (AII).
– S aureus[64]	MSSA: oxacillin/nafcillin IV, IM for ≥5–7 days (shorter course for superficial funisitis without invasive infection) (AIII) MRSA: vancomycin (AIII)	Assess for bacteremia and other focus of infection. Alternatives for MRSA: linezolid, clindamycin (if susceptible).
– Clostridium spp[66]	Clindamycin OR penicillin G IV for ≥10 days, with additional agents based on culture results (AII)	Crepitance and rapidly spreading cellulitis around umbilicus Mixed infection with other gram-positive and gram-negative bacteria common
Osteomyelitis, suppurative arthritis[67–69] Obtain cultures (aerobic; fungal if NICU) of bone or joint fluid before antibiotic therapy. Duration of therapy dependent on causative organism and normalization of erythrocyte sedimentation rate and C-reactive protein; minimum for osteomyelitis 3 wk and arthritis therapy 2–3 wk if no organism identified (AIII). Surgical drainage of pus (AIII); physical therapy may be needed (BIII).		
– Empiric therapy	Nafcillin/oxacillin IV (or vancomycin if MRSA is a concern) AND cefotaxime or gentamicin IV, IM (AIII)	
– Coliform bacteria (eg, Escherichia coli, Klebsiella spp, Enterobacter spp)	For E coli and Klebsiella: cefotaxime OR gentamicin OR ampicillin (if susceptible) (AIII). For Enterobacter, Serratia, or Citrobacter: ADD gentamicin IV, IM to cefotaxime or ceftriaxone, OR use cefepime or meropenem alone (AIII).	Meropenem for ESBL-producing coliforms (AIII). Pip/tazo or cefepime are alternatives for susceptible bacilli (BII).

Condition	Therapy	Comments
– Gonococcal arthritis and tenosynovitis[11-14]	Ceftriaxone IV, IM OR cefotaxime IV AND azithromycin 10 mg/kg PO q24h for 5 days (AIII)	Ceftriaxone no longer recommended as single agent therapy due to increasing cephalosporin resistance; therefore, addition of azithromycin recommended (no data in neonates; azithromycin dose is that recommended for pertussis). Cefotaxime is preferred for neonates with hyperbilirubinemia.
– S aureus	MSSA: oxacillin/nafcillin IV (AII) MRSA: vancomycin IV (AIII)	Alternative for MSSA: cefazolin (AIII) Alternatives for MRSA: linezolid, clindamycin (if susceptible) (BIII) Addition of rifampin if persistently positive cultures
– Group B streptococcus	Ampicillin or penicillin G IV (AII)	
– Haemophilus influenzae	Ampicillin IV OR cefotaxime IV, IM if ampicillin resistant	Start with IV therapy and switch to oral therapy when clinically stable. Amox/clav PO OR amoxicillin PO if susceptible (AIII).
Otitis media[70]	No controlled treatment trials in newborns; if no response, obtain middle ear fluid for culture.	In addition to Pneumococcus and Haemophilus, coliforms and S aureus may also cause AOM in neonates (AIII).
– Empiric therapy[71]	Oxacillin/nafcillin AND cefotaxime or gentamicin	Start with IV therapy and switch to oral therapy when clinically stable. Amox/clav (AIII).
– E coli (therapy of other coliforms based on susceptibility testing)	Cefotaxime OR gentamicin	Start with IV therapy and switch to oral therapy when clinically stable. For ESBL-producing strains, use meropenem (AII). Amox/clav if susceptible (AIII).
– S aureus	MSSA: oxacillin/nafcillin IV MRSA: vancomycin or clindamycin IV (if susceptible)	Start with IV therapy and switch to oral therapy when clinically stable. MSSA: cephalexin PO for 10 days or cloxacillin PO (AIII). MRSA: linezolid PO or clindamycin PO (BII).
– Group A or B streptococci	Penicillin G or ampicillin IV, IM	Start with IV therapy and switch to oral therapy when clinically stable. Amoxicillin 30–40 mg/kg/day PO div q8h for 10 days.
Parotitis, suppurative[72]	Oxacillin/nafcillin IV AND gentamicin IV, IM for 10 days; consider vancomycin if MRSA suspected (AIII).	Usually staphylococcal but occasionally coliform. Antimicrobial regimen without incision/drainage is adequate in >75% of cases.

5

A. RECOMMENDED THERAPY FOR SELECTED NEWBORN CONDITIONS (continued)

Condition	Therapy (evidence grade) See Tables 5B–D for neonatal dosages.	Comments
Pulmonary infections		
– Empiric therapy of the neonate with early onset of pulmonary infiltrates (within the first 48–72 h of life)	Ampicillin IV, IM AND gentamicin or cefotaxime IV, IM for 10 days; many neonatologists treat low-risk neonates for ≤7 days (see Comments).	For newborns with no additional risk factors for bacterial infection (eg, maternal chorioamnionitis) who (1) have negative blood cultures, (2) have no need for >8 h of oxygen, and (3) are asymptomatic at 48 h into therapy, 4 days may be sufficient therapy, based on limited data.[73]
– Aspiration pneumonia[74]	Ampicillin IV, IM AND gentamicin IV, IM for 7–10 days (AIII)	Early onset neonatal pneumonia may represent aspiration of amniotic fluid, particularly if fluid is not sterile. Mild aspiration episodes may not require antibiotic therapy.
– *Chlamydia trachomatis*[75]	Azithromycin PO, IV q24h for 5 days OR erythromycin ethylsuccinate PO for 14 days (AII)	Association of erythromycin and azithromycin with pyloric stenosis in infants treated <6 wk of age[76]
– *Mycoplasma hominis*[77,78]	Clindamycin PO, IV for 10 days (Organisms are resistant to macrolides.)	Pathogenic role in pneumonia not well defined and clinical efficacy unknown; no association with bronchopulmonary dysplasia (BIII)
– Pertussis[79]	Azithromycin 10 mg/kg PO, IV q24h for 5 days OR erythromycin ethylsuccinate PO for 14 days (AII)	Association of erythromycin and azithromycin with pyloric stenosis in infants treated <6 wk of age Alternatives: for >1 mo of age, clarithromycin for 7 days; for >2 mo of age, TMP/SMX 14 days
– *P aeruginosa*[80]	Ceftazidime IV, IM AND tobramycin IV, IM for 10–14 days (AIII)	Alternatives: cefepime or meropenem, OR pip/tazo AND tobramycin
– Respiratory syncytial virus[81]	Treatment: see Comments. Prophylaxis: palivizumab (Synagis, a monoclonal antibody) 15 mg/kg IM monthly (maximum: 5 doses) for these high-risk infants (AI).	Aerosol ribavirin (6-g vial to make 20-mg/mL solution in sterile water), aerosolized over 18–20 h daily for 3–5 days (BII), provides little benefit and should only be used for life-threatening infection with RSV. Difficulties in administration, complications with airway reactivity, and concern for potential toxicities to health care workers preclude routine use.

	In first y of life, palivizumab prophylaxis is recommended for infants born before 29 wk 0 days' gestation. Palivizumab prophylaxis is not recommended for otherwise healthy infants born at ≥29 wk 0 days' gestation. In first y of life, palivizumab prophylaxis is recommended for preterm infants with CLD of prematurity, defined as birth at <32 wk 0 days' gestation and a requirement for >21% oxygen for at least 28 days after birth. Clinicians may administer palivizumab prophylaxis in the first y of life to certain infants with hemodynamically significant heart disease.	Palivizumab does not provide benefit in the treatment of an active RSV infection. Palivizumab prophylaxis may be considered for children <24 mo who will be profoundly immunocompromised during the RSV season. Palivizumab prophylaxis is not recommended in the second y of life except for children who required at least 28 days of supplemental oxygen after birth and who continue to require medical support (supplemental oxygen, chronic corticosteroid therapy, or diuretic therapy) during the 6-mo period before the start of the second RSV season. Monthly prophylaxis should be discontinued in any child who experiences a breakthrough RSV hospitalization. Children with pulmonary abnormality or neuromuscular disease that impairs the ability to clear secretions from the upper airways may be considered for prophylaxis in the first y of life. Insufficient data are available to recommend palivizumab prophylaxis for children with cystic fibrosis or Down syndrome. The burden of RSV disease and costs associated with transport from remote locations may result in a broader use of palivizumab for RSV prevention in Alaska Native populations and possibly in selected other American Indian populations. Palivizumab prophylaxis is not recommended for prevention of health care–associated RSV disease.
– S aureus[17,82–84]	MSSA: oxacillin/nafcillin IV (AIII). MRSA: vancomycin IV OR clindamycin IV if susceptible (AIII). Duration of therapy depends on extent of disease (pneumonia vs empyema vs pulmonary abscesses vs empyema) and should be individualized with therapy up to 21 days or longer.	Alternative for MSSA: cefazolin IV Addition of rifampin or linezolid if persistently positive cultures (AIII) Thoracostomy drainage of empyema
– Group B streptococcus[85,86]	Penicillin G IV OR ampicillin IV, IM for 10 days (AIII)	For serious infections, ADD gentamicin for synergy until clinically improved. No prospective, randomized data on the efficacy of a 7-day treatment course.

Antimicrobial Therapy for Newborns

A. RECOMMENDED THERAPY FOR SELECTED NEWBORN CONDITIONS (continued)

Condition	Therapy (evidence grade) See Tables 5B–D for neonatal dosages.	Comments
– *Ureaplasma* spp (*urea-lyticum or parvum*)[87]	Azithromycin PO, IV for 5 days or clarithro-mycin PO for 10 days (BIII)	Pathogenic role of *Ureaplasma* not well defined and no prophylaxis recommended for CLD Many *Ureaplasma* spp resistant to erythromycin Association of erythromycin and pyloric stenosis in young infants
Sepsis and meningitis[84,88,89]	**NOTE:** Duration of therapy: 10 days for sepsis without a focus (AIII); minimum of 21 days for gram-negative meningitis (or at least 14 days after CSF is sterile) and 14–21 days for GBS meningitis and other gram-positive bacteria (AIII)	There are no prospective, controlled studies on 5- or 7-day courses for mild or presumed sepsis.
– Initial therapy, organism unknown	Ampicillin IV AND a second agent, either cefotaxime IV or gentamicin IV, IM (AII)	Cefotaxime preferred if meningitis suspected or cannot be excluded clinically or by lumbar puncture (AIII). For locations with a high rate (10% or greater) of ESBL-producing *E coli*, and meningitis is suspected, empiric therapy with meropenem (or cefepime) is preferred over cefotaxime. For empiric therapy of sepsis without meningitis, in areas with a high rate of ESBL *E coli*, gentamicin is preferred. Initial empiric therapy of nosocomial infection should be based on each hospital's pathogens and susceptibilities. Always narrow antibiotic coverage once susceptibility data are available.
– *Bacteroides fragilis*	Metronidazole or meropenem IV, IM (AIII)	Alternative: clindamycin, but increasing resistance reported
– *Enterococcus* spp	Ampicillin IV, IM AND gentamicin IV, IM (AIII); for ampicillin-resistant organisms: vanco-mycin AND gentamicin (AIII)	Gentamicin needed with ampicillin or vancomycin for bactericidal activity; continue until clinical and microbiological response documented (AIII). For vancomycin-resistant enterococci that are also ampicillin resistant: linezolid (AIII).
– Enterovirus	Supportive therapy: no antivirals currently FDA approved	Pocapavir PO is currently under investigation for enterovirus (poliovirus). Pleconaril PO is currently under consideration for approval at FDA for treatment of neonatal enteroviral sepsis syndrome.[90]

– E coli[88,89]	Cefotaxime IV or gentamicin IV, IM (AII)	Cefotaxime preferred if meningitis suspected or cannot be excluded clinically or by lumbar puncture (AIII). For locations with a high rate (10% or greater) of ESBL-producing E coli, and meningitis is suspected, empiric therapy with meropenem (or cefepime) is preferred over cefotaxime.
– Gonococcal[11–14]	Ceftriaxone IV, IM OR cefotaxime IV, IM, AND azithromycin 10 mg/kg PO q24h for 5 days (AIII)	Ceftriaxone no longer recommended as single agent therapy due to increasing cephalosporin resistance; therefore, addition of azithromycin is recommended (no data in neonates; azithromycin dose is that recommended for pertussis). Cefotaxime is preferred for neonates with hyperbilirubinemia.
– Listeria monocytogenes[91]	Ampicillin IV, IM AND gentamicin IV, IM (AIII)	Gentamicin is synergistic in vitro with ampicillin. Continue until clinical and microbiological response documented (AIII).
– P aeruginosa	Ceftazidime IV, IM AND tobramycin IV, IM (AIII)	Meropenem, cefepime, and tobramycin are suitable alternatives (AIII). Pip/tazo should not be used for CNS infection.
– S aureus[17,82–84,92,93]	MSSA: oxacillin/nafcillin IV, IM or cefazolin IV, IM (AII) MRSA: vancomycin IV (AIII)	Alternatives for MRSA: clindamycin, linezolid
– Staphylococcus epidermidis (or any coagulase-negative staphylococci)	Vancomycin IV (AIII)	If organism susceptible and infection not severe, oxacillin/nafcillin or cefazolin are alternatives for methicillin-susceptible strains. Cefazolin does not enter CNS. Add rifampin if cultures persistently positive.[94] Alternative: linezolid.
– Group A streptococcus	Penicillin G or ampicillin IV (AII)	
– Group B streptococcus[85]	Ampicillin or penicillin G IV AND gentamicin IV, IM (AI)	Continue gentamicin until clinical and microbiological response documented (AIII). Duration of therapy: 10 days for bacteremia/sepsis (AII); minimum of 14 days for meningitis (AII).

A. RECOMMENDED THERAPY FOR SELECTED NEWBORN CONDITIONS (continued)

Condition	Therapy (evidence grade) See Tables 5B–D for neonatal dosages.	Comments
Skin and soft tissues		
– Breast abscess[95]	Oxacillin/nafcillin, IM (for MSSA) or vancomycin IV (for MRSA). ADD cefotaxime OR gentamicin if gram-negative rods seen on Gram stain (AIII).	Gram stain of expressed pus guides empiric therapy; vancomycin if MRSA prevalent in community; alternative to vancomycin: clindamycin, linezolid, may need surgical drainage to minimize damage to breast tissue. Treatment duration individualized until clinical findings have completely resolved (AIII).
– Congenital cutaneous candidiasis[96]	Amphotericin B for 14 days, or 10 days if CSF culture negative (AII). Fluconazole alternative if *C albicans* or known sensitive *Candida*.	Treat promptly when rash presents with full IV dose, not prophylactic dosing or topical therapy. Diagnostic workup includes aerobic cultures of rash surface, blood, and CSF. Pathology examination of placenta and umbilical cord if possible.
– Erysipelas (and other group A streptococcal infections)	Penicillin G IV for 5–7 days, followed by oral therapy (if bacteremia not present) to complete a 10-day course (AIII).	Alternative: ampicillin. GBS may produce similar cellulitis or nodular lesions.
– Impetigo neonatorum	MSSA: oxacillin/nafcillin IV, IM OR cephalexin (AIII) MRSA: vancomycin IV for 5 days (AIII)	Systemic antibiotic therapy usually not required for superficial impetigo; local chlorhexidine cleansing may help with or without topical mupirocin (MRSA) or bacitracin (MSSA). Alternatives for MRSA: clindamycin IV, PO or linezolid IV, PO.
– *S aureus*[17,82,84,97]	MSSA: oxacillin/nafcillin IV, IM (AII) MRSA: vancomycin IV (AIII)	Surgical drainage may be required. MRSA may cause necrotizing fasciitis. Alternatives for MRSA: clindamycin IV or linezolid IV. Convalescent oral therapy if infection responds quickly to IV therapy.
– Group B streptococcus[85]	Penicillin G IV OR ampicillin IV, IM	Usually no pus formed Treatment course dependent on extent of infection, 7–14 days
Syphilis, congenital (<1 mo of age)[98]	During periods when availability of penicillin is compromised, contact CDC.	Evaluation and treatment do not depend on mother's HIV status. Obtain follow-up serology every 2–3 mo until nontreponemal test nonreactive or decreased 4-fold.

If CSF positive, repeat spinal tap with CSF VDRL at 6 mo and, if abnormal, re-treat.

– Proven or highly probable disease: (1) abnormal physical examination; (2) serum quantitative nontreponemal serologic titer 4-fold higher than mother's titer; or (3) positive dark field or fluorescent antibody test of body fluid(s).	Aqueous penicillin G 50,000 U/kg/dose q12h (day of life 1–7), q8h (>7 days) IV OR procaine penicillin G 50,000 U/kg IM q24h for 10 days (AII)	Evaluation to determine type and duration of therapy: CSF analysis (VDRL, cell count, protein), CBC and platelet count. Other tests as clinically indicated, including long-bone radiographs, chest radiograph, liver function tests, cranial ultrasound, ophthalmologic examination, and hearing test (ABR). If >1 day of therapy is missed, entire course is restarted.
– Normal physical examination, serum quantitative nontreponemal serologic titer ≤ maternal titer, and maternal treatment was (1) none, inadequate, or undocumented; (2) erythromycin, azithromycin, or other non-penicillin regimen; or (3) <4 wk before delivery.	Evaluation abnormal or not done completely: aqueous penicillin G 50,000 U/kg/dose q12h (day of life 1–7), q8h (>7 days) IV OR procaine penicillin G 50,000 U/kg IM q24h for 10 days (AII) Evaluation normal: aqueous penicillin G 50,000 U/kg/dose q12h (day of life 1–7), q8h (>7 days) IV OR procaine penicillin G 50,000 U/kg IM q24h for 10 days; OR benzathine penicillin G 50,000 units/kg/dose IM in a single dose (AIII)	Evaluation: CSF analysis, CBC with platelets, long-bone radiographs. If >1 day of therapy is missed, entire course is restarted. Reliable follow-up important if only a single dose of benzathine penicillin given.

5

A. RECOMMENDED THERAPY FOR SELECTED NEWBORN CONDITIONS (continued)

Condition	Therapy (evidence grade) See Tables 5B–D for neonatal dosages.	Comments
– Normal physical examination, serum quantitative nontreponemal serologic titer ≤ maternal titer, mother treated adequately during pregnancy and >4 wk before delivery; no evidence of reinfection or relapse in mother	Benzathine penicillin G 50,000 units/kg/dose IM in a single dose (AIII)	No evaluation required. Some experts would not treat but provide close serologic follow-up.
– Normal physical examination, serum quantitative nontreponemal serologic titer ≤ maternal titer, mother's treatment adequate before pregnancy	No treatment	No evaluation required. Some experts would treat with benzathine penicillin G 50,000 U/kg as a single IM injection, particularly if follow-up is uncertain.
Syphilis, congenital (>1 mo of age)[98]	Aqueous crystalline penicillin G 200,000–300,000 U/kg/day IV div q4–6h for 10 days (AII)	Evaluation to determine type and duration of therapy: CSF analysis (VDRL, cell count, protein), CBC and platelet count. Other tests as clinically indicated, including long-bone radiographs, chest radiograph, liver function tests, neuroimaging, ophthalmologic examination, and hearing evaluation. If no clinical manifestations of disease, CSF examination is normal, and CSF VDRL test result is nonreactive, some specialists would treat with up to 3 weekly doses of benzathine penicillin G 50,000 U/kg IM. Some experts would provide a single dose of benzathine penicillin G 50,000 U/kg IM after 10 days of parenteral treatment, but value of this additional therapy is not well documented.

Tetanus neonatorum[99]	Metronidazole IV, PO (alternative: penicillin G IV) for 10–14 days (AIII) Human TIG 3,000–6,000 U IM for 1 dose (AIII)	Wound cleaning and debridement vital; IVIG (200–400 mg/kg) is an alternative if TIG not available; equine tetanus antitoxin not available in the United States but is alternative to TIG.
Toxoplasmosis, congenital[100,101]	Sulfadiazine 100 mg/kg/day PO div q12h AND pyrimethamine 2 mg/kg PO daily for 2 days (loading dose), then 1 mg/kg PO q24h for 2–6 mo, then 3 times weekly (M-W-F) up to 1 y (AII) Folinic acid (leucovorin) 10 mg 3 times weekly (AII)	Corticosteroids (1 mg/kg/day div q12h) if active chorioretinitis or CSF protein >1 g/dL (AIII). Start sulfa after neonatal jaundice has resolved. Therapy is only effective against active trophozoites, not cysts.
Urinary tract infection[102]	Initial empiric therapy with ampicillin AND gentamicin; OR ampicillin AND cefotaxime pending culture and susceptibility test results for 7–10 days	Investigate for kidney disease and abnormalities of urinary tract: VCUG indicated if renal ultrasound abnormal or after first UTI. Oral therapy acceptable once neonate asymptomatic and culture sterile. No prophylaxis for grades 1–3 reflux.[103] In neonates with reflux, prophylaxis reduces recurrences but increases likelihood of recurrences being due to resistant organisms. Prophylaxis does not affect renal scarring.[98]
– Coliform bacteria (eg, E coli, Klebsiella, Enterobacter, Serratia)	Cefotaxime IV, IM OR, in absence of renal or perinephric abscess, gentamicin IV, IM for 7–10 days (AII)	Ampicillin used for susceptible organisms
– Enterococcus	Ampicillin IV, IM for 7 days for cystitis, may need 10–14 days for pyelonephritis, add gentamicin until cultures are sterile (AIII); for ampicillin resistance, use vancomycin, add gentamicin until cultures are sterile.	Aminoglycoside needed with ampicillin or vancomycin for synergistic bactericidal activity (assuming organisms susceptible to an aminoglycoside)
– P aeruginosa	Ceftazidime IV, IM OR, in absence of renal or perinephric abscess, tobramycin IV, IM for 7–10 days (AII)	Meropenem or cefepime are alternatives.

Antimicrobial Therapy for Newborns

A. RECOMMENDED THERAPY FOR SELECTED NEWBORN CONDITIONS (continued)

Condition	Therapy (evidence grade) See Tables 5B–D for neonatal dosages.	Comments
– Candida spp[31-33]	AmB-D (1 mg/kg/day) is recommended therapy (AII). Lipid formulation AmB is an alternative but carries a theoretic risk of less urinary tract penetration compared with AmB-D (CIII). Fluconazole (12 mg/kg/day q24h, after a load of 25 mg/kg/day) is an alternative if patient has not been on fluconazole prophylaxis (AII).[45] Duration of therapy for candidemia without obvious metastatic complications is for 2 wk after documented clearance and resolution of symptoms. Echinocandins should be used with caution and generally limited to salvage therapy or to situations in which resistance or toxicity preclude the use of AmB-D or fluconazole (CIII). Role of flucytosine in neonates with meningitis is questionable and not routinely recommended due to toxicity concerns. The addition of flucytosine (100 mg/kg/day div q6h) may be considered as salvage therapy in patients who have not had a clinical response to initial AmB therapy, but adverse effects are frequent (CIII).	Neonatal Candida disease is most often systemic with isolated UTI less likely to occur. Treat Candida identified in the urine as systemic infection until proven otherwise. See Fungal infections earlier in Table. Echinocandins are not renally eliminated and should not be used to treat isolated neonatal UTI. Central venous catheter removal strongly recommended. Length of therapy dependent on disease (BIII), usually 2 wk after all clearance. Antifungal susceptibility testing is suggested with persistent disease. (C krusei inherently resistant to fluconazole; C parapsilosis may be less susceptible to echinocandins; C glabrata demonstrates increasing resistance to fluconazole and echinocandins.) No proven benefit for combination antifungal therapy in candidiasis. Change from AmB or fluconazole to micafungin/caspofungin if cultures persistently positive (BIII). Although fluconazole prophylaxis has been shown to reduce colonization, it has not reduced mortality.[29] Lumbar puncture and dilated retinal examination recommended in neonates with cultures positive for Candida spp from blood (AIII). Same recommended for all infants with birth weight <1,500 g with candiduria with or without candidemia (AIII). CT or ultrasound imaging of genitourinary tract, liver, and spleen should be performed if blood cultures are persistently positive (AIII). Meningoencephalitis in the neonate occurs at a higher rate than in older children/adults. Infected CNS devices, including ventriculostomy drains and shunts, should be removed, if possible.

B. ANTIMICROBIAL DOSAGES FOR NEONATES—Lead author Jason Sauberan, assisted by the editors and John van den Anker

NOTE: This table contains empiric dosage recommendations for each agent listed. See Table 5A (Recommended Therapy for Selected Newborn Conditions) for more details of dosages for specific pathogens in specific tissue sites and for information on anti-influenza and antiretroviral drug dosages.

Antibiotic	Route	Dosages (mg/kg/day) and Intervals of Administration				
		Chronologic Age ≤28 days				Chronologic Age 29-60 days
		Body Weight ≤2,000 g		Body Weight >2,000 g		
		0–7 days old	8–28 days old	0–7 days old	8–28 days old	
Acyclovir	IV	40 div q12h	60 div q8h	60 div q8h	60 div q8h	60 div q8h
	PO	–	900/m²/day div q8h	–	900/m²/day div q8h	900/m²/day div q8h

Only parenteral acyclovir should be used for the treatment of acute neonatal HSV disease. Oral suppression therapy for 6 mo duration after completion of initial neonatal HSV treatment. See text in Table 5A, Herpes simplex infection.

Antibiotic	Route	0–7 days old	8–28 days old	0–7 days old	8–28 days old	29-60 days
Amoxicillin-clavulanate[a]	PO	–	–	–	–	30 div q12h
Amphotericin B						
– deoxycholate	IV	1 q24h	1 q24h	1 q24h	1 q24h	1 q24h
– lipid complex	IV	5 q24h	5 q24h	5 q24h	5 q24h	5 q24h
– liposomal	IV	5 q24h	5 q24h	5 q24h	5 q24h	5 q24h
Ampicillin[b]	IV, IM	100 div q12h	150 div q12h	150 div q8h	150 div q8h	200 div q6h
Anidulafungin[c]	IV	1.5 q24h	1.5 q24h	1.5 q24h	1.5 q24h	1.5 q24h
Azithromycin[d]	PO	10 q24h	10 q24h	10 q24h	10 q24h	10 q24h
	IV	10 q24h	10 q24h	10 q24h	10 q24h	10 q24h
Aztreonam	IV, IM	60 div q12h	90 div q8h[e]	90 div q8h	120 div q6h	120 div q6h
Caspofungin[f]	IV	25/m² q24h	25/m² q24h	25/m² q24h	25/m² q24h	25/m² q24h
Cefazolin	IV, IM	50 div q12h	75 div q8h[e]	50 div q12h	75 div q8h	75 div q8h

5

Antimicrobial Therapy for Newborns

Antimicrobial Therapy for Newborns

5

B. ANTIMICROBIAL DOSAGES FOR NEONATES (continued)—Lead author Jason Sauberan, assisted by the editors and John van den Anker

Dosages (mg/kg/day) and Intervals of Administration

Antibiotic	Route	Chronologic Age ≤28 days				Chronologic Age 29–60 days
		Body Weight ≤2,000 g		Body Weight >2,000 g		
		0–7 days old	8–28 days old	0–7 days old	8–28 days old	
Cefepime	IV, IM	60 div q12h	60 div q12h	100 div q12h	100 div q12h	150 div q8h[g]
Cefotaxime	IV, IM	100 div q12h	150 div q8h[e]	100 div q12h	150 div q8h	200 div q6h
Cefoxitin	IV, IM	70 div q12h	100 div q8h[e]	100 div q8h	100 div q8h	120 div q6h
Ceftazidime	IV, IM	100 div q12h	150 div q8h[e]	100 div q12h	150 div q8h	150 div q8h
Ceftriaxone[h]	IV, IM	—	—	50 q24h	50 q24h	50 q24h
Cefuroxime	IV, IM	100 div q12h	150 div q8h[e]	100 div q12h	150 div q8h	150 div q8h
Chloramphenicol[i]	IV, IM	25 q24h	50 div q12h[e]	25 q24h	50 div q12h	50–100 div q6h
Clindamycin	IV, IM, PO	15 div q8h	15 div q8h	21 div q8h	30 div q8h	30 div q8h
Daptomycin (potential neurotoxicity; use cautiously if no other options)	IV	12 div q12h	12 div q12h	12 div q12h	12 div q12h	12 div q12h
Erythromycin	PO	20 div q12h	30 div q8h	20 div q12h	30 div q8h	40 div q6h
Fluconazole						
– treatment[j]	IV, PO	12 q24h	12 q24h	12 q24h	12 q24h	12 q24h
– prophylaxis	IV, PO	6 mg/kg/dose twice weekly	6 mg/kg/dose twice weekly	6 mg/kg/dose twice weekly	6 mg/kg/dose twice weekly	6 mg/kg/dose twice weekly

Flucytosine^k	PO	75 div q8h	100 div q6h^e	100 div q6h	100 div q6h	100 div q6h
Ganciclovir	IV	Insufficient data	Insufficient data	12 div q12h	12 div q12h	12 div q12h
Linezolid	IV, PO	20 div q12h	30 div q8h	30 div q8h	30 div q8h	30 div q8h
Meropenem						
– sepsis, IAI^l	IV	40 div q12h	60 div q8h^l	60 div q8h	90 div q8h^m	90 div q8h
– meningitis	IV	120 div q8h	120 div q8h	120 div q8h	120 div q8h	120 div q8h
Metronidazole^m	IV, PO	15 div q12h	15 div q12h	22.5 div q8h	30 div q8h	30 div q8h
Micafungin	IV	10 q24h	10 q24h	10 q24h	10 q24h	10 q24h
Nafcillin,^n oxacillin^n	IV, IM	50 div q12h	75 div q8h^e	75 div q8h	100 div q6h	150 div q6h
Penicillin G benzathine	IM	50,000 U	50,000 U	50,000 U	50,000 U	50,000 U
Penicillin G crystalline (GBS sepsis, congenital syphilis)	IV	100,000 U div q12h	150,000 U^e div q8h	100,000 U div q12h	150,000 U div q8h	200,000 U div q6h
Penicillin G crystalline (GBS meningitis)	IV	200,000 U div q12h	300,000 U^e div q8h	300,000 U div q8h	400,000 U div q6h	400,000 U div q6h
Penicillin G procaine	IM	50,000 U q24h	50,000 U q24h	50,000 U q24h	50,000 U q24h	50,000 U q24h
Piperacillin/tazobactam	IV	300 div q8h	320 div q6h	320 div q6h	320 div q6h	320 div q6h
Rifampin	IV, PO	10 q24h	10 q24h	10 q24h	10 q24h	10 q24h
Valganciclovir	PO	Insufficient data	Insufficient data	32 div q12h	32 div q12h	32 div q12h
Voriconazole^o	IV	16 div q12h	16 div q12h	16 div q12h	16 div q12h	16 div q12h

5

B. ANTIMICROBIAL DOSAGES FOR NEONATES (continued)—Lead author Jason Sauberan, assisted by the editors and John van den Anker

		Dosages (mg/kg/day) and Intervals of Administration					
		Chronologic Age ≤28 days					Chronologic Age 29–60 days
		Body Weight ≤2,000 g		Body Weight >2,000 g			
Antibiotic	Route	0–7 days old	8–28 days old	0–7 days old	8–28 days old		
Zidovudine	IV	3 div q12h[p]	3 div q12h[p]	6 div q12h	6 div q12h	See Table 5A, HIV.	
	PO	4 div q12h[p]	4 div q12h[p]	8 div q12h	8 div q12h	See Table 5A, HIV.	

[a] 25- or 50-mg/mL concentration.

[b] 300 mg/kg/day for GBS meningitis div q8h for all neonates ≤7 days of age and q6h >7 days of age.

[c] Loading dose 3 mg/kg followed 24 h later by maintenance dose listed.

[d] Azithromycin oral dose for pertussis should be 10 mg/kg once daily for the entire 5-day treatment course, while for other upper respiratory tract infections, 10 mg/kg is given on the first day, followed by 5 mg/kg once daily for 4 days. For CNS infection, 10 mg/kg once daily for entire course.

[e] Use 0–7 days old dosing until 14 days old if birth weight <1,000 g.

[f] Higher dosage of 50 mg/m² may be needed for Aspergillus.

[g] May require infusion over 3 h, or 200 mg/kg/day div q6h, to treat organisms with MIC ≥8 mg/L.

[h] Usually avoided in over 3 h, or 200 mg/kg/day div q6h, to treat organisms with MIC ≥8 mg/L.
[h] Usually avoided for transitioning to outpatient treatment of GBS bacteremia in well-appearing neonates at low risk for hyperbilirubinemia. Contraindicated if concomitant intravenous calcium; see Pediatrics. 2009;123(4):e609–e613.

[i] Desired serum concentration 15–25 mg/L.

[j] Loading dose 25 mg/kg followed 24 h later by maintenance dose listed.

[k] Desired serum concentrations peak 50–100 mg/L, trough 25–50 mg/L. Dose range 50–100 mg/kg/day.

[l] Adjust dosage after 14 days of age instead of after 7 days of age.

[m] Loading dose 15 mg/kg.

[n] Increase to 50 mg/kg/dose for meningitis.

[o] Initial loading dose of 18 mg/kg div q12h on day 1. Desired serum concentrations, trough 2–5 mg/L. See Table 5A, Aspergillosis.

[p] Starting dose if gestational age <35–+0 wk and postnatal ≤14 days. HIV, for ZDV dosage after 2 wk of age and for NVP and 3TC recommendations. See Table 5A, HIV, for ZDV dosage after 2 wk of age and for NVP and 3TC recommendations.

C. AMINOGLYCOSIDES

Empiric Dosage (mg/kg/dose) by Gestational and Postnatal Age

Medication	Route	<30 wk		30–34 wk		≥35 wk	
		0–14 days	>14 days	0–10 days	>10 days[a]	0–7 days	>7 days[a]
Amikacin[b]	IV, IM	15 q48h	15 q24h	15 q24h	15 q24h	15 q24h	17.5 q24h
Gentamicin[c]	IV, IM	5 q48h	5 q36h	4.5 q36h	5 q36h	4 q24h	5 q24h
Tobramycin[c]	IV, IM	5 q48h	5 q36h	4.5 q36h	5 q36h	4 q24h	5 q24h

[a] If >60 days of age, see Chapter 11.
[b] Desired serum concentrations: 20–35 mg/L or 10 × MIC (peak), <7 mg/L (trough).
[c] Desired serum concentrations: 6–12 mg/L or 10 × MIC (peak), <2 mg/L (trough).

D. VANCOMYCIN[A,B,C]

Empiric Dosage (mg/kg/dose) by Gestational Age and Serum Creatinine (Begin with a 20 mg/kg loading dose.)

≤28 wk			>28 wk		
Serum Creatinine	Dose	Frequency	Serum Creatinine	Dose	Frequency
<0.5	15	q12h	<0.7	15	q12h
0.5–0.7	20	q24h	0.7–0.9	20	q24h
0.8–1	15	q24h	1–1.2	15	q24h
1.1–1.4	10	q24h	1.3–1.6	10	q24h
>1.4	15	q48h	>1.6	15	q48h

[a] Serum creatinine concentrations normally fluctuate and are partly influenced by transplacental maternal creatinine in the first wk of age. Cautious use of creatinine-based dosing strategy with frequent reassessment of renal function and vancomycin serum concentrations are recommended in neonates ≤7 days old.

[b] Desired serum concentrations; for invasive MRSA infections, a 24-h AUC:MIC of 400 mg•h/L is recommended on adult studies. The AUC is best calculated from 2 concentrations (ie, peak and trough) rather than 1 trough concentration measurement. In situations in which AUC calculation is not feasible, a trough concentration 10–12 mg/L is very highly likely (>90%) to achieve the goal AUC target in neonates when the MIC is 1 mg/L. For coagulase-negative staphylococci and Enterococcus, troughs of 5–10 mg/L are likely to be effective.

[c] If >60 days of age, see Chapter 11.

E. Use of Antimicrobials During Pregnancy or Breastfeeding

The use of antimicrobials during pregnancy should be balanced by the risk of fetal toxicity, including anatomic anomalies. A number of factors determine the degree of transfer of antibiotics across the placenta: lipid solubility, degree of ionization, molecular weight, protein binding, placental maturation, and placental and fetal blood flow. The FDA provides 5 categories to indicate the level of risk to the fetus: (1) Category A: fetal harm seems remote, as controlled studies have not demonstrated a risk to the fetus; (2) Category B: animal reproduction studies have not shown a fetal risk, but no controlled studies in pregnant women have been done, or animal studies have shown an adverse effect that has not been confirmed in human studies (penicillin, amoxicillin, ampicillin, cephalexin/cefazolin, azithromycin, clindamycin, vancomycin, zanamivir); (3) Category C: studies in animals have shown an adverse effect on the fetus, but there are no studies in women; the potential benefit of the drug may justify the possible risk to the fetus (chloramphenicol, ciprofloxacin, gentamicin, levofloxacin, oseltamivir, rifampin); (4) Category D: evidence exists of human fetal risk, but the benefits may outweigh such risk (doxycycline); (5) Category X: the drug is contraindicated because animal or human studies have shown fetal abnormalities or fetal risk (ribavirin). Prescription drugs approved after June 30, 2015, are required to conform to a new pregnancy risk labeling format. See www.federalregister.gov/a/2014-28241 (accessed September 15, 2016).

Fetal serum antibiotic concentrations (or cord blood concentrations) following maternal administration have not been systematically studied.[104] The following commonly used drugs appear to achieve fetal concentrations that are equal to or only slightly less than those in the mother: penicillin G, amoxicillin, ampicillin, sulfonamides, trimethoprim, and tetracyclines, as well as oseltamivir.[105] The aminoglycoside concentrations in fetal serum are 20% to 50% of those in maternal serum. Cephalosporins, carbapenems, nafcillin, oxacillin, clindamycin, and vancomycin[106] penetrate poorly (10%–30%), and fetal concentrations of erythromycin and azithromycin are less than 10% of those in the mother.

The most current, updated information on the safety of antimicrobials and other agents in human milk can be found at the National Library of Medicine LactMed Web site (http://toxnet.nlm.nih.gov/newtoxnet/lactmed.htm, accessed September 15, 2016).[107]

In general, neonatal exposure to antimicrobials in human milk is minimal or insignificant. Aminoglycosides, beta-lactams, ciprofloxacin, clindamycin, macrolides, fluconazole, and agents for tuberculosis are considered safe for the mother to take during breastfeeding.[108] The most common reported neonatal side effect of maternal antimicrobial use during breastfeeding is increased stool output. Clinicians should recommend mothers alert their pediatric health care professional if stool output changes occur. Maternal treatment with sulfa-containing antibiotics should be approached with caution in the breastfed infant who is jaundiced or ill.

6. Antimicrobial Therapy According to Clinical Syndromes

NOTES

- This chapter should be considered a rough guidance for a typical patient. Dosage recommendations are for patients with relatively normal hydration, renal function, and hepatic function. Because the dose required is based on the exposure of the antibiotic to the pathogen at the site of infection, higher dosages may be necessary if the antibiotic does not penetrate well into the infected tissue (eg, meningitis) or if the child eliminates the antibiotic from the body more quickly than average. Higher dosages may also be needed if the child is immunocompromised and the immune system cannot help clear the infection.

- Duration of treatment should be individualized. Those recommended are based on the literature, common practice, and general experience. Critical evaluations of duration of therapy have been carried out in very few infectious diseases. In general, a longer duration of therapy should be used (1) for tissues in which antibiotic concentrations may be relatively low (eg, undrained abscess, central nervous system [CNS] infection); (2) for tissues in which repair following infection-mediated damage is slow (eg, bone); (3) when the organisms are less susceptible; (4) when a relapse of infection is unacceptable (eg, CNS infections); or (5) when the host is immunocompromised in some way. An assessment after therapy will ensure that your selection of antibiotic, dose, and duration of therapy were appropriate.

- Diseases in this chapter are arranged by body systems. Please consult the index for the alphabetized listing of diseases and chapters 7 through 10 for the alphabetized listing of pathogens and for uncommon organisms not included in this chapter.

- A more detailed description of treatment of methicillin-resistant *Staphylococcus aureus* infections is provided in Chapter 4.

- Therapy of *Pseudomonas aeruginosa* systemic infections is evolving from intravenous (IV) ceftazidime plus tobramycin to single drug IV therapy with cefepime due to the relative stability of cefepime to beta-lactamases, compared with ceftazidime. Oral therapy with ciprofloxacin has replaced IV therapy in otherwise normal children who are compliant and able to take oral therapy, particularly for "step-down" therapy of invasive infections.

- **Abbreviations:** AAP, American Academy of Pediatrics; ADH, antidiuretic hormone; AFB, acid-fast bacilli; AHA, American Heart Association; ALT, alanine transaminase; AmB, amphotericin B; amox/clav, amoxicillin/clavulanate; AOM, acute otitis media; ARF, acute rheumatic fever; AST, aspartate transaminase; AUC:MIC, area under the serum concentration vs time curve: minimum inhibitory concentration; bid, twice daily; CA-MRSA, community-associated methicillin-resistant *Staphylococcus aureus;* CDC, Centers for Disease Control and Prevention; CMV, cytomegalovirus; CNS, central nervous system; CRP, C-reactive protein; CSD, cat-scratch disease; CSF, cerebrospinal fluid; CT, computed tomography; DAT, diphtheria antitoxin; div, divided;

DOT, directly observed therapy; EBV, Epstein-Barr virus; ESBL, extended spectrum beta-lactamase; ESR, erythrocyte sedimentation rate; ETEC, enterotoxin-producing *Escherichia coli;* FDA, US Food and Drug Administration; GI, gastrointestinal; HACEK, *Haemophilus aphrophilus, Aggregatibacter* (formerly *Actinobacillus*) *actinomycetemcomitans, Cardiobacterium hominis, Eikenella corrodens, Kingella* spp; HIV, human immunodeficiency virus; HSV, herpes simplex virus; HUS, hemolytic uremic syndrome; I&D, incision and drainage; IDSA, Infectious Diseases Society of America; IM, intramuscular; INH, isoniazid; IV, intravenous; IVIG, intravenous immune globulin; KPC, *Klebsiella pneumoniae* carbapenemase; L-AmB, liposomal amphotericin B; LFT, liver function test; LP, lumbar puncture; MDR, multidrug resistant; MRSA, methicillin-resistant *S aureus;* MRSE, methicillin-resistant *Staphylococcus epidermidis;* MSSA, methicillin-susceptible *S aureus;* MSSE, methicillin-sensitive *S epidermidis;* NIH, National Institutes of Health; ophth, ophthalmic; PCR, polymerase chain reaction; PCV13, Prevnar 13-valent pneumococcal conjugate vaccine; pen-R, penicillin-resistant; pen-S, penicillin-susceptible; PIDS, Pediatric Infectious Diseases Society; pip/tazo, piperacillin/tazobactam; PO, oral; PPD, purified protein derivative; PZA, pyrazinamide; qd, once daily; qid, 4 times daily; qod, every other day; RIVUR, Randomized Intervention for Children with Vesicoureteral Reflux; RSV, respiratory syncytial virus; SPAG-2, small particle aerosol generator-2; spp, species; STEC, Shiga toxin-producing *E coli;* STI, sexually transmitted infection; TB, tuberculosis; Td, tetanus, diphtheria; Tdap, tetanus, diphtheria, acellular pertussis; ticar/clav, ticarcillin/clavulanate; tid, 3 times daily; TIG, tetanus immune globulin; TMP/SMX, trimethoprim/sulfamethoxazole; ULN, upper limit of normal; UTI, urinary tract infection; VDRL, Venereal Disease Research Laboratories; WBC, white blood cell.

A. SKIN AND SOFT TISSUE INFECTIONS

Clinical Diagnosis	Therapy (evidence grade)	Comments
NOTE: CA-MRSA (see Chapter 4) is prevalent in most areas of the world. Recommendations for staphylococcal infections are given for 2 scenarios: standard and CA-MRSA. Antibiotic recommendations for CA-MRSA should be used for empiric therapy in regions with greater than 5% to 10% of invasive staphylococcal infections caused by MRSA, in situations where CA-MRSA is suspected, and for documented CA-MRSA infections, while standard recommendations refer to treatment of MSSA. During the past few years, clindamycin resistance in MRSA has increased to 40% in some areas but remained stable at 5% in others, although this increase may be an artifact of changes in reporting, with many laboratories now reporting all clindamycin-susceptible but D-test–positive strains as resistant. Please check your local susceptibility data for S aureus before using clindamycin for empiric therapy. For MSSA, oxacillin/nafcillin are considered equivalent agents.		
Adenitis, acute bacterial[1-7] (S aureus, including CA-MRSA, and group A streptococcus; consider Bartonella [CSD] for subacute adenitis)[8]	Empiric therapy Standard: oxacillin/nafcillin 150 mg/kg/day IV div q6h OR cefazolin 100 mg/kg/day IV div q8h (AI), OR cephalexin 50–75 mg/kg/day PO div tid CA-MRSA: clindamycin 30 mg/kg/day IV or PO (AI) div q8h OR ceftaroline: 2 mo–<2 y, 24 mg/kg/day IV div q8h; ≥2 y, 36 mg/kg/day IV div q8h (max single dose 400 mg); >33 kg, either 400 mg/dose IV q8h or 600 mg/dose IV q12h (BI), OR vancomycin 40 mg/kg/day IV q8h (BII) CSD: azithromycin 12 mg/kg qd (max 500 mg) for 5 days (BII)	May need surgical drainage for staph/strep infection; not usually needed for CSD. Following drainage of mild to moderate suppurative adenitis caused by staph or strep, additional antibiotics may not be required. For oral therapy for MSSA: cephalexin or amox/clav; for CA-MRSA: clindamycin, TMP/SMX, or linezolid. For oral therapy of group A strep: amoxicillin or penicillin V. Total IV plus PO therapy for 7–10 days. For CSD: this is the same high dose of azithromycin that is recommended routinely for strep pharyngitis.
Adenitis, nontuberculous (atypical) mycobacterial[9-12]	Excision usually curative (BII); azithromycin PO OR clarithromycin PO for 6–12 wk (with or without rifampin) if susceptible (BII)	Antibiotic susceptibility patterns are quite variable; cultures should guide therapy: excision >97% effective; medical therapy 60%–70% effective. Newer data suggest toxicity of antimicrobials may not be worth the small clinical benefit of medical therapy over surgery.

Antimicrobial Therapy According to Clinical Syndromes

A. SKIN AND SOFT TISSUE INFECTIONS (continued)

Clinical Diagnosis	Therapy (evidence grade)	Comments
Adenitis, tuberculous[13,14] (*M tuberculosis* and *M bovis*)	INH 10–15 mg/kg/day PO, IV qd, for 6 mo AND rifampin 10–20 mg/kg/day (max 600 mg) PO, IV qd, for 6 mo AND PZA 20–40 mg/kg/day PO qd for first 2 mo therapy (BI); if suspected multidrug resistance, add ethambutol 20 mg/kg/day PO qd.	Surgical excision usually not indicated because organisms are treatable. Adenitis caused by *Mycobacterium bovis* (unpasteurized dairy product ingestion) is uniformly resistant to PZA. Treat 9–12 mo with INH and rifampin, if susceptible (BII). No contraindication to fine needle aspirate of node for diagnosis.
Anthrax, cutaneous[15]	Empiric therapy: ciprofloxacin 20–30 mg/kg/day PO div bid OR doxycycline 4 mg/kg/day (max 200 mg) PO div bid (regardless of age) (AIII)	If susceptible, amoxicillin or clindamycin (BIII). Ciprofloxacin and levofloxacin are FDA approved for inhalational anthrax (BIII).
Bites, dog and cat[1,16–20] (*Pasteurella multocida*; *S aureus*, including CA-MRSA; *Streptococcus* spp, anaerobes; *Capnocytophaga canimorsus*, particularly in asplenic hosts)	Amox/clav 45 mg/kg/day PO div tid (amox/clav 7:1; see Chapter 1, Aminopenicillins) for 5–10 days (AII); for hospitalized children, use ampicillin AND clindamycin (BII) OR ceftriaxone AND clindamycin (BII) OR cefazoline: 2 mo to <2 y, 24 mg/kg/day IV div q8h; ≥2 y, 36 mg/kg/day IV div q8h (max single dose 400 mg); >33 kg, either 400 mg/dose IV q8h or 600 mg/dose IV q12h (BII).	Amox/clav has good *Pasteurella*, MSSA, and anaerobic coverage but lacks MRSA coverage Ceftaroline has good *Pasteurella*, MSSA, and MRSA coverage but lacks *B fragilis* anaerobic coverage.[21] Ticar/clav 200 mg ticarcillin/kg/day div q6h and ampicillin/sulbactam also lack MRSA coverage. Consider rabies prophylaxis[22] for bites from at-risk animals (observe animal for 10 days, if possible) (AI); consider tetanus prophylaxis. For penicillin allergy, ciprofloxacin (for *Pasteurella*) plus clindamycin (BIII). Doxycycline may be considered for *Pasteurella* coverage.
Bites, human[1,19,23] (*Eikenella corrodens*; *S aureus*, including CA-MRSA; *Streptococcus* spp, anaerobes)	Amox/clav 45 mg/kg/day PO div tid (amox/clav 7:1; see Chapter 1, Aminopenicillins) for 5–10 days (AII); for hospitalized children, use ampicillin and clindamycin (BII) OR ceftriaxone and clindamycin (BII).	Human bites have a very high rate of infection (do not close open wounds). Amox/clav has good *Eikenella*, MSSA, and anaerobic coverage but lacks MRSA coverage. Ticar/clav 200 mg ticarcillin/kg/day div q6h and ampicillin/sulbactam also lack MRSA coverage.

		For penicillin allergy, ciprofloxacin (for *Pasteurella*) plus clindamycin (BIII). Doxycycline and TMP-SMX may be considered for *Pasteurella* coverage.
Bullous impetigo[1–3,5–7] (usually *S aureus*, including CA-MRSA)	Standard: cephalexin 50–75 mg/kg/day PO div tid OR amox/clav 45 mg/kg/day PO div tid (CII) CA-MRSA: clindamycin 30 mg/kg/day PO div tid OR TMP/SMX 8 mg/kg/day of TMP PO div bid; for 5–7 days (CI)	For topical therapy if mild infection: mupirocin or retapamulin ointment
Cellulitis of unknown etiology (usually *S aureus*, including CA-MRSA, or group A streptococcus)[1–7,24,25]	Empiric IV therapy Standard: oxacillin/nafcillin 150 mg/kg/day IV div q6h OR cefazolin 100 mg/kg/day IV div q8h (BII) CA-MRSA: clindamycin 30 mg/kg/day IV div q8h OR ceftaroline: 2 mo–<2 y, 24 mg/kg/day IV div q8h; ≥2 y, 36 mg/kg/day IV div q8h (max single dose 400 mg); >33 kg, either 400 mg/dose IV q8h or 600 mg/dose IV q12h (BI) OR vancomycin 40 mg/kg/day IV q8h (BII) For oral therapy for MSSA: cephalexin (AII) OR amox/clav 45 mg/kg/day PO div tid (BII); for CA-MRSA: clindamycin (BII), TMP/SMX (AII), or linezolid (BII)	For periorbital or buccal cellulitis, also consider *Streptococcus pneumoniae* or *Haemophilus influenzae* type b in unimmunized infants. Total IV plus PO therapy for 7–10 days.
Cellulitis, buccal (for unimmunized infants and preschool-aged children, *H influenzae* type b)[26]	Cefotaxime 100–150 mg/kg/day IV div q8h OR ceftriaxone 50 mg/kg/day IV, IM q24h; for 2–7 days parenteral therapy before switch to oral (BII)	Rule out meningitis (larger dosages may be needed). For penicillin allergy, levofloxacin IV/PO covers pathogens, but no clinical data available; safer than chloramphenicol. Oral therapy: amoxicillin if beta-lactamase negative; amox/clav or oral 2nd- or 3rd-generation cephalosporin if beta-lactamase positive.
Cellulitis, erysipelas (streptococcal)[1,2,7]	Penicillin G 100,000–200,000 U/kg/day IV div q4–6h (BII) initially, then penicillin V 100 mg/kg/day PO div qid (BIII) or tid OR amoxicillin 50 mg/kg/day PO div tid (BIII) for 10 days	These dosages may be unnecessarily large, but little clinical experience exists for smaller dosages.

6

Antimicrobial Therapy According to Clinical Syndromes

Antimicrobial Therapy According to Clinical Syndromes

6

A. SKIN AND SOFT TISSUE INFECTIONS (continued)

Clinical Diagnosis	Therapy (evidence grade)	Comments
Gas gangrene (See Necrotizing fasciitis.)		
Impetigo (*S aureus*, including CA-MRSA; occasionally group A streptococcus)[1,2,6,7,27,28]	Mupirocin OR retapamulin topically (BII) to lesions tid; OR for more extensive lesions, oral therapy Standard: cephalexin 50–75 mg/kg/day PO div tid OR amox/clav 45 mg/kg/day PO div tid (AII) CA-MRSA: clindamycin 30 mg/kg/day (CII) PO div tid OR TMP/SMX 8 mg/kg/day TMP PO div bid (AII); for 5–7 days	Cleanse infected area with soap and water.
Ludwig angina[29]	Penicillin G 200,000–250,000 U/kg/day IV div q6h AND clindamycin 40 mg/kg/day IV div q8h (CIII)	Alternatives: meropenem, imipenem, ticar/clav, pip/tazo if gram-negative aerobic bacilli also suspected (CIII); high risk of respiratory tract obstruction from inflammatory edema
Lymphadenitis. (See Adenitis, acute bacterial.)		
Lymphangitis (usually group A streptococcus)[1,2,7]	Penicillin G 200,000 U/kg/day IV div q6h (BII) initially, then penicillin V 100 mg/kg/day PO div qid OR amoxicillin 50 mg/kg/day PO div tid for 10 days	For mild disease, penicillin V 50 mg/kg/day PO qid for 10 days Some recent reports of *S aureus* as a cause Cefazolin IV (for group A strep or MSSA) or clindamycin IV (for group A strep, most MSSA and MRSA)
Myositis, suppurative[30] (*S aureus*, including CA-MRSA; synonyms: tropical myositis, pyomyositis)	Standard: oxacillin/nafcillin 150 mg/kg/day IV div q6h OR cefazolin 100 mg/kg/day IV div q8h (CII) CA-MRSA: clindamycin 40 mg/kg/day IV div q8h OR ceftaroline: 2 mo–<2 y, 24 mg/kg/day IV div q8h; ≥2 y, 36 mg/kg/day IV div q8h (max single dose 400 mg); >33 kg, either 400 mg/dose IV q8h or 600 mg/dose IV q12h (BI) OR vancomycin 40 mg/kg/day IV q8h (CIII)	Surgical debridement is usually necessary. Aggressive, emergent debridement; use clindamycin to help decrease toxin production (BIII); consider IVIG to bind bacterial toxins for life-threatening disease (CIII); abscesses may develop with CA-MRSA while on therapy.

Necrotizing fasciitis (Pathogens vary depending on the age of the child and location of infection. Single pathogen: group A streptococcus; *Clostridia* spp, *S aureus* [including CA-MRSA], *Pseudomonas aeruginosa*, *Vibrio* spp, *Aeromonas*. Multiple pathogen, mixed aerobic/anaerobic synergistic fasciitis: any organism[s] above, plus gram-negative bacilli, plus *Bacteroides* spp, and other anaerobes.)[1,31-34]	Empiric therapy: ceftazidime 150 mg/kg/day IV div q8h, or cefepime 150 mg/kg/day IV div q8h or cefotaxime 200 mg/kg/day IV div q6h AND clindamycin 40 mg/kg/day IV div q8h (BIII); OR meropenem 60 mg/kg/day IV div q8h; OR pip/tazo 400 mg/kg/day pip component IV div q6h (AIII). ADD vancomycin OR ceftaroline for suspect CA-MRSA, pending culture results (AIII). Group A streptococcal: penicillin G 200,000–250,000 U/kg/day div q6h AND clindamycin 40 mg/kg/day div q8h (AIII). Mixed aerobic/anaerobic/gram-negative: meropenem or pip/tazo AND clindamycin (AIII). Aggressive emergent wound debridement (AII). ADD clindamycin to inhibit synthesis of toxins during the first few days of therapy (AIII). If CA-MRSA identified and susceptible to clindamycin, additional vancomycin is not required. Consider IVIG to bind bacterial toxins for life-threatening disease (BIII). Value of hyperbaric oxygen is not established (CIII). Focus definitive antimicrobial therapy based on culture results.
Pyoderma, cutaneous abscesses (*S aureus*, including CA-MRSA; group A streptococcus)[2,5-7,24,35-37]	Standard: cephalexin 50–75 mg/kg/day PO div tid OR amox/clav 45 mg/kg/day PO div tid (BII) CA-MRSA: clindamycin 30 mg/kg/day PO div tid (BII) OR TMP/SMX 8 mg/kg/day of TMP PO div bid (AI) I&D when indicated; IV for serious infections. For prevention of recurrent CA-MRSA infection, use bleach baths twice weekly (½ cup of bleach per full bathtub) (BII), OR bathe with chlorhexidine soap daily or qod (BIII). Decolonization with mupirocin may also be helpful.
Rat-bite fever (*Streptobacillus moniliformis*, *Spirillum minus*)[38]	Penicillin G 100,000–200,000 U/kg/day IV div q6h (BII) for 7–10 days; for endocarditis, ADD gentamicin for 4–6 wk (CIII). For mild disease, oral therapy with amox/clav (CIII). Organisms are normal oral flora for rodents. High rate of associated endocarditis. Alternatives: doxycycline; 2nd- and 3rd-generation cephalosporins (CIII).
Staphylococcal scalded skin syndrome[6,39,40]	Standard: oxacillin 150 mg/kg/day IV div q6h OR cefazolin 100 mg/kg/day IV div q8h (CII). CA-MRSA: clindamycin 30 mg/kg/day IV div q8h (CIII) OR ceftaroline: 2 mo–<2 y, 24 mg/kg/day IV div q8h; ≥2 y, 36 mg/kg/day IV div q8h (max single dose 400 mg); >33 kg, either 400 mg/dose IV q8h or 600 mg/dose IV q12h (BI), OR vancomycin 40 mg/kg/day IV div q8h (CIII) Burow or Zephiran compresses for oozing skin and intertriginous areas. Corticosteroids are contraindicated.

6

B. SKELETAL INFECTIONS

Clinical Diagnosis	Therapy (evidence grade)	Comments
NOTE: CA-MRSA (see Chapter 4) is prevalent in most areas of the world. Recommendations for empiric therapy should include CA-MRSA and MSSA. Antibiotic recommendations for empiric therapy should include CA-MRSA when it is suspected or documented, while treatment for MSSA with beta-lactam antibiotics (eg, cephalexin) is preferred over clindamycin. During the past few years, clindamycin resistance in MRSA has increased to 40% in some areas but remained stable at 5% in others, although this increase may be an artifact of changes in reporting, with many laboratories now reporting all clindamycin-susceptible but D-test-positive strains as resistant. Please check your local susceptibility data for *S aureus* before using clindamycin for empiric therapy. For MSSA, oxacillin/nafcillin are considered equivalent agents. The first pediatric-specific PIDS/IDSA guidelines for bacterial osteomyelitis and bacterial arthritis are currently being written.		
Arthritis, bacterial[41–46]	Switch to appropriate high-dose oral therapy when clinically improved, CRP decreasing (see Chapter 13).[47]	
– Newborns	See Chapter 5.	
– Infants (*S aureus*, including CA-MRSA; group A streptococcus; *Kingella kingae*; in unimmunized or immunocompromised children: pneumococcus, *H influenzae* type b) **– Children** (*S aureus*, including CA-MRSA; group A streptococcus; *K kingae*) For Lyme Disease and Brucellosis, see Chapter 6, Miscellaneous Systemic Infections.	Empiric therapy: clindamycin (to cover CA-MRSA unless clindamycin resistance locally is >10%, then use vancomycin). For serious infections, ADD cefazolin to provide better MSSA coverage and add *Kingella* coverage. See comments for discussion of dexamethasone adjunctive therapy. For CA-MRSA: clindamycin 30 mg/kg/day IV div q8h (AI) OR ceftaroline: 2 mo–<2 y, 24 mg/kg/day IV div q8h; ≥2 y, 36 mg/kg/day IV div q8h (max single dose 400 mg); >33 kg, either 400 mg/dose IV q8h or 600 mg/dose IV q12h (BI) OR vancomycin 40 mg/kg/day IV q8h (BI). For MSSA: oxacillin/nafcillin 150 mg/kg/day IV div q6h OR cefazolin 100 mg/kg/day IV div q8h (AI). For *Kingella*: cefazolin 100 mg/kg/day IV div q8h OR ampicillin 150 mg/kg/day IV div q6h, OR ceftriaxone 50 mg/kg/day IV, IM q24h (AII). For pen-S pneumococci or group A streptococcus: penicillin G 200,000 U/kg/day IV div q6h (BII).	Dexamethasone adjunctive therapy (0.15 mg/kg per dose every 6 h for 4 days in one study) demonstrated significant benefit in decreasing symptoms and earlier hospital discharge (but with some "rebound" symptoms).[48,49] Given the sensitivity of cartilage to injury, these data now support cautious use of concurrent therapy with dexamethasone in children with bacterial arthritis (BII), at least while inpatients. NOTE: children with rheumatologic, postinfectious fungal/mycobacterial infections, or malignant conditions are also likely to improve with antibiotic/steroid therapy. Oral step-down therapy options For CA-MRSA: clindamycin OR linezolid[45] For MSSA: cephalexin OR dicloxacillin caps for older children For *Kingella*, most penicillins or cephalosporins (but not clindamycin)

For pen-R pneumococci or *Haemophilus*: ceftriaxone 50–75 mg/kg/day IV, IM q24h, OR cefotaxime (BII). Total therapy (IV plus PO) for up to 21 days with normal ESR; low-risk, non-hip MSSA arthritis may respond to a 10-day course (AII).[42,43]

– Gonococcal arthritis or tenosynovitis[50,51]	Ceftriaxone 50 mg/kg IV, IM q24h (BII) for 7 days AND azithromycin 20 mg/kg PO as a single dose	Combination therapy with azithromycin to decrease risk of development of resistance. Cefixime 8 mg/kg/day PO as a single daily dose may not be effective due to increasing resistance. Ceftriaxone IV, IM is preferred over cefixime PO.
– Other bacteria	See Chapter 7 for preferred antibiotics.
Osteomyelitis[41,44,45,52-58]	Step down to appropriate high-dose oral therapy when clinically improved (see Chapter 13).[45,55]
– Newborns	See Chapter 5.
– Infants and children, acute infection (usually *S aureus*, including CA-MRSA; group A streptococcus; *K kingae*)	Empiric therapy: clindamycin (for coverage of MSSA and MRSA in most locations). For serious infections, ADD cefazolin to provide better MSSA coverage and add *Kingella* coverage (CIII). For CA-MRSA: clindamycin 30 mg/kg/day IV div q8h OR vancomycin 40 mg/kg/day IV q8h (BII). For MSSA: oxacillin/nafcillin 150 mg/kg/day IV div q6h OR cefazolin 100 mg/kg/day IV div q8h (AII). For *Kingella*: cefazolin 100 mg/kg/day IV div q8h OR ampicillin 150 mg/kg/day IV div q6h, OR ceftriaxone 50 mg/kg/day IV, IM q24h (BII). Total therapy (IV plus PO) usually 4–6 wk for MSSA (with end-of-therapy normal ESR, radiograph to document healing) but may be as short as 3 wk for mild infection. May need longer than 4–6 wk for CA-MRSA (BII). Follow closely for clinical response to empiric therapy.	In children with open fractures secondary to trauma, add ceftazidime for extended aerobic gram-negative bacilli activity. *Kingella* is often resistant to clindamycin and vancomycin. For MSSA (BI) and *Kingella* (BIII), step-down oral therapy with cephalexin 100 mg/kg/day PO div tid. Oral step-down therapy options for CA-MRSA include clindamycin and linezolid,[59] with insufficient clinical data to recommend TMP/SMX. For prosthetic devices, biofilms may impair microbial eradication, requiring the addition of rifampin or other agents.[56]

Antimicrobial Therapy According to Clinical Syndromes

B. SKELETAL INFECTIONS (continued)

Clinical Diagnosis	Therapy (evidence grade)	Comments
– Acute, other organisms	See Chapter 7 for preferred antibiotics.	
– Chronic (staphylococcal)	For MSSA: cephalexin 100 mg/kg/day PO tid OR dicloxacillin caps 75–100 mg/kg/day PO div qid for 3–6 mo or longer (CIII) For CA-MRSA: clindamycin or linezolid (CIII)	Surgery to debride sequestrum is usually required for cure. For prosthetic joint infection caused by staphylococci, add rifampin (CIII).[56] Watch for beta-lactam–associated neutropenia with high-dose, long-term therapy and linezolid-associated neutropenia/thrombocytopenia with long-term (>2 wk) therapy.[59]
Osteomyelitis of the foot[60] (osteochondritis after a puncture wound) P aeruginosa (occasionally S aureus, including CA-MRSA)	Cefepime 150 mg/kg/day IV div q8h (BIII); OR meropenem 60 mg/kg/day IV div q8h (BIII); OR ceftazidime 150 mg/kg/day IV, IM div q8h AND tobramycin 6–7.5 mg/kg/day IM, IV div q8h (BIII); ADD vancomycin 40 mg/kg/day IV q8h for serious infection (for CA-MRSA), pending culture results.	Cefepime and meropenem will provide coverage for MSSA in addition to Pseudomonas. Thorough surgical debridement required for Pseudomonas (second drainage procedure needed in at least 20% of children); oral convalescent therapy with ciprofloxacin (BIII).[61] Treatment course 7–10 days after surgery.

C. EYE INFECTIONS

Clinical Diagnosis	Therapy (evidence grade)	Comments
Cellulitis, orbital[62-64] (also called post-septal cellulitis; may be associated with orbital abscess; usually secondary to sinus infection; caused by respiratory tract flora and S aureus, including CA-MRSA)	Cefotaxime 150 mg/kg/day div q8h or ceftriaxone 50 mg/kg/day q24h; ADD clindamycin 30 mg/kg/day IV div q8h (for S aureus, including CA-MRSA) OR ceftaroline: 2 mo–<2 y, 24 mg/kg/day IV div q8h; ≥2 y, 36 mg/kg/day IV div q8h (max single dose 400 mg); >33 kg, either 400 mg/dose IV q8h or 600 mg/dose IV q12h (BIII) OR vancomycin 40 mg/kg/day IV q8h (AIII). If MSSA isolated, use oxacillin/nafcillin IV OR cefazolin IV.	Surgical drainage of larger collections of pus, if present by CT scan in orbit or subperiosteal tissue. Try medical therapy alone for small abscess (BIII).[65] Treatment course for 10–14 days after surgical drainage, up to 21 days. CT scan to confirm cure (BIII).

6

Cellulitis, periorbital[66] (preseptal infection)

– Associated with entry site lesion on skin (*S aureus*, including CA-MRSA, group A streptococcus) in the fully immunized child	Standard: oxacillin/nafcillin 150 mg/kg/day IV div q6h OR cefazolin 100 mg/kg/day IV div q8h (BII) CA-MRSA: clindamycin 30 mg/kg/day IV div q8h or ceftaroline: 2 mo–<2 y, 24 mg/kg/day IV div q8h; ≥2 y, 36 mg/kg/day IV div q8h (max single dose 400 mg); >33 kg, either 400 mg/dose IV q8h or 600 mg/dose IV q12h (BII)	Oral antistaphylococcal antibiotic (eg, clindamycin) for empiric therapy of less severe infection; treatment course for 7–10 days
– No associated entry site (in febrile, unimmunized infants); pneumococcal or *H influenzae* type b	Ceftriaxone 50 mg/kg/day q24h OR cefotaxime 100–150 mg/kg/day IV, IM div q8h OR cefuroxime 150 mg/kg/day IV div q8h (AII).	Treatment course for 7–10 days; rule out meningitis; alternative: other 2nd-, 3rd-, or 4th-generation cephalosporins or amoxicillin/clavulanate.
– Periorbital, non-tender erythematous swelling (not true cellulitis, usually associated with sinusitis); sinus pathogens *rarely* may erode anteriorly, causing cellulitis.	Ceftriaxone 50 mg/kg/day q24h OR cefotaxime 100–150 mg/kg/day IV, IM div q8h OR cefuroxime 150 mg/kg/day IV div q8h (BIII). ADD clindamycin 30 mg/kg/day IV div q8h for more severe infection with suspect *S aureus* including CA-MRSA or for chronic sinusitis (covers anaerobes) (AIII).	For oral convalescent antibiotic therapy, see Sinusitis, acute; total treatment course of 14–21 days or 7 days after resolution of symptoms.
Conjunctivitis, acute (*Haemophilus* and pneumococcus predominantly)[67–69]	Polymyxin/trimethoprim ophth solution OR polymyxin/bacitracin ophth ointment OR ciprofloxacin ophth solution (BII), for 7–10 days. For neonatal infection, see Chapter 5. Steroid-containing therapy only if HSV ruled out.	Other topical antibiotics (gentamicin, tobramycin ophth solution erythromycin, besifloxacin, moxifloxacin, norfloxacin, ofloxacin, levofloxacin) may offer advantages for particular pathogens (CII). High rates of resistance to sulfacetamide.

6

Antimicrobial Therapy According to Clinical Syndromes

C. EYE INFECTIONS (continued)

Clinical Diagnosis	Therapy (evidence grade)	Comments
Conjunctivitis, herpetic[70–72]	1% trifluridine or 0.15% ganciclovir ophth gel (AIII) AND acyclovir PO (80 mg/kg/day div qid; max daily dose: 3,200 mg/day) has been effective in limited studies (BIII). Oral valacyclovir (60 mg/kg/day div tid) has superior pharmacokinetics to oral acyclovir and can be considered for systemic treatment, as can parenteral (IV) acyclovir if extent of disease is severe (CII).	Refer to ophthalmologist. Recurrences common; corneal scars may form. Topical steroids for keratitis concurrent with topical antiviral solution. Long-term prophylaxis (≥1 y) for suppression of recurrent infection with oral acyclovir 300 mg/m²/dose PO tid (max 400 mg/dose) (little long-term safety data in children). Assess for neutropenia on long-term therapy; potential risks must balance potential benefits to vision (BIII).
Dacryocystitis	No antibiotic usually needed; oral therapy for more symptomatic infection, based on Gram stain and culture of pus; topical therapy as for conjunctivitis may be helpful.	Warm compresses; may require surgical probing of naso-lacrimal duct.

Endophthalmitis[73,74]

NOTE: Subconjunctival/sub-tenon antibiotics are likely to be required (vancomycin/ceftazidime or clindamycin/gentamicin); steroids commonly used; requires anterior chamber or vitreous tap for microbiological diagnosis. Listed systemic antibiotics to be used in addition to ocular injections.

Clinical Diagnosis	Therapy (evidence grade)	Comments
– Empiric therapy following open globe injury	Vancomycin 40 mg/kg/day IV div q8h AND cefepime 150 mg/kg/day IV div q8h (AIII)	Refer to ophthalmologist; vitrectomy may be necessary for advanced endophthalmitis. No prospective, controlled studies.
– Staphylococcal	Vancomycin 40 mg/kg/day IV div q8h pending susceptibility testing; oxacillin/nafcillin 150 mg/kg/day IV div q6h if susceptible (AIII)	Consider ceftaroline for MRSA treatment as it may penetrate the vitreous better than vancomycin.
– Pneumococcal, meningococcal, Haemophilus	Ceftriaxone 100 mg/kg/day IV q24h; penicillin G 250,000 U/kg/day IV div q4h if susceptible (AIII)	Rule out meningitis; treatment course for 10–14 days.
– Gonococcal	Ceftriaxone 50 mg/kg q24h IV, IM (AIII)	ADD azithromycin. Treatment course 7 days or longer.

6

Pseudomonas	Cefepime 150 mg/kg/day IV div q8h for 10–14 days (AIII)	Cefepime is preferred over ceftazidime for _Pseudomonas_ based on decreased risk of development of resistance on therapy; meropenem IV or imipenem IV are alternatives (no clinical data). Very poor outcomes.
Candida	Intravitreal amphotericin 5–10 µg/0.1 mL sterile water OR voriconazole 100 µg/0.1 mL sterile water or normal saline AND fluconazole 12 mg/kg/day IV (load fluconazole with 25 mg/kg IV on day 1) (AIII). Use L-AmB with or without flucytosine for fluconazole-resistant isolates (AIII). Duration of therapy is at least 4–6 wk (AIII).	Echinocandins given IV may not be able to achieve adequate antifungal activity in the eye.[75]
Hordeolum (sty) or chalazion	None (topical antibiotic not necessary)	Warm compresses; I&D when necessary
Retinitis		
– CMV[76–78] For neonatal, see Chapter 5. For HIV-infected children, visit NIH Web site at http://aidsinfo.nih.gov/guidelines/html/5/-pediatric-oi-prevention-and-treatment-guidelines/0.	Ganciclovir 10 mg/kg/day IV div q12h for 2 wk (BIII); if needed, continue at 5 mg/kg/day q24h to complete 6 wk total (BIII).	Neutropenia risk increases with duration of therapy. Foscarnet IV and cidofovir IV are alternatives but demonstrate significant toxicities. Oral valganciclovir has not been evaluated in HIV-infected children with CMV retinitis but is an option primarily for older children who weigh enough to receive the adult dose of valganciclovir (CIII). Intravitreal ganciclovir and combination therapy for non-responding, immunocompromised hosts.

Antimicrobial Therapy According to Clinical Syndromes

D. EAR AND SINUS INFECTIONS

Clinical Diagnosis	Therapy (evidence grade)	Comments
Bullous myringitis (See Otitis media, acute.)	Believed to be a clinical presentation of acute bacterial otitis media	
Mastoiditis, acute (pneumococcus, S aureus, including CA-MRSA; group A streptococcus; increasing Pseudomonas in adolescents, Haemophilus rare)[79–81]	Cefotaxime 150 mg/kg/day IV div q8h or ceftriaxone 50 mg/kg/day q24h AND clindamycin 40 mg/kg/day IV div q8h (BIII) For adolescents: cefepime 150 mg/kg/day IV div q8h AND clindamycin 40 mg/kg/day IV div q8h (BII)	Rule out meningitis; surgery as needed for mastoid and middle ear drainage. Change to appropriate oral therapy after clinical improvement.
Mastoiditis, chronic (See also Otitis, chronic suppurative.) (anaerobes, Pseudomonas, S aureus [including CA-MRSA])[80]	Antibiotics only for acute superinfections (according to culture of drainage); for Pseudomonas: meropenem 60 mg/kg/day IV div q8h, OR pip/tazo 240 mg/kg/day IV div q4–6h for only 5–7 days after drainage stops (BIII)	Daily cleansing of ear important; if no response to antibiotics, surgery. Alternatives: cefepime IV or ceftazidime IV (poor anaerobic coverage with either antibiotic). Be alert for CA-MRSA.
Otitis externa		
Bacterial, swimmer's ear (P aeruginosa, S aureus, including CA-MRSA)[82–85]	Topical antibiotics: fluoroquinolone (ciprofloxacin or ofloxacin) with steroid, OR neomycin/polymyxin B/hydrocortisone (BII) Irrigation and cleaning canal of detritus important	Wick moistened with Burow solution, used for marked swelling of canal; to prevent swimmer's ear, 2% acetic acid to canal after water exposure will restore acid pH.
– Bacterial, malignant otitis externa (P aeruginosa)[84]	Cefepime 150 mg/kg/day IV div q8h (AIII)	Other antipseudomonal antibiotics should also be effective: ceftazidime IV AND tobramycin IV, OR meropenem IV or imipenem IV, pip/tazo IV. For more mild infection, ciprofloxacin PO.
– Bacterial furuncle of canal (S aureus, including CA-MRSA)	Standard: oxacillin/nafcillin 150 mg/kg/day IV div q6H OR cefazolin 100 mg/kg/day IV div q8h (BIII) CA-MRSA: clindamycin 30 mg/kg/day IV div q8h or vancomycin 40 mg/kg/day IV q8h (BIII)	I&D; antibiotics for cellulitis Oral therapy for mild disease, convalescent therapy: for MSSA: cephalexin; for CA-MRSA: clindamycin, TMP/SMX, OR linezolid (BIII)

6

– Candida	Fluconazole 6–12 mg/kg/day PO qd for 5–7 days (CIII)	May occur following antibiotic therapy of bacterial external otitis; debride canal.

Otitis media, acute

A note on AOM: The natural history of AOM in different age groups by specific pathogens has not been well defined; therefore, the actual contribution of antibiotic therapy on resolution of disease had also been poorly defined until 2 amox/clav vs placebo, blinded, prospective studies were published in 2011,[86,87] although neither study required tympanocentesis to define a pathogen. The benefits and risks (including development of antibiotic resistance) of antibiotic therapy for AOM need to be further evaluated before the most accurate advice on the "best" antibiotic can be provided. However, based on available data, for most children, amoxicillin or amox/clav can be used initially. Considerations for the need for extended antimicrobial activity of amox/clav include severity of disease, young age of the child, previous antibiotic therapy within 6 months, and child care attendance, which address the issues of types of pathogens and antibiotic resistance patterns to expect. However, with universal PCV13 immunization, data suggest that the percent of antibiotic-resistant pneumococcal otitis has decreased but the percent of *Haemophilus* responsible for AOM have increased; therefore, some experts recommend use of amox/clav as first-line therapy for well-documented AOM. The most current AAP guidelines[88] and meta-analyses[89] suggest the greatest benefit with therapy occurs in children with bilateral AOM who are younger than 2 years; for other children, close observation is also an option. AAP guidelines provide an option to treatment in non-severe cases, particularly disease in older children, to provide a prescription to parents but have them only fill the prescription if the child deteriorates.[88] Although prophylaxis is only rarely indicated, amoxicillin or other antibiotics can be used in half the therapeutic dose once or twice daily to prevent infections if the benefits outweigh the risks of development of resistant organisms for that child.[88]

– Newborns	See Chapter 5.

Antimicrobial Therapy According to Clinical Syndromes

6

D. EAR AND SINUS INFECTIONS (continued)

Clinical Diagnosis	Therapy (evidence grade)	Comments
— Infants and children (pneumococcus, H influenzae non–type b, Moraxella most common)[90–92]	Usual therapy: amoxicillin 90 mg/kg/day PO bid, with or without clavulanate; failures will be caused by highly pen-R pneumococcus or, if amoxicillin is used alone, by beta-lactamase–producing Haemophilus (or Moraxella). a) For Haemophilus strains that are beta-lactamase positive, the following oral antibiotics offer better in vitro activity than amoxicillin: amox/clav, cefdinir, cefpodoxime, cefuroxime, ceftriaxone IM, levofloxacin. b) For pen-R pneumococci: high-dosage amoxicillin achieves greater middle ear activity than oral cephalosporins. Options include ceftriaxone IM 50 mg/kg/day q24h for 1–3 doses; OR levofloxacin 20 mg/kg/day PO div bid for children ≤5 y and 10 mg/kg PO qd for children >5 y; OR a macrolide-class antibiotic*: (1) 10 mg/kg on day 1, followed by 5 mg/kg qd on days 2–5; (2) 10 mg/kg qd for 3 days; or (3) 30 mg/kg once. * Caution: Up to 40% of pen-R pneumococci are also macrolide resistant.	See Chapter 11 for dosages. Until published data document the lack of penicillin resistance in pneumococci isolated from infants with AOM in the post-PCV13 era,[91] high-dose amoxicillin (90 mg/kg/day) should still be used for empiric therapy. The high serum and middle ear fluid concentrations achieved with 45 mg/kg/dose of amoxicillin, combined with a long half-life in middle ear fluid, allow for a therapeutic antibiotic exposure in the middle ear with only twice-daily dosing; high-dose amoxicillin (90 mg/kg/day) with clavulanate (Augmentin ES) is also available. As published data document decreasing resistance to amoxicillin, standard dosage (45 mg/kg/day) can again be recommended. Tympanocentesis should be performed in children who fail second-line therapy.
Otitis, chronic suppurative (P aeruginosa, S aureus, including CA-MRSA, and other respiratory tract/skin flora)[85,93,94]	Topical antibiotics: fluoroquinolone (ciprofloxacin, ofloxacin, besifloxacin) with or without steroid (BIII) Cleaning of canal, view of tympanic membrane, for patency; cultures important	Presumed middle ear drainage through open tympanic membrane; possible aminoglycoside toxicity if neomycin-containing topical therapy used[95] Other topical fluoroquinolones with/without steroids available

Sinusitis, acute (H influenzae non–type b, pneumococcus, group A streptococcus, Moraxella)[96–100]	Same antibiotic therapy as for AOM as pathogens similar: amoxicillin 90 mg/kg/day PO div bid, OR for children at higher risk of Haemophilus, amox/clav 14:1 ratio, with amoxicillin component at 90 mg/kg/day PO div bid (BIII). Therapy of 14 days may be necessary while mucosal swelling resolves and ventilation is restored.	IDSA sinusitis guidelines recommend amox/clav as first-line therapy,[99] while AAP guidelines (same pediatric authors) recommend amoxicillin.[97] Lack of data prevents a definitive evidence-based recommendation. The same antibiotic therapy considerations used for AOM apply to acute bacterial sinusitis. Sinus irrigations for severe disease or failure to respond.

E. OROPHARYNGEAL INFECTIONS

Clinical Diagnosis	Therapy (evidence grade)	Comments
Dental abscess[101,102]	Clindamycin 30 mg/kg/day PO, IV, IM div q6–8h OR penicillin G 100–200,000 U/kg/day IV div q6h (AIII)	Amox/clav PO; amoxicillin PO; ampicillin AND metronidazole IV are other options. Tooth extraction usually necessary. Erosion of abscess may occur into facial, sinusitis, deep head, and neck compartments.
Diphtheria[103]	Erythromycin 40–50 mg/kg/day PO div qid for 14 days OR penicillin G 150,000 U/kg/day IV div q6h; PLUS antitoxin (AIII)	DAT, a horse antisera, is investigational and only available from CDC Emergency Operations Center at 770/488-7100. The investigational protocol and dosages of DAT are provided on the CDC Web site at www.cdc.gov/diphtheria/downloads/protocol.pdf (protocol version 3/26/14; accessed September 15, 2016).
Epiglottitis (aryepiglottitis, supraglottitis; H influenzae type b in an unimmunized child; rarely pneumococcus, S aureus)[104,105]	Ceftriaxone 50 mg/kg/day IV, IM q24h OR cefotaxime 150 mg/kg/day IV div q8h for 7–10 days	Emergency; provide airway. For S aureus (causes only 5% of epiglottitis), consider adding clindamycin 40 mg/kg/day IV div q8h.

6

Antimicrobial Therapy According to Clinical Syndromes

Antimicrobial Therapy According to Clinical Syndromes

E. OROPHARYNGEAL INFECTIONS (continued)

Clinical Diagnosis	Therapy (evidence grade)	Comments
Gingivostomatitis, herpetic[106-108]	Acyclovir 80 mg/kg/day PO div qid for 7 days (for severe disease, use IV therapy at 30 mg/kg/day div q8h) (BIII); OR for infants ≥3 mo, valacyclovir 20 mg/kg/dose PO bid (instructions for preparing liquid formulation with 28-day shelf life included in package insert) (CIII).[108]	Early treatment is likely to be the most effective. Start treatment as soon as oral intake is compromised. Extended duration of therapy may be needed for immunocompromised children. This oral acyclovir dose is safe and effective for varicella; 75 mg/kg/day div into 5 equal doses has been studied for HSV.[107] Limited pediatric valacyclovir pharmacokinetic data and preparation of an extemporaneous suspension are included in the valacyclovir FDA-approved package label.
Lemierre syndrome (Fusobacterium necrophorum primarily, new reports with MRSA)[109-113] (pharyngitis with internal jugular vein septic thrombosis, postanginal sepsis, necrobacillosis)	Empiric: meropenem 60 mg/kg/day div q8h (or 120 mg/kg/day div q8h for CNS metastatic foci) (AIII) OR ceftriaxone 100 mg/kg/day q24h AND metronidazole 40 mg/kg/day div q8h or clindamycin 40 mg/kg/day div q6h (BIII). ADD empiric vancomycin if MRSA suspected.	Anecdotal reports suggest metronidazole may be effective for apparent failures with other agents. Often requires anticoagulation. Metastatic and recurrent abscesses often develop while on active, appropriate therapy, requiring multiple debridements and prolonged antibiotic therapy. Treat until CRP and ESR are normal (AIII).
Peritonsillar cellulitis or abscess (group A streptococcus with mixed oral flora, including anaerobes, CA-MRSA)[114]	Clindamycin 30 mg/kg/day PO, IV, IM div q8h AND cefotaxime 150 mg/kg/day IV div q8h or ceftriaxone 50 mg/kg/day IV q24h (BIII)	Consider incision and drainage for abscess. Alternatives: meropenem or imipenem; pip/tazo; amox/clav for convalescent oral therapy (BIII). No useful data on benefits of steroids.
Pharyngitis (group A streptococcus primarily)[7,115-117]	Amoxicillin 50–75 mg/kg/day PO, either qd, bid, or tid for 10 days OR penicillin V 50–75 mg/kg/day PO div bid or tid, OR benzathine penicillin 600,000 units IM for children <27 kg, 1.2 million units IM if >27 kg, as a single dose (AII)	Amoxicillin displays better GI absorption than oral penicillin V; the suspension is better tolerated. These advantages should be balanced by the unnecessary increased spectrum of activity. Once-daily amoxicillin dosage: for children 50 mg/kg (max 1,000–1,200 mg).[7] Meta-analysis suggests that oral cephalosporins are more effective than penicillin for treatment of strep.[118]

	For penicillin-allergic children: erythromycin (estolate at 20–40 mg/kg/day PO div bid to qid; or ethylsuccinate at 40 mg/kg/day PO div bid to qid) for 10 days; or azithromycin 12 mg/kg qd for 5 days (AII)	Clindamycin is also effective. A 5-day treatment course is FDA approved for some oral cephalosporins (cefdinir, cefpodoxime), with rapid clinical response to treatment that can be seen with other antibiotics; a 10-day course is preferred for the prevention of ARF, particularly in areas where ARF is prevalent. No data exist on efficacy of 5 days of therapy for prevention of ARF.[117,119]
Retropharyngeal, parapharyngeal, or lateral pharyngeal cellulitis or abscess (mixed aerobic/anaerobic flora, now including CA-MRSA)[114,120–122]	Clindamycin 40 mg/kg/day IV div q8h AND cefotaxime 150 mg/kg/day IV div q8h or ceftriaxone 50 mg/kg/day IV q24h	Consider I&D; possible airway compromise, mediastinitis. Alternatives: meropenem or imipenem (BIII); pip/tazo; amox/clav for convalescent oral therapy (BIII).
Tracheitis, bacterial (S aureus, including CA-MRSA; group A streptococcus; pneumococcus; H influenzae type b, rarely Pseudomonas)[123,124]	Vancomycin 40 mg/kg/day IV div q8h or clindamycin 40 mg/kg/day IV div q8h AND ceftriaxone 50 mg/kg/day div q24h or cefotaxime 150 mg/kg/day div q8h (BIII) OR ceftaroline: 2 mo–<2 y, 24 mg/kg/day IV div q8h; ≥2 y, 36 mg/kg/day IV div q8h (max single dose 400 mg); >33 kg, either 400 mg/dose IV q8h or 600 mg/dose IV q12h (BIII)	For susceptible S aureus, oxacillin/nafcillin or cefazolin. May represent bacterial superinfection of viral laryngotracheobronchitis, including influenza.

6

Antimicrobial Therapy According to Clinical Syndromes

Antimicrobial Therapy According to Clinical Syndromes

F. LOWER RESPIRATORY TRACT INFECTIONS

Clinical Diagnosis	Therapy (evidence grade)	Comments
Abscess, lung		
– Primary (severe, necrotizing community-acquired pneumonia caused by pneumococcus, S aureus, including CA-MRSA, group A streptococcus)[125–127]	Empiric therapy with ceftriaxone 50–75 mg/kg/day q24h or cefotaxime 150 mg/kg/day div q8h AND clindamycin 40 mg/kg/day div q8h or vancomycin 45 mg/kg/day IV div q8h for 14–21 days or longer (AIII) OR (for MRSA) ceftaroline: 2–<6 mo, 30 mg/kg/day IV div q8h (each dose given over 2 h); ≥6 mo, 45 mg/kg/day IV div q8h (each dose given over 2 h) (max single dose 600 mg) (BII)	For severe CA-MRSA infections, see Chapter 4. Bronchoscopy may be necessary if abscess fails to drain; surgical excision rarely necessary for pneumococcus but more important for CA-MRSA and MSSA. Focus antibiotic coverage based on culture results. For MSSA: oxacillin/nafcillin or cefazolin.
– Secondary to aspiration (ie, foul smelling; polymicrobial infection with oral aerobes and anaerobes)[128]	Clindamycin 40 mg/kg/day IV div q8h or meropenem 60 mg/kg/day IV div q8h for 10 days or longer (AIII)	Alternatives: imipenem IV or pip/tazo IV or ticar/clav IV (BIII) Oral step-down therapy with clindamycin or amox/clav (BIII)
Allergic bronchopulmonary aspergillosis[129]	Prednisone 0.5 mg/kg qd for 1–2 wk and then taper (BII) AND voriconazole 18 mg/kg/day PO div q12h load followed by 16 mg/kg/day div q12h (AIII) OR itraconazole 10 mg/kg/day PO div q12h (BII)	Larger steroid dosages may lead to tissue invasion by *Aspergillus*. Voriconazole not as well studied in allergic bronchopulmonary aspergillosis but is more active than itraconazole. Voriconazole or itraconazole require trough concentration monitoring.
Aspiration pneumonia (polymicrobial infection with oral aerobes and anaerobes)[128]	Clindamycin 40 mg/kg/day IV div q8h; ADD ceftriaxone 50–75 mg/kg/day q24h or cefotaxime 150 mg/kg/day div q8h for additional *Haemophilus* activity OR meropenem 60 mg/kg/day IV div q8h; for 10 days or longer (BIII).	Alternatives: imipenem IV or pip/tazo IV or ticar/clav IV (BIII) Oral step-down therapy with clindamycin or amox/clav (BIII)
Atypical pneumonia (See *M pneumoniae*, Legionnaires disease.)		

Bronchitis (bronchiolitis), acute[130]	For bronchitis/bronchiolitis in children, no antibiotic needed for most cases, as disease is usually viral.	Multicenter global studies with anti-RSV therapy are currently underway.

Community-acquired pneumonia
(See Pneumonia: Community-acquired, bronchopneumonia; Pneumonia: Community-acquired, lobar consolidation.)

Cystic fibrosis: Seek advice from those expert in acute and chronic management. Larger than standard dosages of beta-lactam antibiotics are required in most patients with cystic fibrosis due to increased renal clearance.[131]

– Acute exacerbation (*P aeruginosa* primarily; also *Burkholderia cepacia*, *Stenotrophomonas maltophilia*, *S aureus*, including CA-MRSA, nontuberculous mycobacteria)[132-136]	Ceftazidime 150–200 mg/kg/day div q6–8h or meropenem 120 mg/kg/day div q6h AND tobramycin 6–10 mg/kg/day IM, IV div q6–8h for treatment of acute infection (AII); alternatives: imipenem, cefepime, or ciprofloxacin 30 mg/kg/day PO, IV div tid. May require vancomycin 60–80 mg/kg/day IV div q8h for MRSA, OR ceftaroline 45 mg/kg/day IV div q8h (each dose given over 2 h) (max single dose 600 mg) (BIII). Duration of therapy not well defined: 10–14 days (BIII).[133]	Monitor concentrations of aminoglycosides, vancomycin. Insufficient evidence to recommend routine use of inhaled antibiotics for acute exacerbations.[137] Cultures with susceptibility testing and synergy testing will help select antibiotics, as multidrug resistance is common, but synergy testing is not well standardized.[138,139] Combination therapy may provide synergistic killing and delay the emergence of resistance (BIII). Attempt at early eradication of new onset *Pseudomonas* may decrease progression of disease.[135,140] Failure to respond to antibacterials should prompt evaluation for invasive/allergic fungal disease.
Chronic inflammation (Minimize long-term damage to lung.)	Inhaled tobramycin 300 mg bid, cycling 28 days on therapy, 28 days off therapy, is effective adjunctive therapy between exacerbation[141] (AI). Inhaled aztreonam[142] provides an alternative to inhaled tobramycin (AI). Azithromycin adjunctive chronic therapy, greatest benefit for those colonized with *Pseudomonas* (AII).[143,144]	Alternative inhaled antibiotics: aztreonam[144]; colistin[137,145] (BIII) Two new powder preparations of inhaled tobramycin now available

Antimicrobial Therapy According to Clinical Syndromes

6

F. LOWER RESPIRATORY TRACT INFECTIONS (continued)

Clinical Diagnosis	Therapy (evidence grade)	Comments
Pertussis[146-148]	Azithromycin 10 mg/kg/day for 5 days, or clarithromycin 15 mg/kg/day div bid for 7 days, or erythromycin (estolate preferable) 40 mg/kg/day PO div qid; for 7–10 days (All) Alternative: TMP/SMX 8 mg/kg/day TMP div bid for 10 days (BIII)	Azithromycin and clarithromycin are better tolerated than erythromycin; azithromycin is preferred in young infants to reduce pyloric stenosis risk (see Chapter 5). The azithromycin dosage that is recommended for very young neonates with the highest risk of mortality (<1 mo) is 10 mg/kg/day for 5 days. This dose should be used up to 6 mo of age. Older children should receive 10 mg/kg on day 1, followed by 5 mg/kg on days 2–5.[146] Provide prophylaxis to family members. Unfortunately, no adjunctive therapy has been shown beneficial in decreasing the cough.[149]
Pneumonia: Community-acquired, bronchopneumonia		
– Mild to moderate illness (overwhelmingly viral, especially in preschool children)[150]	No antibiotic therapy unless epidemiologic, clinical, or laboratory reasons to suspect bacteria or Mycoplasma.	Broad-spectrum antibiotics may increase risk of subsequent infection with antibiotic-resistant pathogens.
– Moderate to severe illness (pneumococcus; group A streptococcus; S aureus, including CA-MRSA; or Mycoplasma pneumoniae[125,126,151-153], and for those with aspiration due to underlying comorbidities; Haemophilus influenzae, nontypable)	Empiric therapy For regions with high PCV13 vaccine use or low pneumococcal resistance to penicillin: ampicillin 200 mg/kg/day div q6h. For regions with low rates of PCV13 use or high pneumococcal resistance to penicillin: ceftriaxone 50–75 mg/kg/day q24h or cefotaxime 150 mg/kg/day div q8h (AI). For suspected CA-MRSA: vancomycin 40–60 mg/kg/day (AIII)[2] OR ceftaroline 2–<6 mo, 30 mg/kg/day IV div q8h (each dose given over 2 h); ≥6 mo, 45 mg/kg/day IV div q8h (each dose given over 2 h) (max single dose 600 mg).[127]	Tracheal aspirate or bronchoalveolar lavage for Gram stain/ culture for severe infection in intubated children. Check vancomycin serum concentrations and renal function, particularly at the higher dosage needed to achieve an AUC:MIC of 400 for CA-MRSA pneumonia. Alternatives to azithromycin for atypical pneumonia include erythromycin IV, PO, or clarithromycin PO, or doxycycline IV, PO for children >7 y, or levofloxacin. New data suggest that combination empiric therapy with a beta-lactam and a macrolide results in shorter hospitalization compared with a beta-lactam alone, but we are not ready to recommend routine empiric combination therapy yet.[154,155]

| | | For suspect *Mycoplasma*/atypical pneumonia agents, particularly in school-aged children, ADD azithromycin 10 mg/kg IV, PO on day 1, then 5 mg/kg qd for days 2–5 of treatment (AII). | Empiric oral outpatient therapy for less severe illness: high-dosage amoxicillin 80–100 mg/kg/day PO div tid (NOT bid) (BIII). |

Pneumonia: Community-acquired, lobar consolidation

Pneumococcus (May occur with non-vaccine strains, even if immunized for pneumococcus.)[125,126,151–153] Consider *H influenzae* type b in the unimmunized child. (*M pneumoniae* may cause lobar pneumonia.)	**Empiric therapy** For regions with high PCV13 vaccine use or low pneumococcal resistance to penicillin: ampicillin 200 mg/kg/day div q6h. For regions with low rates of PCV13 use or high pneumococcal resistance to penicillin: ceftriaxone 50–75 mg/kg/day q24h or cefotaxime 150 mg/kg/day div q8h (AI); for more severe disease ADD clindamycin 40 mg/kg/day div q8h or vancomycin 40–60 mg/kg/day div q8h for suspect *S aureus* (AIII).[2] For suspect *Mycoplasma*/atypical pneumonia agents, particularly in school-aged children, ADD azithromycin 10 mg/kg IV, PO on day 1, then 5 mg/kg qd for days 2–5 of treatment (AII). Empiric oral outpatient therapy for less severe illness: high-dosage amoxicillin 80–100 mg/kg/day PO div tid (NOT bid); for *Mycoplasma*, ADD a macrolide as above (BIII).	Change to PO after improvement (decreased fever, no oxygen needed); treat until clinically asymptomatic and chest radiography significantly improved (7–21 days) (BIII). No reported failures of ceftriaxone/cefotaxime for pen-R pneumococcus; no need to add empiric vancomycin for this reason (CIII). Oral therapy for pneumococcus and *Haemophilus* may also be successful with amox/clav, cefdinir, cefixime, cefpodoxime, or cefuroxime. Levofloxacin is an alternative, particularly for those with severe allergy to beta-lactam antibiotics (BI),[156] but, due to theoretical cartilage toxicity concerns, should not be first-line therapy.
– Pneumococcal, pen-S	Penicillin G 250,000–400,000 U/kg/day IV div q4–6h for 10 days (BII) or ampicillin 200 mg/kg/day IV divided q6h	After improvement, change to PO amoxicillin 50–75 mg/kg/day PO div tid, or penicillin V 50–75 mg/kg/day div qid.

Antimicrobial Therapy According to Clinical Syndromes

6

F. LOWER RESPIRATORY TRACT INFECTIONS (continued)

Clinical Diagnosis	Therapy (evidence grade)	Comments
– Pneumococcal, pen-R	Ceftriaxone 75 mg/kg/day q24h, or cefotaxime 150 mg/kg/day div q8h for 10–14 days (BII)	Addition of vancomycin has not been required for eradication of pen-R strains. For oral convalescent therapy, high-dosage amoxicillin (100–150 mg/kg/day PO div tid), clindamycin (30 mg/kg/day PO div tid), linezolid (30 mg/kg/day PO div tid), or levofloxacin PO.
S aureus (including CA-MRSA)[26,125,151,157]	For MSSA: oxacillin/nafcillin 150 mg/kg/day IV div q6h or cefazolin 100 mg/kg/day IV div q8h (AII). For CA-MRSA: vancomycin 60 mg/kg/day IV div q8h; 2–<6 mo, 30 mg/kg/day IV div q8h OR ceftaroline: 2–<6 mo, 45 mg/kg/day IV div q8h; ≥6 mo, 45 mg/kg/day IV div q8h (max single dose 600 mg) (BII)[127]; may need addition of rifampin, clindamycin, or gentamicin (AIII) (see Chapter 4).	Check vancomycin serum concentrations and renal function, particularly at the higher dosage designed to attain an AUC:MIC of 400, or serum trough concentrations of 15 µg/mL for invasive CA-MRSA disease. For life-threatening disease, optimal therapy of CA-MRSA is not defined; add gentamicin and/or rifampin for combination therapy (CIII). Linezolid 30 mg/kg/day IV, PO div q8h is another option, more effective in adults than vancomycin for MRSA nosocomial pneumonia[158] (follow platelets and WBC count weekly).
Pneumonia: Immunosuppressed, neutropenic host[159] (P aeruginosa, other community-associated or nosocomial gram-negative bacilli, S aureus, fungi, AFB, Pneumocystis, viral [adenovirus, CMV, EBV, influenza, RSV, others])	Cefepime 150 mg/kg/day IV div q8h and tobramycin 6.0–7.5 mg/kg/day IM, IV div q8h (AII), OR meropenem 60 mg/kg/day div q8h (AII) ± tobramycin (BIII); AND if S aureus (including MRSA) is suspected clinically, ADD vancomycin 40–60 mg/kg/day IV div q8h (AIII) OR ceftaroline: 2–<6 mo, 30 mg/kg/day IV div q8h; ≥6 mo, 45 mg/kg/day IV div q8h (max single dose 600 mg) (BII).	Biopsy or bronchoalveolar lavage usually needed to determine need for antifungal, antiviral, antimycobacterial treatment. Antifungal therapy usually started if no response to antibiotics in 48–72 h (AmB, voriconazole, or caspofungin/micafungin—see Chapter 8). Amikacin 15–22.5 mg/kg/day is an alternative aminoglycoside. Use 2 active agents for definitive therapy for neutropenic hosts, as neutrophils cannot assist clearing the pathogen; may also decrease risk of emergence of resistance (BII).

Condition	Therapy	Comments
– **Pneumonia: Interstitial pneumonia syndrome of early infancy**	If *Chlamydia trachomatis* suspected, azithromycin 10 mg/kg/day qd day 1, followed by 5 mg/kg/day qd days 2–5 OR erythromycin 40 mg/kg/day PO qid for 14 days (BII)	Most often respiratory viral pathogens, CMV, or chlamydial; role of *Ureaplasma* uncertain
– **Pneumonia, nosocomial (health care–associated/ ventilator-associated)** (*P aeruginosa*, gram-negative enteric bacilli [*Enterobacter, Klebsiella, Serratia, Escherichia coli*], *Acinetobacter, Stenotrophomonas,* and gram-positive organisms including CA-MRSA and *Enterococcus*)[160-163]	Commonly used regimens Meropenem 60 mg/kg/day div q8h, OR pip/tazo 240–300 mg/kg/day div q6–8h, OR cefepime 150 mg/kg/day div q8h; ± gentamicin 6.0–7.5 mg/kg/day div q8h (AIII); ADD vancomycin 40–60 mg/kg/day div q8h for suspect CA-MRSA (AIII).	Empiric therapy should be institution specific, based on your hospital's nosocomial pathogens and susceptibilities. Pathogens that cause nosocomial pneumonia often have multidrug resistance. Cultures are critical. Empiric therapy also based on child's prior colonization/infection. For multidrug-resistant gram-negative bacilli, IV therapy options include ceftazidime/avibactam, ceftolozane/tazobactam, or colistin. Aerosol delivery of antibiotics may be required for multi-drug-resistant pathogens, but little high-quality controlled data available for children.[164]
– **Pneumonia: With pleural fluid/empyema** (same regimens as for community-acquired bronchopneumonia) (Based on extent of fluid and symptoms, may benefit from chest tube drainage with fibrinolysis or video-assisted thoracoscopic surgery).[151,165-168]	Empiric therapy: ceftriaxone 50–75 mg/kg/day q24h or cefotaxime 150 mg/kg/day div q8h AND vancomycin 40–60 mg/kg/day IV div q8h (BIII) OR ceftaroline as single drug therapy: 2–<6 mo, 30 mg/kg/day IV div q8h (each dose given over 2 h); ≥6 mo, 45 mg/kg/day IV div q8h (each dose given over 2 h) (max single dose 600 mg) (BII)	Initial therapy based on Gram stain of empyema fluid; typically clinical improvement is slow, with persisting but decreasing "spiking" fever for 2–3 wk.
– Group A streptococcal	Penicillin G 250,000 U/kg/day IV div q4–6h for 10 days (BII)	Change to PO amoxicillin 75 mg/kg/day div tid or penicillin V 50–75 mg/kg/day div qid to tid after clinical improvement (BIII).
– Pneumococcal	(See Pneumonia: Community-acquired, lobar consolidation.)	

Antimicrobial Therapy According to Clinical Syndromes

F. LOWER RESPIRATORY TRACT INFECTIONS (continued)

Clinical Diagnosis	Therapy (evidence grade)	Comments
S aureus (including CA-MRSA)[2,6,125,157]	For MSSA: oxacillin/nafcillin or cefazolin (AII). For CA-MRSA: use vancomycin 60 mg/kg/day (AII) (designed to attain an AUC:MIC of 400, or serum trough concentrations of 15 µg/mL); follow serum concentrations and renal function; OR ceftaroline: 2–<6 mo, 30 mg/kg/day IV div q8h (each dose given over 2 h); ≥6 mo, 45 mg/kg/day IV div q8h (each dose given over 2 h) (max single dose 600 mg) (BII)[127]; may need additional antibiotics (see Chapter 4).	For life-threatening disease, optimal therapy of CA-MRSA is not defined: add gentamicin and/or rifampin. Oral convalescent therapy for MSSA: cephalexin PO; for CA-MRSA: clindamycin or linezolid PO. Total course for 21 days or longer (AIII). For children infected who do not tolerate high-dose vancomycin, alternatives include ceftaroline, clindamycin, and linezolid.

Pneumonias of other established etiologies (See Chapter 7 for treatment by pathogen.)

Clinical Diagnosis	Therapy (evidence grade)	Comments
– Chlamydophila[169] (formerly Chlamydia) pneumoniae, C psittaci, or C trachomatis	Azithromycin 10 mg/kg on day 1, followed by 5 mg/kg/day qd days 2–5 or erythromycin 40 mg/kg/day PO div qid; for 14 days	Doxycycline (patients >7 y)
– CMV (immunocompromised host)[170,171] (See chapters 5 and 9 for CMV infection in newborns.)	Ganciclovir IV 10 mg/kg IV div q12h for 2 wk (BIII); if needed, continue at 5 mg/kg/day q24h to complete 4–6 wk total (BIII).	Some experts add CMV immune globulin to provide a possible small incremental benefit in bone marrow transplant patients[172] (BII). Oral valganciclovir may be used for convalescent therapy (BIII). Foscarnet for ganciclovir-resistant strains.
– E coli	Ceftriaxone 50–75 mg/kg/day q24h or cefotaxime 150 mg/kg/day div q8h (AII)	For cephalosporin-resistant strains (ESBL producers), use meropenem, imipenem, or ertapenem (AIII).
– Enterobacter spp	Cefepime 100 mg/kg/day div q12h or meropenem 60 mg/kg/day div q8h; OR ceftriaxone 50–75 mg/kg/day q24h or cefotaxime 150 mg/kg/day div q8h AND gentamicin 6.0–7.5 mg/kg/day IM, IV div q8h (AIII)	Addition of aminoglycoside to 3rd-generation cephalosporins may retard the emergence of ampC-mediated constitutive high-level resistance, but concern exists for inadequate aminoglycoside concentration in airways[164]; not needed with cefepime, meropenem, or imipenem.

6

Organism/Condition	Therapy	Comments
– *Francisella tularensis*[173]	Gentamicin 6.0–7.5 mg/kg/day IM, IV div q8h for 10 days or longer for more severe disease (AIII); for less severe disease, doxycycline PO for 14–21 days (AIII)	Alternatives for oral therapy of mild disease: ciprofloxacin or levofloxacin (BIII)
– Fungi (See Chapter 8.) – Community-associated pathogens, vary by region (eg, *Coccidioides*,[174,175] *Histoplasma*)[176,177] – *Aspergillus*, mucormycosis, other mold infections in immunocompromised hosts (See Chapter 8.)	For detailed pathogen-specific recommendations, see Chapter 8. For suspected endemic fungi or mucormycosis in immunocompromised host, treat empirically with a lipid AmB and not voriconazole; biopsy needed to guide therapy. For suspected invasive aspergillosis, treat with voriconazole (AI) (load 18 mg/kg/day div q12h on day 1, then continue 16 mg/kg/day div q12h).	For normal hosts, triazoles (fluconazole, itraconazole, voriconazole, posaconazole, isavuconazole) are better tolerated than AmB and equally effective for many community-associated pathogens (see Chapter 2). For dosage, see Chapter 8. Check voriconazole trough concentrations; need to be at least >2 µg/mL. For refractory *Coccidioides* infection, posaconazole or combination therapy with voriconazole and caspofungin may be effective[174] (AIII).
– Influenza virus[178,179] – Recent seasonal influenza A and influenza B strains continue to be resistant to adamantanes.	Empiric therapy, or documented influenza A or influenza B Oseltamivir[179,180] (AII): <12 mo: Term infants 0–8 mo: 3 mg/kg/dose bid 9–11 mo: 3.5 mg/kg/dose bid ≥12 mo: ≤15 kg: 30 mg PO bid >15–23 kg: 45 mg PO bid >23–40 kg: 60 mg PO bid >40 kg: 75 mg PO bid Zanamivir inhaled (AII): for those ≥7 y 10 mg (two 5-mg inhalations) bid	Check for antiviral susceptibility each season at www.cdc.gov/flu/professionals/antivirals/index.htm (accessed September 15, 2016). For children 12–23 mo, the unit dose of 30 mg/dose may provide inadequate drug exposure. 3.5 mg/kg/dose PO bid has been studied,[180] but sample sizes have been inadequate to recommend weight-based dosing at this time. The adamantanes (amantadine and rimantadine) had activity against influenza A prior to the late 1990s, but all circulating A strains of influenza have been resistant for many years. Influenza B is intrinsically resistant to adamantanes. Limited data for premature neonates.[179] <38 wk postmenstrual age (gestational plus chronologic age): 1.0 mg/kg/dose, PO bid 38–40 wk postmenstrual age: 1.5 mg/kg/dose, PO bid Parenteral peramivir and parenteral zanamivir being evaluated in clinical trials in children.

Antimicrobial Therapy According to Clinical Syndromes

6

F. LOWER RESPIRATORY TRACT INFECTIONS (continued)

Clinical Diagnosis	Therapy (evidence grade)	Comments
– *Klebsiella pneumoniae*[181,182]	Ceftriaxone 50–75 mg/kg/day IV, IM q24h OR cefotaxime 150 mg/kg/day IV, IM div q8h (AIII); for ceftriaxone-resistant strains (ESBL strains), use meropenem 60 mg/kg/day IV div q8h (AIII) or other carbapenem.	For *K pneumoniae* that contain ESBLs, fluoroquinolones are an alternative therapy. For *K pneumoniae* carbapenemase-producing strains that are resistant to meropenem: alternatives include ceftazidime/avibactam (FDA-approved for adults, pediatric studies in progress), fluoroquinolones, or colistin (BIII).
– Legionnaires disease (*Legionella pneumophila*)	Azithromycin 10 mg/kg IV, PO q24h for 5 days (AIII)	Alternatives: clarithromycin, erythromycin, ciprofloxacin, levofloxacin, doxycycline
– Mycobacteria, nontuberculous (*M avium* complex most common)[11,183]	In a normal host: azithromycin PO or clarithromycin PO for 6–12 wk if susceptible For more extensive disease: a macrolide AND rifampin AND ethambutol; ± amikacin or streptomycin (AIII)	Highly variable susceptibilities of different nontuberculous mycobacterial species Check if immunocompromised: HIV or gamma-interferon receptor deficiency
– *Mycobacterium tuberculosis* (See Tuberculosis.)		
– *M pneumoniae*[151,184]	Azithromycin 10 mg/kg on day 1, followed by 5 mg/kg/day qd days 2–5, or clarithromycin 15 mg/kg/day div bid for 7–14 days, or erythromycin 40 mg/kg/day PO div qid for 14 days	*Mycoplasma* often causes self-limited infection and does not require treatment (AIII). Little prospective, well-controlled data exist for treatment of documented mycoplasma pneumonia specifically in children.[184] Doxycycline (patients >7 y), or levofloxacin. Macrolide-resistant strains have recently appeared worldwide.[185]
– *Paragonimus westermani*	See Chapter 10.	
– *Pneumocystis jiroveci* (formerly *Pneumocystis carinii*)[186]. disease in immuno-suppressed children and those with HIV	Severe disease: preferred regimen is TMP/SMX, 15–20 mg TMP component/kg/day IV div q8h for 3 wk (AI).	Alternatives for TMP/SMX intolerant, or clinical failure: pentamidine 3–4 mg IV qd, infused over 60–90 min (AII); TMP AND dapsone; OR primaquine AND clindamycin; OR atovaquone.

	Mild-moderate disease: may start with IV therapy, then after acute pneumonitis is resolving, TMP/SMX 20 mg of TMP/kg/day PO div qid for 21 days (AII). Use steroid adjunctive treatment for more severe disease (AII).	Prophylaxis: TMP/SMX as 5 mg TMP/kg/day PO, divided in 2 doses, q12h, daily or 3 times/wk on consecutive days (AII); OR TMP/SMX 5 mg TMP/kg/day PO as a single dose, once daily, given 3 times/wk on consecutive days (AI); once-weekly regimens have also been successful[187]; OR dapsone 2 mg/kg (max 100 mg) PO qd, or 4 mg/kg (max 200 mg) once weekly; OR atovaquone: 30 mg/kg/day for infants 1–3 mo, 45 mg/kg/day for infants 4–24 mo, and 30 mg/kg/day for children >24 mo.
– *P aeruginosa*[164,167,188,189]	Cefepime 150 mg/kg/day IV div q8h ± tobramycin 6.0–7.5 mg/kg/day IM, IV div q8h (AII). Alternatives: meropenem 60 mg/kg/day div q8h, OR pip/tazo 240–300 mg/kg/day div q6–8h (AII) ± tobramycin (BIII).	Ciprofloxacin IV, or colistin IV for multidrug-resistant strains[190]
RSV infection (bronchiolitis, pneumonia)[191]	For immunocompromised hosts, the only FDA-approved treatment is ribavirin aerosol: 6-g vial (20 mg/mL in sterile water), by SPAG-2 generator, over 18–20 h daily for 3–5 days. Two RSV antivirals, ALS-008176 by Alios/J&J and the other GS-5806 by Gilead, are currently under investigation in children.	Treat only for severe disease, immunocompromised, severe underlying cardiopulmonary disease, as aerosol ribavirin only provides a small benefit. Airway reactivity with inhalation precludes routine use. Palivizumab (Synagis) is not effective for treatment of an active RSV infection, only effective for prevention of hospitalization in high-risk patients.

Antimicrobial Therapy According to Clinical Syndromes

F. LOWER RESPIRATORY TRACT INFECTIONS (continued)

Clinical Diagnosis	Therapy (evidence grade)	Comments
– Tuberculosis		
– Primary pulmonary disease[13,14]	INH 10–15 mg/kg/day (max 300 mg) PO qd for 6 mo AND rifampin 10–20 mg/kg/day (max 600 mg) PO qd for 6 mo AND PZA 30–40 mg/kg/day (max 2 g) PO qd for first 2 mo therapy only (AII). If risk factors present for multidrug resistance, ADD ethambutol 20 mg/kg/day PO qd OR streptomycin 30 mg/kg/day IV, IM div q12h initially.	Contact TB specialist for therapy of drug-resistant TB. Fluoroquinolones may play a role in treating multidrug-resistant strains. Bedaquiline, in a new drug class for TB therapy, was recently approved for adults with multidrug-resistant TB, when used in combination therapy. Toxicities and lack of pediatric data preclude routine use in children. Directly observed therapy preferred; after 2 wk of daily therapy, can change to twice-weekly dosing double dosage of INH (max 900 mg), PZA (max 2 g), and ethambutol (max 2.5 g); rifampin remains same dosage (10–20 mg/kg/day, max 600 mg) (AII). LP ± CT of head for children ≤2 y to rule out occult, concurrent CNS infection; consider testing for HIV infection (AIII). *Mycobacterium bovis* from unpasteurized dairy products can rarely cause pulmonary disease; also called "tuberculosis," but all strains of *M bovis* are PZA resistant.
– Latent TB infection[14] (skin test conversion)	INH 10–15 mg/kg/day (max 300 mg) PO daily for 9 mo (12 mo for immunocompromised patients) (AIII); treatment with INH at 20–30 mg/kg twice weekly for 9 mo is also effective (AIII). Alternative[192] (BII): for children ≥2 y, once-weekly DOT for 12 wk: INH (15 mg/kg/dose, max 900 mg). AND rifapentine: 10.0–14.0 kg: 300 mg 14.1–25.0 kg: 450 mg 25.1–32.0 kg: 600 mg 32.1–49.9 kg: 750 mg ≥50.0 kg: 900 mg (max)	Obtain baseline LFTs. Consider monthly LFTs or as needed for symptoms. Stop INH-rifapentine if AST or ALT ≥5 times the ULN even in the absence of symptoms or ≥3 times the ULN in the presence of symptoms. For children ≥2–12 y, 12 wk of INH and rifapentine may be used, but less data on safety and efficacy. Insufficient data for children <2 y. For exposure to known INH-R but rifampin-S strains, use rifampin 6 mo (AIII).

– Exposed child <4 y, or immunocompromised patient (high risk of dissemination)	INH 10–15 mg/kg PO daily for 2–3 mo after last exposure with repeat skin test or interferon-gamma release assay test negative (AIII)	If PPD remains negative at 2–3 mo and child well, consider stopping empiric therapy. PPD may not be reliable in immunocompromised patients. Not much data to assess reliability of interferon-gamma release assays in very young infants or immunocompromised hosts, but not likely to be much better than the PPD skin test.

G. CARDIOVASCULAR INFECTIONS

Clinical Diagnosis	Therapy (evidence grade)	Comments
Bacteremia		
– Occult bacteremia (late-onset neonatal sepsis; fever without focus), infants <2 mo (group B streptococcus, E coli, Listeria, pneumococcus, meningococcus)[193-197]	In general, hospitalization for late-onset neonatal sepsis, with cultures of blood, urine, and CSF; start ampicillin 200 mg/kg/day IV div q6h AND cefotaxime 150 mg/kg/day IV div q8h (AII); higher dosages if meningitis is documented.	Current data document the importance of ampicillin-resistant E coli in bacteremia in infants <90 days.[195,196,198] For a nontoxic, febrile infant with good access to medical care: cultures may be obtained of blood, urine, and CSF; ceftriaxone 50 mg/kg IM (lacks Listeria activity) given with outpatient follow-up the next day (Boston criteria) (BII); alternative is home without antibiotics if evaluation is negative (Rochester; Philadelphia criteria).[193,197] (BI).
– Occult bacteremia (fever without focus) in ages 2–3 mo to 36 mo (H influenzae, pneumococcus, meningococcus; increasingly S aureus)[196-198]	Empiric therapy: if unimmunized, febrile, mild-moderate toxic: after blood culture: ceftriaxone 50 mg/kg IM (BII). If fully immunized (Haemophilus and Pneumococcus) and nontoxic, routine empiric therapy of fever with antibiotics is no longer recommended, but follow closely in case of vaccine failure or meningococcal bacteremia (BII).	Oral convalescent therapy is selected by susceptibility of blood isolate, following response to IM/IV treatment, with CNS and other foci ruled out by examination ± laboratory tests ± imaging.

Antimicrobial Therapy According to Clinical Syndromes

6

G. CARDIOVASCULAR INFECTIONS (continued)

Clinical Diagnosis	Therapy (evidence grade)	Comments
– H influenzae type b, non-CNS infections	Ceftriaxone IM/IV OR, if beta-lactamase negative, ampicillin IV, followed by oral convalescent therapy (AII)	If beta-lactamase negative: amoxicillin 75–100 mg/kg/day PO div tid (AII) If positive: high-dosage cefixime, ceftibuten, cefdinir PO, or levofloxacin PO (CIII)
– Meningococcus	Ceftriaxone IM/IV or penicillin G IV, followed by oral convalescent therapy (AII)	Amoxicillin 75–100 mg/kg/day PO div tid (AIII)
– Pneumococcus, non-CNS infections	Ceftriaxone IM/IV or penicillin G IV (if pen-S), followed by oral convalescent therapy (AII) Ampicillin IM/IV is another option (AII).	If pen-S: amoxicillin 75–100 mg/kg/day PO div tid (AII). If pen-R: continue ceftriaxone IM, or switch to clindamycin if susceptible (CIII); linezolid or levofloxacin PO may also be options (CIII).
– S aureus[2,6,199-202] usually associated with focal infection	MSSA: nafcillin or oxacillin/nafcillin IV 150–200 mg/kg/day div q6h ± gentamicin 6 mg/kg/day div q8h (AII). MRSA: vancomycin 40–60 mg/kg/day IV div q8h OR ceftaroline: 2 mo–<2 y, 24 mg/kg/day IV div q8h; ≥2 y, 36 mg/kg/day IV div q8h (max single dose 400 mg) (BIII) ± gentamicin 6 mg/kg/day div q8h ± rifampin 20 mg/kg/day div q12h (AIII). Treat for 2 wk (IV plus PO) from negative blood cultures unless endocarditis/endovascular thrombus present, which may require 6 wk of therapy (BII).	For persisting bacteremia caused by MRSA, consider adding gentamicin, or changing from vancomycin to ceftaroline or daptomycin (but will not treat pneumonia), particularly for MRSA with vancomycin MIC of >2 μg/mL. For toxic shock syndrome, clindamycin should be added for the initial 48–72 h of therapy to decrease toxin production (linezolid may also act in this way); IVIG may be added to bind circulating toxin (linezolid may also act in this way); no controlled data exist for these measures. Watch for the development of metastatic foci of infection, including endocarditis. If catheter-related, remove catheter.

Endocarditis: Surgical indications: intractable heart failure; persistent infection; large mobile vegetations; peripheral embolism; and valve dehiscence, perforation, rupture or fistula, or a large perivalvular abscess.[203-206] Consider community versus nosocomial pathogens based on recent surgeries, prior antibiotic therapy, and possible entry sites for bacteremia (skin, oropharynx and respiratory tract, gastrointestinal tract). Children with congenital heart disease are more likely to have more turbulent cardiovascular blood flow, which increases risk of endovascular infection. Immune-compromised hosts may become bacteremic with a wide range of bacteria, fungi, and mycobacteria.

— Native valve[203,204]

– Empiric therapy for presumed endocarditis (viridans streptococci, *Staphylococcus aureus*, HACEK group)	Ceftriaxone IV 100 mg/kg q24h AND gentamicin IV, IM 6 mg/kg/day div q8h (AII). For more acute, severe infection, ADD vancomycin 40–60 mg/kg/day IV div q8h to cover *S aureus* (AII).	Combination (ceftriaxone + gentamicin) provides bactericidal activity against most strains of viridans streptococci, the most common pathogens in infective endocarditis. Cefepime is recommended for adults,[206] but resistance in enteric bacilli in children suggests that ceftriaxone remains a reasonable choice. May administer gentamicin with a qd regimen (CIII). For beta-lactam allergy, use vancomycin 45 mg/kg/day IV div q8h AND gentamicin 6 mg/kg/day IV div q8h.

Culture negative native valve endocarditis: treat 4–6 wk (please obtain advice from an infectious diseases specialist for an appropriate regimen that is based on likely pathogens).[203]

– Viridans streptococci: Follow echocardiogram for resolution of vegetation (BIII); for beta-lactam allergy: vancomycin.

Fully susceptible to penicillin	Ceftriaxone 50 mg/kg IV, IM q24h for 4 wk OR penicillin G 200,000 U/kg/day IV div q4–6h for 4 wk (BII); OR penicillin G or ceftriaxone AND gentamicin 6 mg/kg/day IM, IV div q8h (AII) for 14 days for adults (4 wk for children per AHA guidelines due to lack of data in children)	AHA recommends higher dosage of ceftriaxone similar to that for penicillin nonsusceptible strains.
Relatively resistant to penicillin	Penicillin G 300,000 U/kg/day IV div q4–6h for 4 wk, or ceftriaxone 100 mg/kg IV q24h for 4 wk; AND gentamicin 6 mg/kg/day IM, IV div q8h for the first 2 wk (AIII)	Gentamicin is used for the first 2 wk of a total of 4 wk of therapy for relatively resistant strains. Vancomycin-containing regimens should use at least a 4-wk treatment course, with gentamicin used for the entire course.

– Enterococcus (dosages for native or prosthetic valve infections)

Antimicrobial Therapy According to Clinical Syndromes

G. CARDIOVASCULAR INFECTIONS (continued)

Clinical Diagnosis	Therapy (evidence grade)	Comments
Ampicillin-susceptible (gentamicin-S)	Ampicillin 300 mg/kg/day IV, IM div q6h or penicillin G 300,000 U/kg/day IV div q4–6h; AND gentamicin 6.0 mg/kg/day IV div q8h; for 4–6 wk (AII)	Combined treatment with cell-wall active antibiotic plus aminoglycoside used to achieve bactericidal activity.
Ampicillin-resistant (gentamicin-S)	Vancomycin 40 mg/kg/day IV div q8h AND gentamicin 6.0 mg/kg/day IV div q8h; for 6 wk (AII)	For beta-lactam allergy: vancomycin. Little data exist in children for daptomycin, linezolid, or quinupristin/dalfopristin.
Vancomycin-resistant (gentamicin-S)	Daptomycin IV if also ampicillin-resistant (dose is age-dependent; see Chapter 11) AND gentamicin 6.0 mg/kg/day IV div q8h; for 4–6 wk (AIII)	For gentamicin-R strains, use streptomycin or other aminoglycoside if susceptible.
– Staphylococci: S aureus, including CA-MRSA; S epidermidis[6,200]	MSSA or MSSE: nafcillin or oxacillin/nafcillin 150–200 mg/kg/day IV div q6h for 4–6 wk AND gentamicin 6 mg/kg/day div q8h for first 14 days.	Surgery may be necessary in acute phase; avoid first-generation cephalosporins (conflicting data on efficacy).
Consider continuing therapy at end of 6 wk if vegetations persist on echocardiogram.	CA-MRSA or MRSE: vancomycin 40–60 mg/kg/day IV div q8h AND gentamicin for 6 wk; consider for slow response, ADD rifampin 20 mg/kg/day IV div q8–12h.
For vancomycin-resistant MRSA, please consult an infectious diseases specialist.	AHA suggests gentamicin for only the first 3–5 days for MSSA or MSSE and optional gentamicin for MRSA. For failures on therapy, or vancomycin-resistant MRSA, consider daptomycin (dose is age-dependent; see Chapter 11) AND gentamicin 6 mg/kg/day div q8h.
– Pneumococcus, gonococcus, group A streptococcus	Penicillin G 200,000 U/kg/day IV div q4–6h for 4 wk (BII); alternatives: ceftriaxone or vancomycin	Ceftriaxone plus azithromycin for suspected gonococcus until susceptibilities known. For penicillin non-susceptible strains of pneumococcus, use high-dosage penicillin G 300,000 U/kg/day IV div q4–6h or high-dosage ceftriaxone 100 mg/kg IV q24h for 4 wk.
HACEK (Haemophilus spp, Aggregatibacter [formerly Actinobacillus], Cardiobacterium, Eikenella, Kingella spp)	Usually susceptible to ceftriaxone 100 mg/kg IV q24h for 4 wk (BIII)	Some organisms will be ampicillin-susceptible. Usually do not require the addition of gentamicin.

6

– Enteric gram-negative bacilli	Antibiotics specific to pathogen (usually ceftriaxone plus gentamicin); duration at least 6 wk (AIII)	ESBL or beta-lactam/beta-lactamase inhibitor combinations will be effective, PLUS gentamicin.
– *Pseudomonas aeruginosa*	Antibiotic specific to susceptibility: cefepime or meropenem PLUS tobramycin	Cefepime and meropenem are both more active against *Pseudomonas* and less likely to allow beta-lactamase–resistant pathogens to emerge than ceftazidime.
– Prosthetic valve/material[203,204]		
– Viridans streptococci		Follow echocardiogram for resolution of vegetation. For beta-lactam allergy: vancomycin.
Fully susceptible to penicillin	Ceftriaxone 100 mg/kg IV, IM q24h for 6 wk OR penicillin G 300,000 U/kg/day IV div q4–6h for 6 wk (AII); OR penicillin G or ceftriaxone AND gentamicin 6.0 mg/kg/day IM, IV div q8h for first 2 wk of 6 wk course (AII)	Gentamicin is optional for the first 2 wk of a total of 6 wk of therapy for prosthetic valve/material endocarditis.
Relatively resistant to penicillin	Penicillin G 300,000 U/kg/day IV div q4–6h for 6 wk, or ceftriaxone 100 mg/kg IV q24h for 6 wk; AND gentamicin 6.0 mg/kg/day IM, IV div q8h for 6 wk (AIII)	Gentamicin is used for all 6 wk of therapy for prosthetic valve/material endocarditis caused by relatively resistant strains.
– Enterococcus (See dosages under native valve.) Treatment course is at least 6 wk, particularly if vancomycin is used.[203]		
– Staphylococci: *S aureus*, including CA-MRSA; *S epidermidis*[6,203] Consider continuing therapy at end of 6 wk if vegetations persist on echocardiogram.	MSSA or MSSE: nafcillin or oxacillin/nafcillin 150–200 mg/kg/day IV div q6h for ≥6 wk AND gentamicin 6 mg/kg/day div q8h for first 14 days. CA-MRSA or MRSE: vancomycin 40–60 mg/kg/day IV div q8h AND gentamicin for ≥6 wk; ADD rifampin 20 mg/kg/day IV div q8–12h.	For failures on therapy, consider daptomycin (dose is age-dependent; see Chapter 11) AND gentamicin 6 mg/kg/day div q8h.

6

Antimicrobial Therapy According to Clinical Syndromes

G. CARDIOVASCULAR INFECTIONS (continued)

Clinical Diagnosis	Therapy (evidence grade)	Comments
– *Candida*[206,207]	AmB preparations have more experience and are preferred (no comparative trials against echino-candins), OR caspofungin 70 mg/m² load on day 1, then 50 mg/m²/day or micafungin 2–4 mg/kg/day (BIII).	Surgery to resect infected valve. Long-term suppressive therapy with fluconazole. Suspect *Candida* vegetations when lesions are large on echocardiography.
– Culture negative prosthetic valve endocarditis: treat at least 6 wks.		
Endocarditis Prophylaxis[204,208,209]: Given that (1) endocarditis is rarely caused by dental/GI procedures and (2) prophylaxis for procedures prevents an exceedingly small number of cases, the risks of antibiotics outweigh the benefits. Highest risk conditions currently recommended for prophylaxis: (1) prosthetic heart valve (or prosthetic material used to repair a valve); (2) previous endocarditis; (3) cyanotic congenital heart disease that is unrepaired (or palliatively repaired with shunts and conduits); (4) congenital heart disease that is repaired but with defects at the site of repair adjacent to prosthetic material; (5) completely repaired congenital heart disease using prosthetic material, for the first 6 mo after repair; or (6) cardiac transplant patients with valvulopathy. Routine prophylaxis no longer is required for children with native valve abnormalities. Assessment of new prophylaxis guidelines documents no significant increase in endocarditis at this time.[209]		
– In highest risk patients: dental procedures that involve manipulation of the gingival or periodontal region of teeth	Amoxicillin 50 mg/kg PO 60 min before procedure OR ampicillin or ceftriaxone or cefazolin, all at 50 mg/kg IM/IV 30–60 min before procedure	If penicillin allergy: clindamycin 20 mg/kg PO (60 min before) or IV (30 min before); OR azithromycin 15 mg/kg or clarithromycin 15 mg/kg, 60 min before
– Genitourinary and GI procedures	None	No longer recommended
Lemierre syndrome (*Fusobacterium necrophorum* primarily, new reports with MRSA)[109–113] (pharyngitis with internal jugular vein septic thrombosis, postanginal sepsis, necrobacillosis)	Empiric: meropenem 60 mg/kg/day div q8h (or 120 mg/kg/day div q8h for CNS metastatic foci) (AIII) OR ceftriaxone 100 mg/kg/day q24h AND metronidazole 40 mg/kg/day div q8h or clindamycin 40 mg/kg/day div q6h (BIII). ADD empiric vancomycin if MRSA suspected.	Anecdotal reports suggest metronidazole may be effective for apparent failures with other agents. Often requires anticoagulation. Metastatic and recurrent abscesses often develop while on active, appropriate therapy, requiring multiple debridements and prolonged antibiotic therapy. Treat until CRP and ESR are normal (AIII).

Purulent pericarditis

– Empiric (acute, bacterial: *S aureus* [including MRSA], group A streptococcus, pneumococcus, meningococcus, *H influenzae* type b)[2,10,211]	Vancomycin 40 mg/kg/day IV div q8h AND ceftriaxone 50–75 mg/kg/day q24h (AIII), OR ceftaroline 2–<6 mo, 30 mg/kg/day IV div q8h; ≥6 mo, 45 mg/kg/day IV div q8h (max single dose 600 mg) (BIII)	For presumed staphylococcal infection, ADD gentamicin (AIII). Increasingly uncommon with immunization against pneumococcus and *H influenzae* type b.[211] Pericardiocentesis is essential to establish diagnosis. Surgical drainage of pus with pericardial window or pericardiectomy is important to prevent tamponade.
– *S aureus*	For MSSA: oxacillin/nafcillin 150–200 mg/kg/day IV div q6h OR cefazolin 100 mg/kg/day IV div q8h. Treat for 2–3 wk after drainage (BIII). For CA-MRSA: continue vancomycin or ceftaroline. Treat for 3–4 wk after drainage (BIII).	Continue therapy with gentamicin; consider use of rifampin in severe cases.
– *H influenzae* type b in unimmunized children	Ceftriaxone 50 mg/kg/day q24h or cefotaxime 150 mg/kg/day div q8h; for 10–14 days (AIII)	Ampicillin for beta-lactamase–negative strains
– Pneumococcus, meningococcus, group A streptococcus	Penicillin G 200,000 U/kg/day IV, IM div q6h for 10–14 days OR ceftriaxone 50 mg/kg qd for 10–14 days (AIII)	Ceftriaxone or cefotaxime for penicillin non-susceptible pneumococci
– Coliform bacilli	Ceftriaxone 50–75 mg/kg/day q24h or cefotaxime 150 mg/kg/day div q8h for 3 wk or longer (AIII)	Alternative drugs depending on susceptibilities; for *Enterobacter*, *Serratia*, or *Citrobacter*, use cefepime or meropenem. For ESBL *E coli* or *Klebsiella*, use a carbapenem.
– Tuberculous[13,14]	INH 10–15 mg/kg/day (max 300 mg) PO, IV qd, for 6 mo AND rifampin 10–20 mg/kg/day (max 600 mg) PO qd, IV for 6 mo. ADD PZA 20–40 mg/kg/day PO qd for first 2 mo therapy; if suspected multidrug resistance, also add ethambutol 20 mg/kg/day PO qd (AIII).	Corticosteroids improve survival in adults. For children: prednisone 2 mg/kg/day PO for 4 wk, then 0.5 mg/kg/day for 4 wk, then 0.25 mg/kg/day for 2 wk, then 0.1 mg/kg/day for 1 wk (AIII).[13,14]

6

Antimicrobial Therapy According to Clinical Syndromes

H. GASTROINTESTINAL INFECTIONS (See Chapter 10 for parasitic infections.)

Clinical Diagnosis	Therapy (evidence grade)	Comments
Diarrhea/Gastroenteritis		
Note on E coli and diarrheal disease: Antibiotic susceptibility of E coli varies considerably from region to region. For mild to moderate disease, TMP/SMX may be started as initial therapy, but for more severe disease and for locations with rates of TMP/SMX resistance greater than 10% to 20%, oral 3rd-generation cephalosporins (eg, cefixime, cefdinir, ceftibuten), azithromycin, or ciprofloxacin should be used (AIII). Cultures and antibiotic susceptibility testing are recommended for significant disease (AIII).		
– Empiric therapy of community-associated diarrhea in the United States (E coli [STEC], including O157:H7 strains, and ETEC], Salmonella, Campylobacter, and Shigella predominate; Yersinia and parasites causing <5%; however, viral pathogens are far more common, especially for children <3 y).[212,213]	Azithromycin 10 mg/kg qd for 3 days (BII), OR cefixime 8 mg/kg/day PO qd (BII) for 5 days; OR ciprofloxacin 30 mg/kg/day PO div bid for 3 days	Alternatives: other oral 3rd-generation cephalosporins (eg, cefdinir, ceftibuten); or rifaximin 600 mg/day div tid for 3 days (for nonfebrile, non-bloody diarrhea for children >11 y). Controversy exists regarding treatment of O157:H7 strains and the prevention or increased incidence of HUS, with retrospective data to support either treatment, or withholding treatment. Some experts treat with antimicrobials and others prefer to use supportive care.[214–217]
– Traveler's diarrhea: empiric therapy (E coli, Campylobacter, Salmonella, Shigella, plus many other pathogens, including protozoa)[218–225]	Azithromycin 10 mg/kg qd for 3 days (AII); OR rifaximin 600 mg/day div tid for 3 days (for nonfebrile, non-bloody diarrhea for children 12 y) (BII); OR ciprofloxacin 8–10 mg/kg qd for 5 days (CII); OR ciprofloxacin 30 mg/kg/day div bid for 3 days (CII)	Susceptibility patterns of E coli, Campylobacter, Salmonella, and Shigella vary widely by country; check country-specific data for departing or returning travelers. Azithromycin preferable to ciprofloxacin for travelers to Southeast Asia given high prevalence of quinolone-resistant Campylobacter. Rifaximin is less effective than ciprofloxacin for invasive bloody bacterial enteritis; rifaximin may also not be as effective for Shigella, Salmonella, and Campylobacter as other agents. Interestingly, for adults who travel and take antibiotics (mostly fluoroquinolones), colonization with ESBL-positive E coli is more frequent on return home.[226] Adjunctive therapy with loperamide (anti-motility) is not recommended for children <2 y and should be used only in nonfebrile, non-bloody diarrhea.[227,228] May shorten symptomatic illness by about 24 h.

– Traveler's diarrhea: prophylaxis[218,219]		– Prophylaxis: Early self-treatment with agents listed previously is preferred over long-term prophylaxis, but may use prophylaxis for a short-term (<14 days) visit to very high-risk region: rifaximin (for older children), azithromycin, or bismuth subsalicylate (BIII).
– *Aeromonas hydrophila*[229]	Ciprofloxacin 30 mg/kg/day PO div bid for 5 days OR azithromycin 10 mg/kg qd for 3 days OR cefixime 8 mg/kg/day PO qd (BIII)	Not all strains produce enterotoxins and diarrhea; role in diarrhea questioned.[229] Resistance to TMP/SMX about 10%–15%. Choose most narrow spectrum agent based on in vitro susceptibilities.
– *Campylobacter jejuni*[230–232]	Azithromycin 10 mg/kg/day for 3 days (BII) or erythromycin 40 mg/kg/day PO div qid for 5 days (BII)	Alternatives: doxycycline or ciprofloxacin (high rate of fluoroquinolone resistance in Thailand, India, and now the United States). Single-dose azithromycin (1 g, once) is effective in adults.
– Cholera[223,233]	Azithromycin 20 mg/kg once; OR erythromycin 50 mg/kg/day PO div qid for 3 days; OR doxycycline 4 mg/kg/day (max 200 mg/day) PO div bid, for all ages	Ciprofloxacin or TMP/SMX (if susceptible)
– *Clostridium difficile* (antibiotic-associated colitis)[234–236]	Metronidazole 30 mg/kg/day PO div qid OR vancomycin 40 mg/kg/day PO div qid for 7 days; for relapsing *C difficile* enteritis, consider pulse therapy (1 wk on/1 wk off for 3–4 cycles) or prolonged tapering therapy.[234]	Vancomycin is more effective for severe infection.[236] Fidaxomicin approved for adults; pediatric studies underway. Many infants and children may have asymptomatic colonization with *C difficile*.[236] Higher risk of relapse in children with multiple comorbidities.
– *E coli*		
Enterotoxigenic (etiology of most traveler's diarrhea)[219,220,222]	Azithromycin 10 mg/kg qd for 3 days; OR cefixime 8 mg/kg/day PO qd for 3 days; OR ciprofloxacin 30 mg/kg/day PO div bid for 3 days	Most illnesses brief and self-limited. Alternatives: rifaximin 600 mg/day div tid for 3 days (for nonfebrile, non-bloody diarrhea for children >11 y, as rifaximin is not absorbed systemically); OR TMP/SMX. Resistance increasing worldwide; check country-specific rates, if possible.[222]

Antimicrobial Therapy According to Clinical Syndromes

6

H. GASTROINTESTINAL INFECTIONS (continued) (See Chapter 10 for parasitic infections.)

Clinical Diagnosis	Therapy (evidence grade)	Comments
Enterohemorrhagic (O157:H7; STEC, etiology of HUS)[214-217]	Controversy on whether treatment of O157:H7 diarrhea results in more or less toxin-mediated renal damage.[214-217] For severe infection, treat as for enterotoxigenic strains above, preferably with azithromycin that is associated with decreased toxin production in animal models.[217]	Injury to colonic mucosa may lead to invasive bacterial colitis.
Enteropathogenic	Neomycin 100 mg/kg PO div q6–8h for 5 days	Most traditional "enteropathogenic" strains are not toxigenic or invasive. Postinfection diarrhea may be problematic.
– Gastritis, peptic ulcer disease (Helicobacter pylori)[238-241]	Either triple agent therapy in areas of low clarithromycin resistance: clarithromycin 7.5 mg/kg/dose 2–3 times each day, AND amoxicillin 40 mg/kg/dose (max 1 g) PO bid AND omeprazole 0.5 mg/kg/dose PO bid 14 days (BII), OR quadruple therapy that includes metronidazole (15 mg/kg/day div bid) added to the regimen above.[242]	Sequential therapy using 5 days of amoxicillin and omeprazole followed by 5 days of clarithromycin, metronidazole, and omeprazole is effective for susceptible strains, but resistance to clarithromycin is as high as 20% in some regions.[240,243] Most data from studies in adults; of effective regimens, no one combination has been shown superior. New, current regimens use 4 drugs (with metronidazole) initially or with relapse due to concerns for clarithromycin resistance.[238,240] Other regimens include bismuth, metronidazole instead of amoxicillin, and other proton pump inhibitors.
– Giardiasis (See Chapter 10.) (Giardia intestinalis, formerly lamblia)[244]	Metronidazole 30–40 mg/kg/day PO div tid for 7–10 days (BII); OR nitazoxanide PO (take with food; age 12–47 mo, 100 mg/dose bid for 7 days; age 4–11 y, 200 mg/dose bid for 7 days; age ≥12 y, 1 tab (500 mg)/dose bid for 7 days (BII); OR tinidazole 50 mg/kg/day (max 2 g) for 1 day (BII)	If therapy is inadequate, another course of the same agent is usually curative. Alternatives: tinidazole OR furazolidone, OR paromomycin; OR albendazole (CII). Prolonged courses may be needed for immunocompromised conditions (eg, hypogammaglobulinemia). Treatment of asymptomatic carriers not usually recommended.

– Salmonellosis[245] (See Chapter 10 for discussion of traveler's diarrhea for typhoid infection outside of North America.)

Non-typhoid strains[246]	Usually none for self-limited diarrhea in immunocompetent child (eg, diarrhea is often much improved by the time culture results are available). Treat those with persisting symptomatic infection; infants <3 mo with increased risk of bacteremia and infection: azithromycin 10 mg/kg PO qd for 3 days (AII); OR ceftriaxone 75 mg/kg/day IV, IM q24h for 5 days (AII); OR cefixime 20–30 mg/kg/day PO for 5 days (BII); OR for susceptible strains: TMP/SMX 8 mg/kg/day of TMP PO div bid for 5 days (AI).	Alternatives: ciprofloxacin 30 mg/kg/day PO bid for 5 days (AI). Carriage of strains may be prolonged in treated children.
Typhoid fever[247–251]	Azithromycin 10 mg/kg qd for 5 days (AII); OR ceftriaxone 75 mg/kg/day IV, IM q24h for 5 days (AII); OR cefixime 20–30 mg/kg/day PO, div q12h for 14 days (BII); OR for susceptible strains: TMP/SMX 8 mg/kg/day of TMP PO div bid for 10 days (AI)	Increasing cephalosporin resistance. For newly emergent MDR strains, may require prolonged IV therapy. Longer treatment courses for focal invasive disease (eg, osteomyelitis). Alternative: ciprofloxacin 30 mg/kg/day PO bid for 5–7 days (AI).
— Shigellosis[252–254]	Cefixime 8 mg/kg/day PO qd for 5 days (AII); OR azithromycin 10 mg/kg/day PO for 3 days (AII); OR ciprofloxacin 30 mg/kg/day PO bid for 3–5 days (BII)	Alternatives for susceptible strains: TMP/SMX 8 mg/kg/day of TMP PO div bid for 5 days; OR ampicillin (*not* amoxicillin). Ceftriaxone 50 mg/kg/day IM, IV if parenteral therapy necessary, for 2–5 days. Avoid antiperistaltic drugs. Treatment for the improving child is not usually necessary to hasten recovery, but some experts would treat to decrease communicability.
— *Yersinia enterocolitica*[255–257]	Antimicrobial therapy probably not of value for mild disease in normal hosts. TMP/SMX PO, IV; OR ciprofloxacin PO, IV (BII).	Alternatives: ceftriaxone or gentamicin. High rates of resistance to ampicillin. May mimic appendicitis in older children. Limited clinical data exist on oral therapy.

Antimicrobial Therapy According to Clinical Syndromes

6

H. GASTROINTESTINAL INFECTIONS (continued) (See Chapter 10 for parasitic infections.)

Clinical Diagnosis	Therapy (evidence grade)	Comments
Intraabdominal Infection (abscess, peritonitis secondary to bowel/appendix contents)		
– Appendicitis; bowel-associated (enteric gram-negative bacilli, *Bacteroides* spp, *Enterococcus* spp, increasingly *Pseudomonas*)[258-263]	Meropenem 60 mg/kg/day IV div q8h or imipenem 60 mg/kg/day IV div q6h; OR pip/tazo 240 mg pip/kg/day div q6h; for 4–5 days for patients with adequate source control,[262] 7–10 days or longer if suspicion of persisting intra-abdominal abscess (AII). Data support IV outpatient therapy or oral step-down therapy[263] when clinically improved, particularly when oral therapy can be focused on the most prominent, invasive cultured pathogens.	Recent studies of the microbiology of appendicitis indicate *Pseudomonas* as a common pathogen (found in up to 30% of children),[258,260,264] mandating the empiric use of an antipseudomonal drug, such as a carbapenem or pip/tazo, unless the surgery was highly effective at drainage/source control. Many other regimens may be effective, including ampicillin 150 mg/kg/day div q8h AND gentamicin 6–7.5 mg/kg/day IV, IM q8h AND metronidazole 40 mg/kg/day IV div q8h; OR ceftriaxone 50 mg/kg q24h AND metronidazole 40 mg/kg/day IV div q8h. Gentamicin demonstrates poor activity at low pH; surgical source control is critical to achieve cure.
– Tuberculosis, abdominal (*Mycobacterium bovis*, from unpasteurized dairy products)[14,265,266]	INH 10–15 mg/kg/day (max 300 mg) PO qd for 6 mo AND rifampin 10–20 mg/kg/day (max 600 mg) PO qd for 6 mo. *M bovis* is resistant to PZA. If risk factors are present for multidrug resistance (eg, poor adherence to previous therapy), add ethambutol 20 mg/kg/day PO qd OR a fluoroquinolone (moxifloxacin or levofloxacin).	Corticosteroids are routinely used as adjunctive therapy to decrease symptoms from inflammation.[267] Directly observed therapy preferred; after 2 + wk of daily therapy, can change to twice-weekly dosing double dosage of INH (max 900 mg); rifampin remains same dosage (10–20 mg/kg/day, max 600 mg) (AII). LP ± CT of head for children ≤2 y with active disease to rule out occult, concurrent CNS infection (AIII).
Perirectal abscess (*Bacteroides* spp, other anaerobes, enteric bacilli, and *S aureus* predominate)[268]	Clindamycin 30–40 mg/kg/day IV div q8h AND cefotaxime or ceftriaxone or gentamicin (BII)	Surgical drainage alone may be curative.

Peritonitis		
– Peritoneal dialysis indwelling catheter infection (staphylococcal; enteric gram-negatives; yeast)[269,270]	Antibiotic added to dialysate in concentrations approximating those attained in serum for systemic disease (eg, 4 μg/mL for gentamicin, 25 μg/mL for vancomycin, 125 μg/mL for cefazolin, 25 μg/mL for ciprofloxacin) after a larger loading dose (AII)[270]	Selection of antibiotic based on organism isolated from peritoneal fluid; systemic antibiotics if there is accompanying bacteremia/fungemia
– Primary (pneumococcus or group A streptococcus)[271]	Ceftriaxone 50 mg/kg/day q24h, or cefotaxime 150 mg/kg/day div q8h; if pen-S, then penicillin G 150,000 U/kg/day IV div q6h; for 7–10 days (AII)	Other antibiotics according to culture and susceptibility tests, as peritonitis with nephrotic syndrome or with some chronic liver disease is not apparently more common than spontaneous peritonitis. A review of the current literature suggests spontaneous pneumococcal peritonitis has become a disease of the past with the widespread use of conjugate pneumococcal vaccine.

I. GENITAL AND SEXUALLY TRANSMITTED INFECTIONS

Clinical Diagnosis	Therapy (evidence grade)	Comments
Consider testing for HIV and other STIs in a child with one documented STI; consider sexual abuse in prepubertal children. The most recent CDC STI treatment guidelines are posted online at www.cdc.gov/std/treatment (accessed September 15, 2016).		
Chancroid (*Haemophilus ducreyi*)[50]	Azithromycin 1 g PO as single dose OR ceftriaxone 250 mg IM as single dose	Alternative: erythromycin 1.5 g/day PO div tid for 7 days OR ciprofloxacin 1,000 mg PO qd, div bid for 3 days
C trachomatis (cervicitis, urethritis)[50,272]	Azithromycin 20 mg/kg (max 1 g) PO for 1 dose; OR doxycycline (patients >7 y) 4 mg/kg/day (max 200 mg/day) PO div bid for 7 days	Alternatives: erythromycin 2 g/day PO div qid for 7 days; OR levofloxacin 500 mg PO q24h for 7 days
Epididymitis (associated with positive urine cultures and STIs)[50,273,274]	Ceftriaxone 50 mg/kg/day q24h for 7–10 days AND (for older children) doxycycline 200 mg/day div bid for 10 days	Microbiology not well studied in children; in infants, also associated with urogenital tract anomalies. Treat infants for *S aureus* and *E coli*; may resolve spontaneously; in STI, caused by *Chlamydia* and gonococcus.

6

Antimicrobial Therapy According to Clinical Syndromes

Antimicrobial Therapy According to Clinical Syndromes

6

I. GENITAL AND SEXUALLY TRANSMITTED INFECTIONS (continued)

Clinical Diagnosis	Therapy (evidence grade)	Comments
Gonorrhea		
– Newborns	See Chapter 5.	
– Genital infections (uncomplicated vulvovaginitis, cervicitis, urethritis, or proctitis)[50,272,275,276]	Ceftriaxone 250 mg IM for 1 dose (regardless of weight) AND azithromycin 1 g PO for 1 dose or doxycycline 200 mg/day div q12h for 7 days	Cefixime no longer recommended due to increasing cephalosporin resistance.[276] Fluoroquinolones are no longer recommended due to resistance.[277] Dual therapy has not been evaluated yet in children but should be effective.
– Pharyngitis[50,276,277]	Ceftriaxone 250 mg IM for 1 dose (regardless of weight) AND azithromycin 1 g PO for 1 dose or doxycycline 200 mg/day div q12h for 7 days	
– Conjuctivitis[50]	Ceftriaxone 1 g IM for 1 dose AND azithromycin 1 g PO for 1 dose	Lavage the eye with saline.
– Disseminated gonococcal infection[50,276,277]	Ceftriaxone 50 mg/kg/day IM, IV q24h (max: 1 g) AND azithromycin 1 g PO for 1 dose; total course for 7 days	No studies in children: increase dosage for meningitis.
Granuloma inguinale (donovanosis, *Klebsiella granulomatis*, formerly *Calymmatobacterium*)[50]	Azithromycin 1 g orally once per week or 500 mg daily for at least 3 weeks and until all lesions have completely healed	Primarily in tropical regions of India, Pacific, and Africa. Options: Doxycycline 4 mg/kg/day PO bid (max 200 mg/day) PO for at least 3 wk OR ciprofloxacin 750 mg PO bid for at least 3 wk, OR erythromycin base 500 mg PO qid for at least 3 wk OR TMP/SMX 1 double-strength (160 mg/800 mg) tablet PO bid for at least 3 wk; all regimens continue until all lesions have completely healed.

Herpes simplex virus, genital infection[50,278,279]	Acyclovir 20 mg/kg/dose (max 400 mg) PO tid for 7–10 days (first episode) (AI); OR valacyclovir 20 mg/kg/dose of extemporaneous suspension (directions on package label), max 1.0 g PO bid for 7–10 days (first episode) (AI); OR famciclovir 250 mg PO tid for 7–10 days (AI); for more severe infection: acyclovir 15 mg/kg/day IV div q8h as 1-h infusion for 7–10 days (All)	For recurrent episodes: treat with acyclovir PO, valacyclovir PO, or famciclovir PO, immediately when symptoms begin, for 5 days. For suppression: acyclovir 20 mg/kg/dose (max 400 mg) PO bid; OR valacyclovir 20 mg/kg/dose PO qd (little long-term safety data in children; no efficacy data in children). Prophylaxis is recommended in pregnant women.[280]
Lymphogranuloma venereum (*C trachomatis*)[50]	Doxycycline 4 mg/kg/day (max 200 mg/day) PO (patients >7 y) div bid for 21 days	Alternatives: erythromycin 2 g/day PO div qid for 21 days; OR azithromycin 1 g PO once weekly for 3 wk
Pelvic inflammatory disease (*Chlamydia*, gonococcus, plus anaerobes)[50,281]	Cefoxitin 2 g IV q6h; AND doxycycline 200 mg/day PO or IV div bid; OR cefotetan 2 g IV q12h AND doxycycline 100 mg orally or IV q12h, OR clindamycin 900 mg IV q8h AND gentamicin 1.5 mg/kg IV, IM q8h until clinical improvement for 24 hr, followed by doxycycline 200 mg/day PO div bid (AND clindamycin 1,800 mg/day PO div qid for tubo-ovarian abscess) to complete 14 days of therapy	Optional regimen: ceftriaxone 250 mg IM for 1 dose AND doxycycline 200 mg/day PO div bid; WITH/WITHOUT metronidazole 1 g/day PO div bid; for 14 days
Syphilis[50,282] (Test for HIV.)		
– Congenital	See Chapter 5.	
– Neurosyphilis (positive CSF VDRL or CSF pleocytosis with serologic diagnosis of syphilis)	Crystalline penicillin G 200–300,000 U/kg/day (max 24,000,000 U/day) div q6h for 10–14 days (AIII)	

Antimicrobial Therapy According to Clinical Syndromes

I. GENITAL AND SEXUALLY TRANSMITTED INFECTIONS (continued)

Clinical Diagnosis	Therapy (evidence grade)	Comments
– Primary, secondary	Benzathine penicillin G 50,000 U/kg (max 2,400,000 U) IM as a single dose (AIII); do not use benzathine-procaine penicillin mixtures.	Follow-up serologic tests at 6, 12, and 24 mo; 15% may remain seropositive despite adequate treatment. If allergy to penicillin: doxycycline (patients >7 y) 4 mg/kg/day (max 200 mg) PO bid for 14 days. CSF examination should be obtained for children being treated for primary or secondary syphilis to rule out asymptomatic neurosyphilis. Test for HIV.
– Syphilis of <1 y duration, without clinical symptoms (early latent syphilis)	Benzathine penicillin G 50,000 U/kg (max 2,400,000 U) IM as a single dose (AIII)	Alternative if allergy to penicillin: doxycycline (patients >7 y) 4 mg/kg/day (max 200 mg/day) PO div bid for 14 days
– Syphilis of >1 y duration, without clinical symptoms (late latent syphilis) or syphilis of unknown duration	Benzathine penicillin G 50,000 U/kg (max 2,400,000 U) IM weekly for 3 doses (AIII)	Alternative if allergy to penicillin: doxycycline (patients >7 y) 4 mg/kg/day (max 200 mg/day) PO div bid for 28 days. Look for neurologic, eye, and aortic complications of tertiary syphilis.
Trichomoniasis[50]	Metronidazole 2 g PO as a single dose, OR tinidazole 50 mg/kg (max 2 g) PO for 1 dose	Metronidazole 500 mg PO bid for 7 days
Urethritis, nongonococcal (See Gonorrhea for gonorrhea therapy.)[50,283]	Azithromycin 20 mg/kg (max 1 g) PO for 1 dose, OR doxycycline (patients >7 y) 40 mg/kg/day (max 200 mg/day) PO div bid for 7 days (AII)	Erythromycin, levofloxacin, or ofloxacin Increasing resistance noted in *Mycoplasma genitalium*
Vaginitis[50]		
– Bacterial vaginosis[50,284]	Metronidazole 500 mg PO twice daily for 7 days OR metronidazole vaginal gel (0.75%) qd for 5 days, OR clindamycin vaginal cream for 7 days	Alternative: tinidazole 1 g PO qd for 5 days, OR clindamycin 300 mg PO bid for 7 days Relapse common Caused by synergy of *Gardnerella* with anaerobes

– Candidiasis, vulvovaginal[50,285]	Topical vaginal cream/tablets/suppositories (alphabetic order): butoconazole, clotrimazole, econazole, fenticonazole, miconazole, sertaconazole, terconazole, or tioconazole for 3–7 days (AI); OR fluconazole 10 mg/kg (max 150 mg) as a single dose (AII)	For uncomplicated vulvovaginal candidiasis, no topical agent is clearly superior. Avoid azoles during pregnancy. For recurring disease, consider 10–14 days of induction with topical agent or fluconazole, followed by fluconazole once weekly for 6 mo (AI).
– Prepubertal vaginitis[286]	No prospective studies	Cultures from symptomatic prepubertal girls are statistically more likely to yield E coli, enterococcus, coagulase-negative staphylococci, and streptococci (viridans strep and group A strep), but these organisms may also be present in asymptomatic girls.
– Shigella[287]	Cefixime 8 mg/kg/day PO qd for 5 days OR ciprofloxacin 30 mg/kg/day PO bid for 5 days	50% have bloody discharge; usually not associated with diarrhea.
– Streptococcus, group A[288]	Penicillin V 50–75 mg/kg/day PO div tid for 10 days	Amoxicillin 50–75 mg/kg/day PO div tid

Antimicrobial Therapy According to Clinical Syndromes

6

J. CENTRAL NERVOUS SYSTEM INFECTIONS

Clinical Diagnosis	Therapy (evidence grade)	Comments
Abscess, brain (respiratory tract flora, skin flora, or bowel flora, depending on the pathogenesis of infection based on underlying comorbid disease and origin of bacteremia)[289,290]	Until etiology established, cover flora of respiratory tract, skin, and/or bowel, based on individual patient evaluation and risk for brain abscess (see Comments for MRSA considerations): meropenem 120 mg/kg/day div q8h (AIII); OR nafcillin 150–200 mg/kg/day IV div q6h AND cefotaxime 200–300 mg/kg/day IV div q6h or ceftriaxone 100 mg/kg/day IV div q24h AND metronidazole 30 mg/kg/day IV div q8h (BIII); for 2–3 wk after successful drainage (depending on pathogen, size of abscess, and response to therapy); longer course if no surgery (3–6 wk) (BIII).	Surgery for abscesses ≥2 cm diameter. If CA-MRSA suspected, ADD vancomycin 60 mg/kg/day IV div q6h ± rifampin 20 mg/kg/day IV div q12h, pending culture results. We have successfully treated MRSA intracranial infections with ceftaroline, but no prospective data exist: ceftaroline: 2–<6 mo, 30 mg/kg/day IV div q8h (each dose given over 2 h); ≥6 mo, 45 mg/kg/day IV div q8h (each dose given over 2 h) (max single dose 600 mg) (BII). If secondary to chronic otitis, include meropenem or cefepime in regimen for anti-*Pseudomonas* activity. For enteric gram-negative bacilli, consider ESBL-producing *E coli* and *Klebsiella* that require meropenem and are resistant to cefotaxime. Follow abscess size by CT.
Encephalitis[291,292]		
– Amebic (*Naegleria fowleri, Balamuthia mandrillaris,* and *Acanthamoeba*)	See Chapter 10, Amebiasis.	
– CMV[291]	See Chapter 9, CMV. Not well studied in children. Consider ganciclovir 10 mg/kg/day IV div q12h; for severe immunocompromised, ADD foscarnet 180 mg/kg/day IV div q8h for 3 wk; follow quantitative PCR for CMV.	High-dose ganciclovir[293] (IV 20 mg/kg/day div q12h) not well studied. Reduce dose for renal insufficiency. Watch for neutropenia.
– Enterovirus	Supportive therapy; no antivirals currently FDA approved.	Pocapavir PO is currently under investigation for enterovirus (poliovirus). Pleconaril PO is currently under consideration for approval at the FDA for treatment of neonatal enteroviral sepsis syndrome.[294]

– EBV[295]	Not studied in a controlled comparative trial. Consider ganciclovir 10 mg/kg/day IV div q12h or acyclovir 60 mg/kg/day IV div q8h for 3 wk; follow quantitative PCR in CSF for EBV.	Efficacy of antiviral therapy not well defined; some experts recommend against antiviral treatment.[291]
– Herpes simplex virus[291,296]	Acyclovir 60 mg/kg/day IV as 1–2 h infusion div q8h for 21 days for infants ≤4 mo; for older infants and children, 30–45 mg/kg/day IV for 21 days (AIII)	See Chapter 5 for neonatal infection. Perform CSF HSV PCR near end of 21 days of therapy and continue acyclovir until PCR negative. Safety of high-dose acyclovir (60 mg/kg/day) not well defined beyond the neonatal period; can be used, but monitor for neurotoxicity and nephrotoxicity; FDA has approved acyclovir at this dosage for encephalitis for children up to 12 y.
– Toxoplasma	See Chapter 10.	
– Arbovirus (flavivirus—Zika, West Nile, St. Louis encephalitis, tick-borne encephalitis; togavirus—western equine encephalitis, eastern equine encephalitis; bunyavirus—La Crosse encephalitis, California encephalitis)[291,292]	Supportive therapy.	Investigational only (antiviral, interferon, immune globulins). No specific antiviral agents are commercially available for any of the arboviruses, including Zika or West Nile.

Meningitis, bacterial, community-associated

NOTES

– In areas where pen-R pneumococci exist (>5% of invasive strains), initial empiric therapy for suspect pneumococcal meningitis should be with vancomycin AND cefotaxime or ceftriaxone until susceptibility test results are available. Although ceftaroline is more active than ceftriaxone against pneumococci and, as a beta-lactam, should be expected to achieve therapeutic CSF concentrations, no pediatric data yet exist on CNS infections.

– Dexamethasone 0.6 mg/kg/day IV div q6h for 2 days as an adjunct to antibiotic therapy decreases hearing deficits and other neurologic sequelae in adults and children (for *Haemophilus* and pneumococcus; not prospectively studied in children for meningococcus or *E coli*). The first dose of dexamethasone is given before or concurrent with the first dose of antibiotic; probably little benefit if given ≥1 h after the antibiotic.[297,298]

6

Antimicrobial Therapy According to Clinical Syndromes

Antimicrobial Therapy According to Clinical Syndromes

6

J. CENTRAL NERVOUS SYSTEM INFECTIONS (continued)

Clinical Diagnosis	Therapy (evidence grade)	Comments
– Empiric therapy[299]	Cefotaxime 200–300 mg/kg/day IV div q6h, or ceftriaxone 100 mg/kg/day IV q24h; AND vancomycin 60 mg/kg/day IV div q8h (AII)	If Gram stain or cultures demonstrate a pathogen other than pneumococcus, vancomycin is not needed; vancomycin used empirically only for possible pen-R pneumococcus; high-dose (MRSA dosing) ceftaroline should also prove effective, but no data exist currently.
– *H influenzae* type b[299]	Cefotaxime 200–300 mg/kg/day IV div q6h, or ceftriaxone 100 mg/kg/day IV q24h; for 10 days (AI)	Alternative: ampicillin 200–400 mg/kg/day IV div q6h (for beta-lactamase–negative strains) OR chloramphenicol 100 mg/kg/day IV div q6h
– Meningococcus (*Neisseria meningitidis*)[299]	Penicillin G 250,000 U/kg/day IV div q4h; or ceftriaxone 100 mg/kg/day IV q24h, or cefotaxime 200 mg/kg/day IV div q6h; treatment course for 7 days (AI)	Meningococcal prophylaxis: rifampin 10 mg/kg PO q12h for 4 doses OR ceftriaxone 125–250 mg IM once OR ciprofloxacin 500 mg PO once (adolescents and adults)
– Neonatal	See Chapter 5.	
– Pneumococcus (*S pneumoniae*)[299]	For pen-S and cephalosporin-susceptible strains: penicillin G 250,000 U/kg/day IV div q4–6h, OR ceftriaxone 100 mg/kg/day IV q24h or cefotaxime 200–300 mg/kg/day IV div q6h; for 10 days (AI). For pen-R pneumococci: continue the combination of vancomycin and cephalosporin IV for total course (AIII).	Some pneumococci may be resistant to penicillin but susceptible to cefotaxime and ceftriaxone and may be treated with the cephalosporin alone. With the efficacy of current pneumococcal conjugate vaccines, primary bacterial meningitis is uncommon, and penicillin resistance has decreased substantially. Test-of-cure LP helpful in those with pen-R pneumococci.
Meningitis, TB (*M tuberculosis*; *M bovis*)[13,14]	For non-immunocompromised children: INH 15 mg/kg/day PO, IV div q12–24h AND rifampin 15 mg/kg/day PO, IV div q12–24h for 12 mo AND PZA 30 mg/kg/day PO div q12–24h for first 2 mo of therapy, AND streptomycin 30 mg/kg/day IV, IM div q12h for first 4–8 wk of therapy until susceptibility test results available. Ethionamide is an alternative to aminoglycosides.	Hyponatremia from inappropriate ADH secretion is common; ventricular drainage may be necessary for obstructive hydrocephalus. Corticosteroids (can use the same dexamethasone dose as for bacterial meningitis, 0.6 mg/kg/day IV div q6h) for 4 wk until neurologically stable, then taper dose for 1–3 mo to decrease neurologic complications and improve prognosis by decreasing the incidence of infarction.[300] Watch for rebound inflammation during taper; increase dose to previously effective level, then taper more slowly.

Shunt infections: The use of antibiotic-impregnated shunts has decreased the frequency of this infection.[303] Shunt removal is usually necessary for cure.[302]

– Empiric therapy pending Gram stain and culture[299,302]	Vancomycin 60 mg/kg/day IV div q8h, AND ceftriaxone 100 mg/kg/day IV q24h (AII)	If Gram stain shows only gram-positive cocci, can use vancomycin alone. Cefepime or meropenem should be used instead of ceftriaxone if Pseudomonas is suspected.
– S epidermidis or S aureus[299,302]	Vancomycin (for S epidermidis and CA-MRSA) 60 mg/kg/day IV div q8h; OR nafcillin (if organisms susceptible) 150–200 mg/kg/day AND (if severe infection or slow response) gentamicin or rifampin; for 10–14 days (AIII)	Shunt removal usually necessary; may need to treat with ventriculostomy until ventricular CSF cultures negative; obtain CSF cultures at time of shunt replacement, continue therapy an additional 48–72 h pending cultures. For children who cannot tolerate vancomycin, ceftaroline has anecdotally been successful: ceftaroline: 2–<6 mo, 30 mg/kg/day IV div q8h (each dose given over 2 h); ≥6 mo, 45 mg/kg/day IV div q8h (each dose given over 2 h) (max single dose 600 mg) (BIII).
– Gram-negative bacilli[299,302]	Empiric therapy with meropenem 120 mg/kg/day IV div q8h OR cefepime 150 mg/kg/day IV div q8h (AIII). For E coli (without ESBLs): ceftriaxone 100 mg/kg/day IV q12h OR cefotaxime 200–300 mg/kg/day IV div q6h; ADD gentamicin 6–7.5 mg/kg/day IV until CSF sterile; for 21 days or longer.	Remove shunt. Select appropriate therapy based on in vitro susceptibilities. Meropenem, ceftriaxone, cefotaxime, and cefepime have all been studied in pediatric meningitis. Intrathecal therapy with aminoglycosides not routinely necessary in children with highly active beta-lactam therapy and shunt removal.

For recommendations for drug-resistant strains and treatment of TB in HIV-infected patients, visit the CDC Web site for TB: www.cdc.gov/tb (accessed September 15, 2016).

Antimicrobial Therapy According to Clinical Syndromes

6

K. URINARY TRACT INFECTIONS

Clinical Diagnosis	Therapy (evidence grade)	Comments
NOTE: Antibiotic susceptibility profiles of *E coli*, the most common cause of UTI, vary considerably. For mild disease, TMP/SMX may be started as initial therapy if local susceptibility ≥80% and a 20% failure rate is acceptable. For moderate to severe disease (possible pyelonephritis), obtain cultures and begin an oral 2nd- or 3rd-generation cephalosporin (cefuroxime, cefaclor, cefprozil, cefixime, ceftibuten, cefdinir, cefpodoxime), ciprofloxacin PO, or ceftriaxone IM. Antibiotic susceptibility testing will help direct your therapy to the most narrow spectrum agent.		
Cystitis, acute (*E coli*)[303,304]	For mild disease: TMP/SMX 8 mg/kg/day of TMP PO div bid for 3 days (See NOTE about resistance to TMP/SMX.) For moderate to severe disease: cefixime 8 mg/kg/day PO qd; OR ceftriaxone 50 mg/kg IM q24h for 3–5 days (with normal anatomy) (BII); follow-up culture after 36–48 h treatment ONLY if still symptomatic	Alternative: amoxicillin 30 mg/kg/day PO div tid OR amoxicillin/clavulanate PO if susceptible (BII); ciprofloxacin 15–20 mg/kg/day PO div bid for suspected or documented resistant organisms
Nephronia, lobar *E coli* and other enteric rods (also called focal bacterial nephritis)[305,306]	Ceftriaxone 50 mg/kg/day IV, IM q24h. Duration depends on resolution of cellulitis vs development of abscess (10–21 days) (AIII). For ESBL-positive *E coli*, carbapenems and fluoroquinolones are often active agents.	Invasive, consolidative parenchymal infection; complication of pyelonephritis, can evolve into renal abscess. Step down therapy with oral cephalosporins once cellulitis/abscess has initially responded to therapy.
Pyelonephritis, acute (*E coli*)[303,304,307-310]	Ceftriaxone 50 mg/kg/day IV, IM q24h OR gentamicin 5–6 mg/kg/day IV, IM q24h. For documented or suspected ceftriaxone-resistant ESBL-positive strains, use meropenem IV, imipenem IV, or ertapenem IV; OR gentamicin IV, IM, OR pip/tazo. Switch to oral therapy following clinical response (BII). If organism resistant to amoxicillin and TMP/SMX, use an oral 2nd- or 3rd-generation cephalosporin (BII); if cephalosporin-R, can use ciprofloxacin PO 30 mg/kg/day div q12h (BIII); for 7–10 days total (depending on response to therapy).	For mild to moderate infection, oral therapy is likely to be as effective as IV/IM therapy for susceptible strains, down to 3 mo of age.[308] If bacteremia documented and infant is <2–3 mo, rule out meningitis and treat 14 days IV + PO (AIII). Aminoglycosides at any dose are more nephrotoxic than beta-lactams but represent effective therapy (AI).

| **Recurrent urinary tract infection, prophylaxis**[303,311–313] | Only for those with grade III–V reflux or with recurrent febrile UTI: TMP/SMX 2 mg/kg/dose of TMP PO qd OR nitrofurantoin 1–2 mg/kg PO qd at bedtime; more rapid resistance may develop using beta-lactams (BII). | Prophylaxis not recommended for patients with grade I–II reflux and no evidence of renal damage (although the RIVUR study[313] included these children, and they may also benefit, but early treatment of new infections is recommended for these children).

Resistance eventually develops to every antibiotic; follow resistance patterns for each patient. The use of periodic urine cultures is controversial, as there are no data to guide management of asymptomatic bacteriuria in a child at high risk of recurrent UTI. |

L. MISCELLANEOUS SYSTEMIC INFECTIONS

Clinical Diagnosis	Therapy (evidence grade)	Comments
Actinomycosis[314,315]	Penicillin G 250,000 U/kg/day IV div q6h, or ampicillin 150 mg/kg/day IV div q8h until improved (often up to 6 wk); then long-term convalescent therapy with penicillin V 100 mg/kg/day (up to 4 g/day) PO for 6–12 mo (AII)	Surgery as indicated Alternatives: amoxicillin, clindamycin, erythromycin; ceftriaxone IM/IV, doxycycline for children >7 y
Anaplasmosis[316] (human granulocytotropic anaplasmosis, *Anaplasma phagocytophilum*)	Doxycycline 4 mg/kg/day IV, PO (max 200 mg/day) div bid for 7–10 days (regardless of age) (AII)	For mild disease, consider rifampin 20 mg/kg/day PO div bid for 7–10 days (BIII).
Anthrax, sepsis/pneumonia, community vs bioterror exposure (inhalation, cutaneous, gastrointestinal, meningoencephalitis)[15]	For community-associated anthrax infection, amoxicillin 75 mg/kg/day div q8h or doxycycline for children >7 y should be effective. For bioterror-associated exposure (regardless of age): ciprofloxacin 20–30 mg/kg/day IV div q12h, OR levofloxacin 16 mg/kg/day IV div q12h not to exceed 250 mg/dose (AIII); OR doxycycline 4 mg/kg/day PO (max 200 mg/day) div bid (regardless of age).	For invasive infection after bioterror exposure, 2 or 3 antibiotics may be required.[15] For oral step-down therapy, can use ciprofloxacin or doxycycline; if susceptible, can use penicillin, amoxicillin, or clindamycin.

Antimicrobial Therapy According to Clinical Syndromes

L. MISCELLANEOUS SYSTEMIC INFECTIONS (continued)

Clinical Diagnosis	Therapy (evidence grade)	Comments
Appendicitis (See Gastrointestinal Infection, Intra-abdominal Infection, Appendicitis.)		
Brucellosis[317–320]	Doxycycline 4 mg/kg/day PO (max 200 mg/day) div bid (for children >7 y) AND rifampin (15–20 mg/kg/day div q12h) (BIII); OR for children <8 y: TMP/SMX 10 mg/kg/day TMP IV, PO div q12h AND rifampin 15–20 mg/kg/day div q12h (BIII); for 4–8 wk	Combination therapy with rifampin will decrease the risk of relapse. ADD gentamicin 6–7.5 mg/kg/day IV, IM div q8h for the first 1–2 wk of therapy to further decrease risk of relapse[319] (BIII), particularly for endocarditis, osteomyelitis, or meningitis. Prolonged treatment for 4–6 mo and surgical debridement may be necessary for deep infections (AIII).
Cat-scratch disease (*Bartonella henselae*)[321,322]	Supportive care for adenopathy (I&D of infected lymph node); azithromycin 12 mg/kg/day PO qd for 5 days shortens the duration of adenopathy (AIII). No prospective data exist for invasive CSD: gentamicin (for 14 days) AND TMP/SMX AND rifampin for hepatosplenic disease and osteomyelitis (AIII). For CNS infection, use cefotaxime AND gentamicin ± TMP/SMX (AIII). Alternatives: ciprofloxacin, doxycycline.	This dosage of azithromycin has been documented to be safe and effective for streptococcal pharyngitis and may offer greater deep tissue exposure than the dosage studied by Bass et al[8] and used for otitis media.
Chickenpox/shingles (varicella-zoster virus)[323–325]	Acyclovir 30 mg/kg/day IV as 1–2 h infusion div q8h; for 10 days (acyclovir doses of 45–60 mg/kg/day in 3 div doses IV should be used for disseminated or CNS infection). Dosing can also be provided as 1,500 mg/m²/day IV div q8h. Duration in immunocompromised children: 7–14 days, based on clinical response (AI). For treatment in normal immunocompetent children, acyclovir 80 mg/kg/day PO div qid, for 5 days, with the most benefit from early treatment. Otherwise healthy children with mild disease do not require routine therapy (AI).	See Chapter 9; therapy for 10 days in immunocompromised children. Famciclovir can be provided as 25- and 100-mg sprinkles (from capsules).[326] See Chapter 9 for dosages by body weight. No treatment data in children (CIII).

6

	Valacyclovir pharmacokinetics have been assessed in an extemporaneously[325] compounded suspension of crushed tablets and simple syrup (60 mg/kg/day div tid) for children 3 mo to 12 y; instructions for preparation provided in package insert, and shelf life is 28 days.
Ehrlichiosis (human monocytic ehrlichiosis, caused by *Ehrlichia chaffeensis*, and *Ehrlichia ewingii*)[327–329]	Doxycycline 4 mg/kg/day IV, PO div bid (max 100 mg/dose) for 7–10 days (regardless of age) (AIII)	For mild disease, consider rifampin 20 mg/kg/day PO div bid (max 300 mg/dose) for 7–10 days (BIII).
Febrile neutropenic patient (empiric therapy of invasive infection: *Pseudomonas*, enteric gram-negative bacilli, staphylococci, streptococci, yeast, fungi)[330,331]	Cefepime 150 mg/kg/day div q8h (AI); or meropenem 60 mg/kg/day div q8h (AII); OR pip/tazo (300-mg piperacillin component/kg/day div q8h for 9 mo; 240 mg/kg/day div q8h for 2–9 mo), OR ceftazidime 150 mg/kg/day IV div q8h AND tobramycin 6 mg/kg/day IV div q8h (AII). ADD vancomycin 40 mg/kg/day IV div q8h if MRSA or coagulation-negative staph suspected (eg, central catheter infection) (AIII). ADD metronidazole to ceftazidime or cefepime if colitis or other deep anaerobic infection suspected (AIII).	Alternatives: other anti-*Pseudomonas* beta-lactams (imipenem) AND anti-staphylococcal antibiotics. If no response in 2–3 days and no alternative etiology demonstrated, begin additional empiric therapy with antifungals (BII); dosages and formulations outlined in Chapter 8. Increasingly resistant pathogens (ESBL *E coli* and *Klebsiella*, KPC) will require alternative empiric therapy if MDR organisms are colonizing or present on the child's hospital unit. For low-risk patients with close follow-up, alternative management strategies are being explored: oral therapy with amox/clav and ciprofloxacin may be used, or early hospital discharge.[332]
Human immunodeficiency virus infection	See Chapter 9.	

Antimicrobial Therapy According to Clinical Syndromes

6

L. MISCELLANEOUS SYSTEMIC INFECTIONS (continued)

Clinical Diagnosis	Therapy (evidence grade)	Comments
Infant botulism[333]	Botulism immune globulin for infants (BabyBIG) 50 mg/kg IV for 1 dose (AI); BabyBIG can be obtained from the California Department of Public Health at www.infantbotulism.org, through your state health department.	www.infantbotulism.org provides information for physicians and parents. Web site organized by the California Department of Public Health (accessed September 15, 2016). Aminoglycosides should be avoided because they potentiate the neuromuscular effect of botulinum toxin.
Kawasaki syndrome[334-338]	No antibiotics; IVIG 2 g/kg as single dose (AI); may need to repeat dose in up to 15% of children for persisting fever that lasts 24 h after completion of the IVIG infusion (AII). For subsequent relapse, many children will respond to a second IVIG infusion, otherwise consult an infectious diseases physician or pediatric cardiologist.	Aspirin 80–100 mg/kg/day qid in acute, febrile phase; once afebrile for 24–48 h, initiate low-dosage (3–5 mg/kg/day) aspirin therapy for 6–8 wk (assuming echocardiogram is normal). Role of corticosteroids,[335,336] infliximab,[338] and calcineurin inhibitors, as well as methotrexate and cyclosporin, for IVIG-resistant Kawasaki syndrome under investigation and may improve outcome in severe cases.
Leprosy (Hansen disease)[339]	Dapsone 1 mg/kg/day PO qd AND rifampin 10 mg/kg/day PO qd (for multibacillary disease) clofazimine 1 mg/kg/day PO qd; for 12 mo for paucibacillary disease; for 24 mo for multibacillary disease (AII).	Consult Health Resources and Services Administration National Hansen's Disease (Leprosy) Program at www.hrsa.gov/hansensdisease (accessed September 15, 2016) for advice about treatment and free antibiotics; 800/642-2477.
Leptospirosis[340,341]	Penicillin G 250,000 U/kg/day IV div q6h, or ceftriaxone 50 mg/kg/day IV, IM q24h; for 7 days (BII) For mild disease, doxycycline (>7 y) 4 mg/kg/day (max 200 mg/day) PO div bid for 7–10 days and for those ≤7 y or intolerant of doxycycline, azithromycin 20 mg/kg on day 1, 10 mg/kg on days 2 and 3 (BII)	Alternative: amoxicillin for children ≤7 y of age with mild disease

Lyme disease (*Borrelia burgdorferi*)[329,342–344]	Neurologic evaluation, including LP, if there is clinical suspicion of CNS involvement	
– Early localized disease	>7 y: doxycycline 4 mg/kg/day (max 200 mg/day) PO div bid for 14 days (AII) ≤7 y: amoxicillin 50 mg/kg/day (max 1.5 g/day) PO tid for 14 days (AII)	Alternative: cefuroxime, 30 mg/kg/day (max 1,000 mg/day) PO, in 2 div doses (or 1 g/day) for 14 days
– Arthritis (no CNS disease)	Oral therapy as outlined above, but for 28 days (AIII). Alternative: ceftriaxone 50–75 mg/kg IV q24h OR penicillin 300,000 U/kg/day IV div q4h; either for 14–28 days.	Persistent or recurrent joint swelling after treatment: repeat a 4-wk course of oral antibiotics or give ceftriaxone 50–75 mg/kg IV q24h OR penicillin 300,000 U/kg/day IV div q4h; either for 14–28 days. For persisting arthritis after 2 defined antibiotic treatment courses, use symptomatic therapy.
– Erythema migrans	Oral therapy as outlined previously; for 14 days (AIII)	
– Isolated facial (Bell) palsy	Oral therapy as outlined previously; for 21–28 days (AIII)	LP is not routinely required unless CNS symptoms present. Treatment to prevent late sequelae; will not provide a quick response for palsy.
– Carditis	Ceftriaxone 50–75 mg/kg IV q24h OR penicillin 300,000 U/kg/day IV div q4h; for 14–21 days (AIII)	For asymptomatic disease, treat with oral regimen as for early localized disease.
– Neuroborreliosis	Ceftriaxone 50–75 mg/kg IV q24h OR penicillin G 300,000 U/kg/day IV div q4h; for 14–28 days (AIII)	
Melioidosis (*Burkholderia pseudomallei*)[345,346]	Acute sepsis: meropenem 75 mg/kg/day div q8h; OR ceftazidime 150 mg/kg/day IV div q8h; followed by TMP/SMX (10 mg/kg/day of TMP) PO bid for 3–6 mo	Alternative convalescent therapy: amox/clav (90 mg/kg/day amox div tid, not bid) for children ≤7 y, or doxycycline for children >7 y; for 20 wk (AII)

6

Antimicrobial Therapy According to Clinical Syndromes

Antimicrobial Therapy According to Clinical Syndromes

L. MISCELLANEOUS SYSTEMIC INFECTIONS (continued)

Clinical Diagnosis	Therapy (evidence grade)	Comments
Mycobacteria, nontuberculous[9,11,12,347]		
– Adenitis in normal host (See Adenitis entries in this table and Table 6A.)	Excision usually curative (BII); azithromycin PO OR clarithromycin PO for 6–12 wk (with or without rifampin) if susceptible (BII)	Antibiotic susceptibility patterns are quite variable; cultures should guide therapy; medical therapy 60%–70% effective. Newer data suggest toxicity of antimicrobials may not be worth the small clinical benefit.
– Pneumonia or disseminated infection in compromised hosts (HIV or gamma-interferon receptor deficiency)[11,347–350]	Usually treated with 3 or 4 active drugs (eg, clarithromycin OR azithromycin, AND amikacin, cefoxitin, meropenem). Also test for ciprofloxacin, TMP/SMX, ethambutol, rifampin, linezolid, clofazimine, and doxycycline (BII).	See Chapter 11 for dosages; cultures are essential, as the susceptibility patterns of nontuberculous mycobacteria are varied.
Nocardiosis (*Nocardia asteroides* and *Nocardia brasiliensis*)[351,352]	TMP/SMX 8 mg/kg/day TMP div bid or sulfisoxazole 120–150 mg/kg/day PO div qid for 6–12 wk or longer. For severe infection, particularly in immunocompromised hosts, use ceftriaxone or imipenem AND amikacin 15–20 mg/kg/day IM, IV div q8h (AIII).	Wide spectrum of disease from skin lesions to brain abscess. Surgery when indicated. Alternatives: doxycycline (for children >7 y), amox/clav, or linezolid.
Plague (*Yersinia pestis*)[353–355]	Gentamicin 7.5 mg/kg/day IV div q8h (AII)	Doxycycline 4 mg/kg/day (max 200 mg/day) PO div bid or ciprofloxacin 30 mg/kg/day PO div bid
Q fever (*Coxiella burnetii*)[356,357]	Acute stage: doxycycline 4.4 mg/kg/day (max 200 mg/day) PO div bid for 14 days (AII) for children of any age. Endocarditis and chronic disease (ongoing symptoms for 6–12 mo): doxycycline for children >7 y AND hydroxychloroquine for 18–36 mo (AIII). Seek advice from pediatric infectious diseases specialist for children ≤7 y; may require TMP-SMX, 8–10 mg TMP/kg/day div q12h with doxycycline; or levofloxacin with rifampin for 18 mo.	Follow doxycycline and hydroxychloroquine serum concentrations during endocarditis/chronic disease therapy. CNS: Use fluoroquinolone (no prospective data) (BIII). Clarithromycin may be an alternative based on limited data (CIII).

Rocky Mountain spotted fever (fever, petechial rash with centripetal spread; *Rickettsia rickettsii*)[358,359]	Doxycycline 4.4 mg/kg/day (max 200 mg/day) PO div bid for 7–10 days (AI) for children of any age	Start empiric therapy early.
Tetanus (*Clostridium tetani*)[360,362]	Metronidazole 30 mg/kg/day IV, PO div q8h or penicillin G 100,000 U/kg/day IV div q6h for 10–14 days AND TIG 3,000–6,000 U IM (AII)	Wound debridement essential; IVIG may provide antibody to toxin if TIG not available. Immunize with Td or Tdap. See Chapter 14 for prophylaxis recommendations.
Toxic shock syndrome (toxin-producing strains of *S aureus* [including MRSA] or group A streptococcus)[1,6,7,362,363]	Empiric: vancomycin 45 mg/kg/day IV div q8h AND oxacillin/nafcillin 150 mg/kg/day IV div q6h, AND clindamycin 30–40 mg/kg/day div q8h ± gentamicin for 7–10 days (AIII)	Clindamycin added for the initial 48–72 h of therapy to decrease toxin production. Ceftaroline is an option for MRSA treatment, particularly with renal insufficiency from shock and vancomycin (BIII). IVIG may provide additional benefit by binding circulating toxin (CIII). For MSSA: oxacillin/nafcillin AND clindamycin ± gentamicin. For CA-MRSA: vancomycin AND clindamycin ± gentamicin. For group A streptococcus: penicillin G AND clindamycin.
Tularemia (*Francisella tularensis*)[173,364]	Gentamicin 6–7.5 mg/kg/day IM, IV div q8h; for 10–14 days (AII)	Alternatives: doxycycline (for 14–21 days) or ciprofloxacin (for 10 days)

7. Preferred Therapy for Specific Bacterial and Mycobacterial Pathogens

NOTES

- For fungal, viral, and parasitic infections, see chapters 8, 9, and 10, respectively.

- Limitations of space do not permit listing of all possible alternative antimicrobials.

- **Abbreviations:** amox/clav, amoxicillin/clavulanate (Augmentin); amp/sul, ampicillin/sulbactam (Unasyn); CA-MRSA, community-associated methicillin-resistant *Staphylococcus aureus;* CDC, Centers for Disease Control and Prevention; CNS, central nervous system; ESBL, extended spectrum beta-lactamase; FDA, US Food and Drug Administration; HRSA, Health Resources and Services Administration; IM, intramuscular; IV, intravenous; KPC, *Klebsiella pneumoniae* carbapenemase; MDR, multidrug resistant; MIC, minimal inhibitory concentration; MRSA, methicillin-resistant *S aureus;* MSSA, methicillin-susceptible *S aureus;* NARMS, National Antimicrobial Resistance Monitoring System for Enteric Bacteria; NDM, New Delhi metallo-beta-lactamase; pen-S, penicillin-susceptible; pip/tazo, piperacillin/tazobactam (Zosyn); PO, oral; PZA, pyrazinamide; spp, species; ticar/clav, ticarcillin/clavulanate (Timentin); TMP/SMX, trimethoprim/sulfamethoxazole; UTI, urinary tract infection.

A. COMMON BACTERIAL PATHOGENS AND USUAL PATTERN OF SUSCEPTIBILITY TO ANTIBIOTICS (GRAM POSITIVE)

	Commonly Used Antibiotics (One Agent per Class Listed)			
	Penicillin	Ampicillin/ Amoxicillin	Amoxicillin/ Clavulanate	Methicillin/ Oxacillin
Enterococcus faecalis[a]	+	+	+	−
Enterococcus faecium[a]	+	+	+	−
Staphylococcus, coagulase negative +/−	−	−	−	+/−
Staphylococcus aureus, methicillin-resistant	−	−	−	−
Staphylococcus aureus, methicillin-susceptible	−	−	−	++
Streptococcus pneumoniae	++	++	++	+
Streptococcus pyogenes	++	++	++	++

NOTE: ++ = very active (>90% of isolates are susceptible in most locations); + = some decreased susceptibility (substantially less active in vitro or resistance in isolates between 10% and 30% in some locations); +/− = significant resistance (30%–80% in some locations); − = not likely to be effective.

[a] Need to add gentamicin or other aminoglycoside to ampicillin/penicillin or vancomycin for in vitro bactericidal activity.

	Commonly Used Antibiotics (One Agent per Class Listed)			Approved for Adults Some Studies in Children	
Cefazolin/ Cephalexin	Vancomycin	Clindamycin	Linezolid	Daptomycin	Ceftaroline
−	+	−	+	++	−
−	+	−	+	+	−
+/−	++	+	++	++	++
−	++	+	++	++	++
++	++	+	++	++	++
++	++	++	++	++	++
++	++	++	++	++	++

B. COMMON BACTERIAL PATHOGENS AND USUAL PATTERN OF SUSCEPTIBILITY TO ANTIBIOTICS (GRAM NEGATIVE)[a]

	Commonly Used Antibiotics (One Agent per Class Listed)				
	Ampicillin/ Amoxicillin	Amoxicillin/ Clavulanate	Cefazolin/ Cephalexin	Cefuroxime	Ceftriaxone/ Cefotaxime
Acinetobacter spp	−	−	−		+
Citrobacter spp	−	−	−	+	+
Enterobacter spp[b]	−	−	−	+/−	+
Escherichia coli[c]	+/−	+	+	++[d]	++[d]
Haemophilus influenzae[f]	++	++	++	++	++
Klebsiella spp[c]	−	−	+	++	++
Neisseria meningitidis	++	++	0	++	++
Pseudomonas aeruginosa	−	−	−	−	−
Salmonella, non-typhoid spp	+	++	0	0	++
Serratia spp[b]	−	−	−	+/−	+
Shigella spp	+	+	0	+	++
Stenotrophomonas maltophilia	−	−	−	−	−

NOTE: ++ = very active (>90% of isolates are susceptible in most locations); + = some decreased susceptibility (substantially less active in vitro or resistance in isolates between 10% and 30% in some locations); +/− = significant resistance (30%–80% in some locations); − = not likely to be effective; 0 = not usually tested for susceptibility for treatment of infections (resistant or has not previously been considered for routine therapy, so little data exist).

[a] CDC (NARMS) statistics and SENTRY surveillance system (JMI Laboratories) as primary references; also using current antibiograms from Children's Medical Center, Dallas, TX, and Rady Children's Hospital San Diego to assess pediatric trends. When sufficient data are available, pediatric community isolate susceptibility data are used. Nosocomial resistance patterns may be quite different, usually with increased resistance, particularly in adults; please check your local/regional hospital antibiogram for your local susceptibility patterns.

[b] AmpC will be constitutively produced in low frequency in every population of organisms and will be selected out during therapy with third-generation cephalosporins if used as single agent therapy.

[c] Rare carbapenem-resistant isolates in pediatrics (KPC, NDM strains).

[d] Will be resistant to virtually all current cephalosporins if ESBL producing.

[e] Follow the MIC, not the report for susceptible (S), intermediate (I), or resistant (R), as some ESBL producers will have low MICs and can be effectively treated with higher dosages.

[f] Will be resistant to ampicillin/amoxicillin if beta-lactamase producing.

		Commonly Used Antibiotics (One Agent per Class Listed)				
Ceftazidime	Cefepime	Meropenem/ Imipenem	Piperacillin/ Tazobactam	TMP/ SMX	Ciprofloxacin	Gentamicin
+	+	++	+	+	+	++
+	++	++	+	++	++	++
+	++	++	+	+	++	++
++[d]	++[e]	++	++	+	++	++
++	++	++	++	++	++	+/−
++	++[e]	++	++	++	++	++
+	++	++	++	0	++	0
+	++	++	++	−	++	+
++	++	++	++	++	++	0
+	++	++	+	++	++	++
++	++	++	++	+/−	++	0
+	+/−	+/−	+	++	++	+/−

C. COMMON BACTERIAL PATHOGENS AND USUAL PATTERN OF SUSCEPTIBILITY TO ANTIBIOTICS (ANAEROBES)

	Commonly Used Antibiotics (One Agent per Class Listed)				
	Penicillin	Ampicillin/ Amoxicillin	Amoxicillin/ Clavulanate	Cefazolin	Cefoxitin
Anaerobic streptococci	++	++	++	++	++
Bacteroides fragilis	+/−	+/−	++	−	+
Clostridia (eg, *tetani, perfringens*)	++	++	++	0	+
Clostridium difficile	−	−	−	0	−

NOTE: + + = very active (>90% of isolates are susceptible in most locations); + = some decreased susceptibility (substantially less active in vitro or resistance in isolates between 10% and 30% in some locations); +/− = significant resistance (30%–80% in some locations); − = not likely to be effective; 0 = not usually tested for susceptibility for treatment of infections (resistant or has not previously been considered for routine therapy, so little data exist).

		Commonly Used Antibiotics (One Agent per Class Listed)			
Ceftriaxone/ Cefotaxime	Meropenem/ Imipenem	Piperacillin/ Tazobactam	Metronidazole	Clindamycin	Vancomycin
++	++	++	++	++	++
−	++	++	++	+	0
+/−	++	++	++	+	++
−	++	0	++	−	++

Preferred Therapy for Specific Bacterial and Mycobacterial Pathogens

7

D. PREFERRED THERAPY FOR SPECIFIC BACTERIAL AND MYCOBACTERIAL PATHOGENS

Organism	Clinical Illness	Drug of Choice (evidence grade)	Alternatives
Acinetobacter baumannii[1-4]	Sepsis, meningitis, nosocomial pneumonia, wound infection	Meropenem (BIII) or other carbapenem	Use culture results to guide therapy: ceftazidime, amp/sul; pip/tazo; TMP/SMX; ciprofloxacin; tigecycline; colistin. Watch for emergence of resistance during therapy, including to colistin. Consider combination therapy for life-threatening infection. Inhaled colistin for pneumonia caused by MDR strains (BIII).
Actinomyces israelii[5]	Actinomycosis (cervicofacial, thoracic, abdominal)	Penicillin G; ampicillin (CIII)	Amoxicillin; doxycycline; clindamycin; ceftriaxone; imipenem
Aeromonas hydrophila[6]	Diarrhea	Ciprofloxacin (CIII)	Azithromycin, cefepime, TMP/SMX
	Sepsis, cellulitis, necrotizing fasciitis	Ceftazidime (BIII)	Cefepime; ceftriaxone, meropenem; ciprofloxacin
Aggregatibacter (formerly Actinobacillus) actinomycetemcomitans[7]	Periodontitis, abscesses (including brain), endocarditis	Ampicillin (amoxicillin) ± gentamicin (CIII)	Doxycycline; TMP/SMX; ciprofloxacin; ceftriaxone
Anaplasma (formerly Ehrlichia) phagocytophilum[8,9]	Human granulocytic anaplasmosis	Doxycycline (all ages) (AII)	Rifampin, levofloxacin
Arcanobacterium haemolyticum[10]	Pharyngitis, cellulitis, Lemierre syndrome	Erythromycin; penicillin (BIII)	Azithromycin, amoxicillin, clindamycin; doxycycline; vancomycin
Bacillus anthracis[11]	Anthrax (cutaneous, gastrointestinal, inhalational, meningoencephalitis)	Ciprofloxacin (regardless of age) (AIII). For invasive, systemic infection, use combination therapy.	Doxycycline; amoxicillin, levofloxacin, clindamycin, penicillin G; vancomycin, meropenem. Bioterror strains may be antibiotic resistant.

Organism		
Bacillus cereus or *subtilis*[12,13]	Sepsis; toxin-mediated gastroenteritis	Vancomycin (BIII)	Ciprofloxacin, linezolid, daptomycin, clindamycin
Bacteroides fragilis[14,15]	Peritonitis, sepsis, abscesses	Metronidazole (AI)	Meropenem or imipenem (AII); ticar/clav; pip/tazo (AI); amox/clav (BII). Recent surveillance suggests resistance of up to 25% for clindamycin.
Bacteroides, other spp[14,15]	Pneumonia, sepsis, abscesses	Metronidazole (BII)	Meropenem or imipenem; penicillin G or ampicillin if beta-lactamase negative
Bartonella henselae[16,17]	Cat-scratch disease	Azithromycin for lymph node disease (BII); gentamicin in combination with TMP/SMX AND rifampin for invasive disease (BIII)	Cefotaxime; ciprofloxacin; doxycycline
Bartonella quintana[18]	Bacillary angiomatosis, peliosis hepatis	Gentamicin plus doxycycline (BIII); erythromycin; ciprofloxacin (BIII)	Azithromycin; doxycycline
Bordetella pertussis, parapertussis[19,20]	Pertussis	Azithromycin (AIII); erythromycin (BII)	Clarithromycin; TMP/SMX; ampicillin
Borrelia burgdorferi, Lyme disease[21–23]	Treatment based on stage of infection (See Lyme disease in Chapter 6.)	Doxycycline if >7 y (AII); amoxicillin or cefuroxime in children ≤7 y (AIII); ceftriaxone IV for meningitis (AII)	
Borrelia hermsii, turicatae, parkeri, tick-borne relapsing fever[24,25]	Relapsing fever	Doxycycline for all ages (AIII)	Penicillin or erythromycin in children intolerant of doxycycline (BIII)
Borrelia recurrentis, louse-borne relapsing fever[24,25]	Relapsing fever	Single-dose doxycycline for all ages (AIII)	Penicillin or erythromycin in children intolerant of doxycycline (BIII)

7

Preferred Therapy for Specific Bacterial and Mycobacterial Pathogens

Preferred Therapy for Specific Bacterial and Mycobacterial Pathogens

7

Organism	Clinical Illness	Drug of Choice (evidence grade)	Alternatives
D. PREFERRED THERAPY FOR SPECIFIC BACTERIAL AND MYCOBACTERIAL PATHOGENS (continued)			
Brucella spp[26-28]	Brucellosis (See Chapter 6.)	Doxycycline AND rifampin (BIII); OR, for children ≤7 y: TMP/SMX AND rifampin (BIII)	For serious infection: doxycycline AND gentamicin AND rifampin; or TMP/SMX AND gentamicin AND rifampin (AIII). May require extended therapy (months).
Burkholderia cepacia complex[29-31]	Pneumonia, sepsis in immunocompromised children; pneumonia in children with cystic fibrosis[32]	Meropenem (BIII); for severe disease, ADD tobramycin AND TMP/SMX (AIII).	Imipenem, doxycycline; ceftazidime; pip/tazo; ciprofloxacin. Aerosolized antibiotics may provide higher concentrations in lung.[31]
Burkholderia pseudomallei[33-35]	Melioidosis	Meropenem (AIII) or ceftazidime (BIII), followed by prolonged TMP/SMX for 12 wk (AII)	TMP/SMX, doxycycline, or amox/clav for chronic disease
Campylobacter fetus[36,37]	Sepsis, meningitis in the neonate	Meropenem (BIII)	Cefotaxime; gentamicin; erythromycin
Campylobacter jejuni[37-39]	Diarrhea	Azithromycin (BII); erythromycin (BII)	Doxycycline; ciprofloxacin (very high rates of ciprofloxacin-resistant strains in Thailand, Hong Kong, and Spain)
Capnocytophaga canimorsus[40,41]	Sepsis after dog bite (increased risk with asplenia)	Pip/tazo OR meropenem; amox/clav (BIII)	Clindamycin; linezolid; penicillin G; ciprofloxacin
Capnocytophaga ochracea[42]	Sepsis, abscesses	Clindamycin (BIII); amox/clav (BIII)	Meropenem; pip/tazo
Chlamydia trachomatis[43-45]	Lymphogranuloma venereum	Doxycycline (AII)	Azithromycin; erythromycin
	Urethritis, cervicitis	Doxycycline (AII)	Azithromycin; erythromycin; ofloxacin

Organism	Condition		
	Inclusion conjunctivitis of newborn	Azithromycin (AIII)	Erythromycin
	Pneumonia of infancy	Azithromycin (AIII)	Erythromycin; ampicillin
	Trachoma	Azithromycin (AI)	Doxycycline; erythromycin
Chlamydophila (formerly *Chlamydia*) *pneumoniae*[43,44,46,47]	Pneumonia	Azithromycin (AII); erythromycin (AII)	Doxycycline; ciprofloxacin
Chlamydophila (formerly *Chlamydia*) *psittaci*[48]	Psittacosis	Doxycycline for >7 y; azithromycin (AIII) OR erythromycin (AIII) for ≤7 y	Doxycycline, levofloxacin
Chromobacterium violaceum[49,50]	Sepsis, pneumonia, abscesses	Meropenem AND ciprofloxacin (AIII)	Imipenem, TMP/SMX
Citrobacter koseri (formerly *diversus*) and *freundii*[51-53]	Meningitis, sepsis	Meropenem (AIII) for ampC beta-lactamase resistance	Cefepime; ciprofloxacin; pip/tazo; ceftriaxone AND gentamicin; TMP/SMX Carbapenem-resistant strains now reported

7

Preferred Therapy for Specific Bacterial and Mycobacterial Pathogens

7

D. PREFERRED THERAPY FOR SPECIFIC BACTERIAL AND MYCOBACTERIAL PATHOGENS (continued)

Organism	Clinical Illness	Drug of Choice (evidence grade)	Alternatives
Clostridium botulinum[54-56]	Botulism: foodborne; wound; potentially bio-terror related	Botulism antitoxin heptavalent (equine) types A–G FDA approved in 2013 (www.fda.gov/downloads/BiologicsBloodVaccines/BloodBloodProducts/ApprovedProducts/LicensedProductsBLAs/FractionatedPlasmaProducts/UCM345147.pdf; accessed September 15, 2016) No antibiotic treatment	For more information, call your state health department or the CDC Emergency Operations Center, 770/488-7100 (http://emergency.cdc.gov/agent/Botulism/clinicians/treatment.asp; accessed September 15, 2016).
	Infant botulism	Human botulism immune globulin for infants (BabyBIG) (AII) No antibiotic treatment	BabyBIG available nationally from the California Department of Public Health at 510/231-7600 (www.infantbotulism.org; accessed September 15, 2016)
Clostridium difficile[57,58]	Antibiotic-associated colitis (See Chapter 6, Table 6H, Gastrointestinal Infections, Clostridium difficile.)	Metronidazole PO (AI)	Vancomycin PO for metronidazole failures; stop the predisposing antimicrobial therapy, if possible. No pediatric data on fidaxomicin PO. No pediatric data on fecal transplantation for recurrent disease.
Clostridium perfringens[59,60]	Gas gangrene/necrotizing fasciitis/sepsis (also caused by C sordellii, C septicum, C novyi) Food poisoning	Penicillin G AND clindamycin for invasive infection (BII); no antimicrobials indicated for foodborne illness	Meropenem, metronidazole, clindamycin monotherapy
Clostridium tetani[61,62]	Tetanus	Metronidazole (AIII); penicillin G (BIII)	Treatment: tetanus immune globulin 3,000 to 6,000 U IM, with part injected directly into the wound.

Organism	Disease	Preferred therapy	Notes
Corynebacterium diphtheriae[63]	Diphtheria	Diphtheria equine antitoxin (available through CDC under an investigational protocol [www.cdc.gov/diphtheria/dat.html]) AND erythromycin or penicillin G (AIII)	Antitoxin from the CDC Emergency Operations Center, 770/488-7100; protocol: www.cdc.gov/diphtheria/downloads/protocol.pdf (accessed September 15, 2016). Prophylaxis for contaminated wounds: 250 U IM for those with <3 tetanus immunizations. Start/continue immunizations for tetanus. Alternative antibiotics: meropenem; doxycycline, clindamycin.
Corynebacterium jeikeium[64]	Sepsis, endocarditis	Vancomycin (AIII)	Penicillin G AND gentamicin, tigecycline, linezolid, daptomycin
Corynebacterium minutissimum[65,66]	Erythrasma; bacteremia in compromised hosts	Erythromycin PO for erythrasma (BIII); vancomycin IV for bacteremia (BIII)	Topical clindamycin for cutaneous infection
Coxiella burnetii[67,68]	Q fever (See Chapter 6, Table 6L, Q fever.)	Acute infection: doxycycline (all ages) (AII) Chronic infection: TMP/SMX AND doxycycline (BII); OR levofloxacin AND rifampin	Alternative for acute infection: TMP/SMX
Ehrlichia chaffeensis[8,9] Ehrlichia muris-like[69]	Human monocytic ehrlichiosis	Doxycycline (all ages) (AII)	Rifampin
Ehrlichia ewingii[8,9]	E ewingii ehrlichiosis	Doxycycline (all ages) (AII)	Rifampin
Eikenella corrodens[70]	Human bite wounds; abscesses, meningitis, endocarditis	Ampicillin; penicillin G (BIII)	Amox/clav; ticar/clav; pip/tazo; amp/sul; ceftriaxone; ciprofloxacin; imipenem Resistant to clindamycin, cephalexin, erythromycin
Elizabethkingia (formerly Chryseobacterium) meningoseptica[71,72]	Sepsis, meningitis	Levofloxacin; TMP/SMX (BIII)	Add rifampin to another active drug; pip/tazo.

Preferred Therapy for Specific Bacterial and Mycobacterial Pathogens

D. PREFERRED THERAPY FOR SPECIFIC BACTERIAL AND MYCOBACTERIAL PATHOGENS (continued)

Organism	Clinical Illness	Drug of Choice (evidence grade)	Alternatives
Enterobacter spp[53,73,74]	Sepsis, pneumonia, wound infection, UTI	Cefepime; meropenem; pip/tazo (BII)	Ertapenem; imipenem; cefotaxime or ceftriaxone AND gentamicin; TMP/SMX; ciprofloxacin. Newly emerging carbapenem-resistant strains worldwide[74,75]
Enterococcus spp[76–78]	Endocarditis, UTI, intra-abdominal abscess	Ampicillin AND gentamicin (AI)	Vancomycin AND gentamicin. For vancomycin-resistant strains that are also ampicillin resistant: linezolid and daptomycin show in vitro susceptibility.
Erysipelothrix rhusiopathiae[79]	Cellulitis (erysipeloid), sepsis, abscesses, endocarditis	Ampicillin (BIII); penicillin G (BII)	Ceftriaxone; clindamycin, meropenem; amoxicillin, ciprofloxacin, erythromycin. Resistant to vancomycin, daptomycin, TMP/SMX
Escherichia coli See Chapter 6 for specific infection entities and references. *Increasing resistance to 3rd-generation cephalosporins due to ESBLs.*	UTI, community acquired, not hospital acquired	A 2nd- or 3rd-generation cephalosporin PO, IM as empiric therapy (BI)	Amoxicillin; TMP/SMX if susceptible. Ciprofloxacin if resistant to other options. For hospital-acquired UTI, review hospital antibiogram for choices.
	Traveler's diarrhea	Azithromycin (AII)	Rifaximin (for nonfebrile, non-bloody diarrhea for children >11 y); cefixime
	Sepsis, pneumonia, hospital-acquired UTI	A 2nd- or 3rd-generation cephalosporin IV (BI)	For ESBL-producing strains: meropenem (AIII) or other carbapenem; pip/tazo and ciprofloxacin if resistant to other antibiotics
	Meningitis	Ceftriaxone; cefotaxime (AIII)	For ESBL-producing strains: meropenem (AIII)
Francisella tularensis[80,81]	Tularemia	Gentamicin (AII)	Doxycycline; ciprofloxacin
Fusobacterium spp[82,83]	Sepsis, soft tissue infection, Lemierre syndrome	Metronidazole (AIII); clindamycin (BIII)	Penicillin G; meropenem; pip/tazo

7

Gardnerella vaginalis[48,84]	Bacterial vaginosis	Metronidazole (BII)	Tinidazole; clindamycin; metronidazole gel; clindamycin cream
Haemophilus (now Aggregatibacter) aphrophilus[85]	Sepsis, endocarditis, abscesses (including brain abscess)	Ceftriaxone (AII); OR ampicillin AND gentamicin (BII)	Ciprofloxacin, amox/clav (for strains resistant to ampicillin)
Haemophilus ducreyi[48]	Chancroid	Azithromycin (AIII); ceftriaxone (BIII)	Erythromycin; ciprofloxacin
Haemophilus influenzae[86]	Nonencapsulated strains; upper respiratory tract infections	Beta-lactamase negative: ampicillin IV (AI); amoxicillin PO (AI) Beta-lactamase positive: ceftriaxone IV, IM (AI) or cefotaxime IV (AI); amox/clav (AI) OR 2nd- or 3rd-generation cephalosporins PO (AI)	Levofloxacin; azithromycin; TMP/SMX
	Type b strains: meningitis, arthritis, cellulitis, epiglottitis, pneumonia	Beta-lactamase negative: ampicillin IV (AI); amoxicillin PO (AI) Beta-lactamase positive: ceftriaxone IV, IM (AI) or cefotaxime IV (AI); amox/clav (AI) OR 2nd- or 3rd-generation cephalosporins PO (AI)	Full IV course (10 days) for meningitis, but oral step-down therapy well documented after response to treatment for non-CNS infections Levofloxacin PO for step-down therapy
Helicobacter pylori[87,88]	Gastritis, peptic ulcer	Clarithromycin AND amoxicillin AND omeprazole (AII)	Other regimens include metronidazole (especially for concerns of clarithromycin resistance)[89] and other proton-pump inhibitors.
Kingella kingae[90,91]	Osteomyelitis, arthritis	Ampicillin; penicillin G (AII)	Ceftriaxone; TMP/SMX; cefuroxime; ciprofloxacin

7

Preferred Therapy for Specific Bacterial and Mycobacterial Pathogens

Preferred Therapy for Specific Bacterial and Mycobacterial Pathogens

D. PREFERRED THERAPY FOR SPECIFIC BACTERIAL AND MYCOBACTERIAL PATHOGENS (continued)

Organism	Clinical Illness	Drug of Choice (evidence grade)	Alternatives
Klebsiella spp (*K pneumoniae*, *K oxytoca*)[92–94]	UTI	A 2nd- or 3rd-generation cephalosporin (AII)	Use most narrow spectrum agent active against pathogen: TMP/SMX; ciprofloxacin, gentamicin. ESBL producers should be treated with a carbapenem (meropenem, ertapenem, imipenem), but KPC (carbapenemase)-containing bacteria may require ciprofloxacin, colistin.[94]
	Sepsis, pneumonia, meningitis	Ceftriaxone; cefotaxime, cefepime (AIII)	Carbapenem or ciprofloxacin if resistant to other routine antibiotics. Meningitis caused by ESBL producer: meropenem. KPC (carbapenemase) producers: ciprofloxacin, colistin, OR ceftazidime/avibactam, approved by FDA for adults in 2015 and should be active against current strains of KPC *Klebsiella*.
Klebsiella granulomatis[48]	Granuloma inguinale	Azithromycin (AII)	Doxycycline; TMP/SMX; ciprofloxacin
Legionella spp[95]	Legionnaires disease	Azithromycin (AI) OR levofloxacin (AII)	Erythromycin, TMP/SMX, doxycycline
Leptospira spp[96]	Leptospirosis	Penicillin G IV (AII); ceftriaxone IV (AII)	Amoxicillin; doxycycline; azithromycin
Leuconostoc[97]	Bacteremia	Penicillin G (AIII); ampicillin (BIII)	Clindamycin; erythromycin; doxycycline (resistant to vancomycin)
Listeria monocytogenes[98]	Sepsis, meningitis in compromised host; neonatal sepsis	Ampicillin (ADD gentamicin for severe infection.) (AII)	Ampicillin AND TMP/SMX; ampicillin AND linezolid
Moraxella catarrhalis[99]	Otitis, sinusitis, bronchitis	Amox/clav (AI)	TMP/SMX; a 2nd- or 3rd-generation cephalosporin
Morganella morganii[100,101]	UTI, sepsis, wound infection	Cefepime (AIII); meropenem (AIII)	Pip/tazo; ceftriaxone AND gentamicin; ciprofloxacin

Mycobacterium abscessus[102,103]	Skin and soft tissue infections; pneumonia in cystic fibrosis	Clarithromycin or azithromycin (AIII); ADD amikacin ± cefoxitin for invasive disease (AIII).	Also test for susceptibility to meropenem, tigecycline, linezolid. May need pulmonary resection.
Mycobacterium avium complex[102,104]	Cervical adenitis	Clarithromycin (AIII); azithromycin (AI)	Surgical excision is more likely to lead to cure than sole medical therapy. May increase cure rate with addition of rifampin or ethambutol.
	Pneumonia	Clarithromycin (AII) or azithromycin (AII) AND ethambutol ± rifampin	Depending on susceptibilities and the severity of illness, ADD amikacin ± ciprofloxacin.
	Disseminated disease in competent host, or disease in immunocompromised host	Clarithromycin or azithromycin AND ethambutol AND rifampin (AIII)	Depending on susceptibilities and the severity of illness, ADD amikacin ± ciprofloxacin.
Mycobacterium bovis[105,106]	Tuberculosis (adenitis; abdominal tuberculosis; meningitis)	Isoniazid AND rifampin (AII); ADD ethambutol for suspected resistance (AIII).	ADD streptomycin for severe infection. *M bovis* is always resistant to PZA.
Mycobacterium chelonae[102,104,107,108]	Abscesses; catheter infection	Clarithromycin or azithromycin (AIII); ADD amikacin ± cefoxitin for invasive disease (AIII).	Also test for susceptibility to cefoxitin; TMP/SMX; doxycycline; tobramycin; imipenem; moxifloxacin, linezolid.
Mycobacterium fortuitum complex[102,108]	Skin and soft tissue infections; catheter infection	Amikacin AND meropenem (AIII) ± ciprofloxacin (AIII)	Also test for susceptibility to clarithromycin, cefoxitin; sulfonamides; doxycycline; linezolid.
Mycobacterium leprae[109]	Leprosy	Dapsone AND rifampin for paucibacillary (1–5 patches) (AII). ADD clarithromycin (or clofazimine) for lepromatous, multibacillary (>5 patches) disease (AII).	Consult HRSA (National Hansen's Disease [Leprosy] Program) at www.hrsa.gov/hansensdisease for advice about treatment and free antibiotics: 800/642-2477 (accessed September 15, 2016).

7

Preferred Therapy for Specific Bacterial and Mycobacterial Pathogens

Preferred Therapy for Specific Bacterial and Mycobacterial Pathogens

D. PREFERRED THERAPY FOR SPECIFIC BACTERIAL AND MYCOBACTERIAL PATHOGENS (continued)

Organism	Clinical Illness	Drug of Choice (evidence grade)	Alternatives
Mycobacterium marinum/balnei[102,110]	Papules, pustules, abscesses (swimming pool granuloma)	Clarithromycin ± rifampin (AIII)	TMP/SMX AND rifampin; doxycycline
Mycobacterium tuberculosis[105,111] See Tuberculosis in Chapter 6, Table 6F, Lower Respiratory Tract Infections, for detailed recommendations for active infection, latent infection, and exposures in high-risk children.	Tuberculosis (pneumonia; meningitis; cervical adenitis; mesenteric adenitis; osteomyelitis)	For active infection: isoniazid AND rifampin AND PZA (AI) For latent infection: isoniazid daily, biweekly, or in combination with rifapentine once weekly (AII)	Add ethambutol for suspect resistance; add streptomycin for severe infection. For MDR tuberculosis, bedaquiline is now FDA approved for adults and available for children. Corticosteroids should be added to regimens for meningitis, mesenteric adenitis, and endobronchial infection (AIII).
Mycoplasma hominis[112,113]	Nongonococcal urethritis; neonatal infection including meningitis	Clindamycin (AIII)	Fluoroquinolones; doxycycline Usually erythromycin resistant
Mycoplasma pneumoniae[114]	Pneumonia	Azithromycin (AI); erythromycin (BI); macrolide resistance emerging worldwide[115]	Doxycycline and fluoroquinolones are active against macrolide-susceptible and macrolide-resistant strains.
Neisseria gonorrhoeae[48]	Gonorrhea; arthritis	Ceftriaxone AND azithromycin or doxycycline (AIII)	Oral cefixime as single drug therapy no longer recommended due to increasing resistance[116] Spectinomycin IM
Neisseria meningitidis[117,118]	Sepsis, meningitis	Ceftriaxone (AI); cefotaxime (AI)	Penicillin G or ampicillin if susceptible For prophylaxis following exposure: rifampin or ciprofloxacin (ciprofloxacin-resistant strains have now been reported). Azithromycin may be less effective.

7

Nocardia asteroides or *brasiliensis*[119,120]	Nocardiosis	TMP/SMX (AII); sulfisoxazole (BII); imipenem AND amikacin for severe infection (AII)	Linezolid, ceftriaxone; clarithromycin, minocycline; levofloxacin, tigecycline, amox/clav
Oerskovia (now known as *Cellulosimicrobium cellulans*)[121]	Wound infection; catheter infection	Vancomycin ± rifampin (AIII)	Linezolid; resistant to beta-lactams, macrolides, clindamycin, aminoglycosides
Pasteurella multocida[122]	Sepsis, abscesses, animal bite wound	Penicillin G (AIII); ampicillin (AIII); amoxicillin (AIII)	Amox/clav; ticar/clav; pip/tazo; doxycycline; ceftriaxone; cefpodoxime; cefuroxime, TMP/SMX. Cephalexin may not demonstrate adequate activity. Not usually susceptible to clindamycin.
Peptostreptococcus[123]	Sepsis, deep head/neck space and intra-abdominal infection	Penicillin G (AIII); ampicillin (AII)	Clindamycin; vancomycin; meropenem, imipenem, metronidazole
Plesiomonas shigelloides[124,125]	Diarrhea, neonatal sepsis, meningitis	Antibiotics may not be necessary to treat diarrhea: 2nd- and 3rd-generation cephalosporins (AIII); azithromycin (BIII); ciprofloxacin (CIII). For meningitis/sepsis: ceftriaxone.	Meropenem; TMP/SMX, amox/clav
Prevotella (*Bacteroides*) spp,[126] *melaninogenica*	Deep head/neck space abscess; dental abscess	Metronidazole (AII); meropenem or imipenem (AII)	Pip/tazo; clindamycin
Propionibacterium acnes[127,128]	In addition to acne, invasive infection: sepsis, post-op wound infection	Penicillin G (AIII); vancomycin (AIII)	Cefotaxime; ceftriaxone, doxycycline; clindamycin; linezolid, daptomycin

Preferred Therapy for Specific Bacterial and Mycobacterial Pathogens

D. PREFERRED THERAPY FOR SPECIFIC BACTERIAL AND MYCOBACTERIAL PATHOGENS (continued)

Organism	Clinical Illness	Drug of Choice (evidence grade)	Alternatives
Proteus mirabilis[129]	UTI, sepsis, meningitis	Ceftriaxone (AII) or cefotaxime (AII); cefepime; ciprofloxacin; gentamicin	Carbapenem; pip/tazo; increasing resistance to ampicillin, TMP/SMX, and fluoroquinolones, particularly in nosocomial isolates Colistin resistant
Proteus vulgaris, other spp (indole-positive strains)[53]	UTI, sepsis, meningitis	Cefepime; ciprofloxacin; gentamicin (BIII)	Meropenem or other carbapenem; pip/tazo; TMP/SMX Colistin resistant
Providencia spp[53,74,130]	Sepsis	Cefepime; ciprofloxacin, gentamicin (BIII)	Meropenem or other carbapenem; pip/tazo; TMP/SMX Colistin resistant
Pseudomonas aeruginosa[74,131-135]	UTI	Cefepime (AIII); other antipseudomonal beta-lactams	Tobramycin; amikacin; ciprofloxacin
	Nosocomial sepsis, pneumonia	Cefepime (AI) or meropenem (AI); OR pip/tazo AND tobramycin (BI); ceftazidime AND tobramycin (BII)	Ciprofloxacin AND tobramycin. Controversy regarding additional clinical benefit in outcomes using newer, more potent beta-lactams over aminoglycoside combinations, but combinations may decrease emergence of resistance. Ceftolozane/tazobactam was approved by FDA for adults in 2015 and may be active against otherwise resistant strains.
	Pneumonia in cystic fibrosis[136-138] See Cystic Fibrosis in Chapter 6, Table 6F, Lower Respiratory Tract Infections.	Cefepime (AII) or meropenem (AI); OR ceftazidime AND tobramycin (BII); ADD aerosol tobramycin (AI). Azithromycin provides benefit in prolonging interval between exacerbations.	Inhalational antibiotics for prevention of acute exacerbations: tobramycin, aztreonam, colistin. Many organisms are MDR; consider ciprofloxacin or colistin parenterally; in vitro synergy testing may suggest effective combinations.[138] For MDR organisms, colistin aerosol (AIII).

Pseudomonas cepacia, mallei, or pseudomallei (See Burkholderia.)		
Rhodococcus equi[139]	Necrotizing pneumonia	Imipenem AND vancomycin (AIII)	Dual drug combination therapy with ciprofloxacin AND azithromycin or rifampin
Rickettsia[68,140,141]	Rocky Mountain spotted fever, Q fever, typhus, rickettsialpox	Doxycycline (all ages) (AII)	Chloramphenicol is less effective than doxycycline.
Salmonella, non-typhi[142-144]	Gastroenteritis (may not require therapy if clinically improving and not immunocompromised or <1 y); focal infections; bacteremia	Ceftriaxone (AII); cefixime (AII); azithromycin (AII)	For susceptible strains: ciprofloxacin; TMP/SMX; ampicillin; resistance to fluoroquinolones detected by nalidixic acid testing
Salmonella typhi[142,145]	Typhoid fever	Azithromycin (AII); ceftriaxone (AII); ciprofloxacin (AII)	For susceptible strains: TMP/SMX; ampicillin
Serratia marcescens[53,74]	Nosocomial sepsis, pneumonia	A carbapenem (AII)	Pip/tazo; cefepime if susceptible; ceftriaxone or cefotaxime AND gentamicin; or ciprofloxacin Resistant to colistin
Shewanella spp[146]	Wound infection, nosocomial pneumonia, peritoneal-dialysis peritonitis, ventricular shunt infection, neonatal sepsis	Ceftazidime (AIII); gentamicin (AIII)	Ampicillin, meropenem, pip/tazo, ciprofloxacin
Shigella spp[147,148]	Enteritis, UTI, prepubertal vaginitis	Ceftriaxone (AII); azithromycin[149] (AII); cefixime (AII); ciprofloxacin[150] (AII)	Resistance to azithromycin now reported. Use most narrow spectrum agent active against pathogen: ampicillin (not amoxicillin for enteritis); TMP/SMX.

Preferred Therapy for Specific Bacterial and Mycobacterial Pathogens

D. PREFERRED THERAPY FOR SPECIFIC BACTERIAL AND MYCOBACTERIAL PATHOGENS (continued)

7

Organism	Clinical Illness	Drug of Choice (evidence grade)	Alternatives
Spirillum minus[151,152]	Rat-bite fever (sodoku)	Penicillin G IV (AIII); for endocarditis, ADD gentamicin or streptomycin (AIII).	Ampicillin; doxycycline; cefotaxime, vancomycin, streptomycin
Staphylococcus aureus (See chapters 4 and 6 for specific infections).[153,154]			
– Mild–moderate infections	Skin infections, mild–moderate	MSSA: a 1st-generation cephalosporin (cefazolin IV, cephalexin PO) (AI); oxacillin/nafcillin IV (AI), dicloxacillin PO (AI) MRSA: vancomycin IV, or clindamycin IV or PO (if susceptible), or TMP/SMX PO (AII)	For MSSA: amox/clav For CA-MRSA: linezolid IV, PO; daptomycin IV
– Moderate–severe infections, treat empirically for CA-MRSA.	Pneumonia, sepsis, myositis, osteomyelitis, etc	MSSA: oxacillin/nafcillin IV (AI); a 1st-generation cephalosporin (cefazolin IV) (AI) ± gentamicin (AIII) MRSA: vancomycin (AII) or clindamycin (AII); ± gentamicin ± rifampin (AIII)	For CA-MRSA: linezolid (AII); OR daptomycin for non-pulmonary infection (AII) (studies published in children); ceftaroline IV (studies published in children) Approved for adults in 2015: dalbavancin, oritavancin, tedizolid (See Chapter 4.)
Staphylococcus, coagulase negative[155,156]	Nosocomial bacteremia (neonatal bacteremia), infected intravascular catheters, CNS shunts, UTI	Vancomycin (AII)	If susceptible: nafcillin (or other anti-staph beta-lactam); rifampin (in combination); clindamycin; linezolid; ceftaroline IV (studies published in children)
Stenotrophomonas maltophilia[157,158]	Sepsis	TMP/SMX (AII)	Ceftazidime; ticar/clav; doxycycline; levofloxacin

Streptobacillus moniliformis[151,152]	Rat-bite fever (Haverhill fever)	Penicillin G (AIII); ampicillin (AIII); for endocarditis, ADD gentamicin or streptomycin (AIII).	Doxycycline; ceftriaxone; carbapenems; clindamycin; vancomycin
Streptococcus, group A[159]	Pharyngitis, impetigo, adenitis, cellulitis, necrotizing fasciitis	Penicillin (AI); amoxicillin (AI)	A 1st-generation cephalosporin (cefazolin or cephalexin) (AI); clindamycin (AI); a macrolide (AI), vancomycin (AIII) For recurrent streptococcal pharyngitis, clindamycin or amox/clav (AIII)
Streptococcus, group B[160]	Neonatal sepsis, pneumonia, meningitis	Penicillin (AII) or ampicillin (AII)	Gentamicin is used initially until group B strep has been identified as the cause of infection and a clinical/microbiologic response has been documented (AIII).
Streptococcus, milleri/ anginosus group (*S intermedius, anginosus,* and *constellatus*; includes some beta-hemolytic group C and group G streptococci)[161–163]	Pneumonia, sepsis, skin and soft tissue infection, sinusitis,[164] arthritis, brain abscess, meningitis	Penicillin G (AIII); ampicillin (AIII); ADD gentamicin for serious infection (AIII). Many strains show decreased susceptibility to penicillin, requiring higher dosages.	Ceftriaxone; clindamycin; vancomycin

Preferred Therapy for Specific Bacterial and Mycobacterial Pathogens

7

D. PREFERRED THERAPY FOR SPECIFIC BACTERIAL AND MYCOBACTERIAL PATHOGENS (continued)

Organism	Clinical Illness	Drug of Choice (evidence grade)	Alternatives
Streptococcus pneumoniae[165-168] With widespread use of conjugate pneumococcal vaccines, antibiotic resistance in pneumococci has decreased substantially.[168]	Sinusitis, otitis[165]	Amoxicillin, high-dose (90 mg/kg/day) (AIII); new data suggest that standard dose (40–45 mg/kg/day) may again be effective.[168]	Amox/clav; cefdinir; cefpodoxime; cefuroxime; clindamycin; OR ceftriaxone IM
	Meningitis	Ceftriaxone (AI) or cefotaxime (AI); AND vancomycin for possible ceftriaxone-resistant strains (AIII)	Penicillin G alone for pen-S strains; ceftriaxone alone for ceftriaxone-susceptible strains
	Pneumonia,[114] osteomyelitis/arthritis, sepsis	Ampicillin (AII); ceftriaxone (AI); cefotaxime (AI)	Penicillin G for pen-S strains (AI)
Streptococcus, viridans group (alpha-hemolytic streptococci, most commonly *S sanguis, S oralis* [*mitis*], *S salivarius, S mutans, S morbillorum*)[169]	Endocarditis	Penicillin G ± gentamicin (AII) OR ceftriaxone ± gentamicin (AII)	Vancomycin
Treponema pallidum[48,170]	Syphilis	Penicillin G (AII)	Desensitize to penicillin preferred to alternate therapies. Doxycycline; ceftriaxone.
Ureaplasma urealyticum[48,171]	Genitourinary infections	Azithromycin (AII)	Erythromycin; doxycycline, ofloxacin (for adolescent genital infections)
	Neonatal pneumonia (Therapy may not be effective.)	Azithromycin (AIII)	

Organism	Clinical Condition	Preferred Therapy	Alternative Therapy
Vibrio cholerae[172,173]	Cholera	Doxycycline (AI) or azithromycin (AII)	If susceptible: ciprofloxacin
Vibrio vulnificus[174,175]	Sepsis, necrotizing fasciitis	Doxycycline AND ceftazidime (AII)	Ciprofloxacin AND cefotaxime or ceftriaxone
Yersinia enterocolitica[176,177]	Diarrhea, mesenteric enteritis, reactive arthritis, sepsis	TMP/SMX for enteritis (AIII); ciprofloxacin or ceftriaxone for invasive infection (AIII)	Gentamicin, doxycycline
Yersinia pestis[178,179]	Plague	Gentamicin (AIII)	Levofloxacin; doxycycline; ciprofloxacin
Yersinia pseudotuberculosis[177,180]	Mesenteric adenitis; Far East scarlet fever; reactive arthritis	TMP/SMX (AIII) or ciprofloxacin (AIII)	Ceftriaxone; gentamicin, doxycycline

8. Preferred Therapy for Specific Fungal Pathogens

NOTES

- See Chapter 2 for discussion of the differences between polyenes, azoles, and echinocandins.

- **Abbreviations:** ABLC, amphotericin B lipid complex (Abelcet); AmB, amphotericin B; AmB-D, amphotericin B deoxycholate, the conventional standard AmB (original trade name Fungizone); bid, twice daily; CNS, central nervous system; CSF, cerebrospinal fluid; CT, computed tomography; div, divided; ECMO, extracorporeal membrane oxygenation; HAART, highly active antiretroviral therapy; HIV, human immuno-deficiency virus; IV, intravenous; L-AmB, liposomal amphotericin B (AmBisome); PO, orally; qd, once daily; qid, 4 times daily; spp, species; TMP/SMX, trimethoprim/sulfamethoxazole.

Preferred Therapy for Specific Fungal Pathogens

A. OVERVIEW OF MORE COMMON FUNGAL PATHOGENS AND THEIR USUAL PATTERN OF ANTIFUNGAL SUSCEPTIBILITIES

Fungal Species	Amphotericin B Formulations	Fluconazole	Itraconazole	Voriconazole	Posaconazole	Isavuconazole	Flucytosine	Caspofungin, Micafungin, or Anidulafungin
Aspergillus calidoustus	++	–	–	–	–	–	–	++
Aspergillus fumigatus	+	–	+/–	++	+	++	–	+
Aspergillus terreus	–	–	+	++	+	++	–	+
Blastomyces dermatitidis	++	+	++	+	+	+	–	–
Candida albicans	+	++	+	+	+	+	+	++
Candida glabrata	+	–	+/–	+/–	+/–	+/–	+	+/–
Candida guilliermondii	+	+/–	+	+	+	+	+	–
Candida krusei	+	–	–	+	+	+	+	++
Candida lusitaniae	–	++	+	+	+	+	+	+
Candida parapsilosis	++	++	+	+	+	+	+	+/–
Candida tropicalis	+	++	+	+	+	+	+	++
Coccidioides immitis	++	+	++	+	++	+	–	–

8

Cryptococcus spp	++	+	+	+	+	+	++	–
Fusarium spp	+/–	–	+	+	++	–	+	–
Histoplasma capsulatum	++	+	++	+	+	+	+	–
Mucor spp	++	–	+/–	–	+/–	+	+	–
Paracoccidioides spp	+	+	++	+	++	+	+	–
Penicillium spp	+/–	–	++	–	+	+	+	–
Rhizopus spp	++	–	–	–	+	+	–	–
Scedosporium apiospermum	–	–	+/–	–	+	+	+	+/–
Scedosporium prolificans	–	–	+/–	–	+/–	+/–	+/–	+/–
Sporothrix spp	+	+	++	+	+	+	+	–
Trichosporon spp	–	+	+	++	+	+	+	–

NOTE: ++ = preferred therapy(ies); + = usually active; +/– = variably active; – = usually not active.

B. SYSTEMIC INFECTIONS

Infection	Therapy (evidence grade)	Comments
Prophylaxis		
Prophylaxis of invasive fungal infection in patients with hematologic malignancies[1-11]	Fluconazole 6 mg/kg/day PO for prevention of infection (AII). Posaconazole for prevention of infection has been well studied in adults (AI) and offers anti-mold coverage.[4]	Fluconazole is not effective against molds and some strains of *Candida*. Posaconazole PO, voriconazole PO, and micafungin IV are effective in adults in preventing yeast and mold infections but are not well studied in children for this indication.[12]
Prophylaxis of invasive fungal infection in patients with solid organ transplants[13-17]	Fluconazole 6 mg/kg/day PO for prevention of infection (AII)	AmB, caspofungin, micafungin, voriconazole, or posaconazole may be effective in preventing infection.
Treatment		
Aspergillosis[1,18-26]	Voriconazole (AI) 18 mg/kg/day IV div q12h for a loading dose on the first day, then 16 mg/kg/day IV div q12h as a maintenance dose for children 2–12 y or 12–14 y and weighing <50 kg. In children ≥15 y or 12–14 y and weighing >50 kg, use adult dosing (load 12 mg/kg/day IV div q12h on the first day, then 8 mg/kg/day div q12h as a maintenance dose) (AII). When stable, may switch from voriconazole IV to voriconazole PO at a dose of 18 mg/kg/day div bid for children 2–12 y and at least 400 mg/day div bid for children >12 y (AII). Dosing in children <2 y is less clear, but doses are generally higher (AIII). These are only initial dosing recommendations; continued dosing in all ages is guided by close monitoring of trough serum voriconazole concentrations in individual patients (AII). Unlike in adults, voriconazole PO bioavailability in children is only approximately 60%, so trough levels are crucial when using PO.[27]	Voriconazole is the preferred primary antifungal therapy for all clinical forms of aspergillosis. Early initiation of therapy in patients with strong suspicion of disease is important while a diagnostic evaluation is conducted. Optimal voriconazole trough serum concentrations (generally thought to be 2–5 μg/mL) are important for success. It is critical to monitor trough concentrations to guide therapy due to high inter-patient variability.[28] Low voriconazole concentrations are a leading cause of clinical failure. Younger children often have lower voriconazole levels and need much higher dosing. Total treatment course is for a minimum of 6–12 wk, largely dependent on the degree and duration of immunosuppression and evidence of disease improvement. Salvage antifungal therapy options after failed primary therapy may include a change of antifungal class (using L-AmB or an echinocandin), switching to isavuconazole, switching to posaconazole (trough concentrations >0.7 μg/mL), or using combination antifungal therapy.

Alternatives for primary therapy when voriconazole cannot be administered: L-AmB 5 mg/kg/day (AII) or isavuconazole (AI). Dosing of isavuconazole in children is unknown. ABLC is another possible alternative. Echinocandin primary monotherapy should not be used for treating invasive aspergillosis (CII). AmB deoxycholate should be used only in resource-limited settings in which no alternative agent is available (AII).

Careful consideration has to be used before beginning azole therapy after a patient has failed azole prophylaxis.

Combination antifungal therapy with voriconazole plus an echinocandin may be considered in select patients. The addition of anidulafungin to voriconazole as combination therapy found some statistical benefit to the combination over voriconazole monotherapy in only certain patients.[29] In vitro data suggest some synergy with 2 (but not 3) drug combinations: an azole plus an echinocandin is the most well studied. If combination therapy is employed, this is likely best done initially when voriconazole trough concentrations may not be appropriate yet.

Routine antifungal susceptibility testing is not recommended but is suggested for patients suspected of having an azole-resistant isolate or who are unresponsive to therapy.

Azole-resistant *Aspergillus fumigatus* is increasing. If local epidemiology suggests >10% azole resistance, empiric initial therapy should be voriconazole + echinocandin OR with L-AmB, and subsequent therapy guided based on antifungal susceptibilities.[30]

Micafungin likely has equal efficacy to caspofungin against aspergillosis.[31]

Return of immune function is paramount to treatment success; for children receiving corticosteroids, decreasing the corticosteroid dosage or changing to steroid-sparing protocols is important.

Preferred Therapy for Specific Fungal Pathogens

8

B. SYSTEMIC INFECTIONS (continued)

Infection	Therapy (evidence grade)	Comments
Bipolaris, Cladophialophora, Curvularia, Exophiala, Alternaria, and other agents of **phaeohyphomycosis** (dematiaceous, pigmented molds)[32-39]	Voriconazole (AI) 18 mg/kg/day IV div q12h for a loading dose on the first day, then 16 mg/kg/day IV div q12h as a maintenance dose for children 2–12 y or 12–14 y and weighing <50 kg. In children ≥15 y or 12–14 y and weighing >50 kg, use adult dosing (load 12 mg/kg/day IV div q12h on the first day, then 8 mg/kg/day div q12h as a maintenance dose) (AII). When stable, may switch from voriconazole IV to voriconazole PO at a dose of 18 mg/kg/day div bid for children 2–12 y and at least 400 mg/day div bid for children >12 y (AII). Dosing in children <2 y is less clear, but doses are generally higher (AIII). These are only initial dosing recommendations; continued dosing in all ages is guided by close monitoring of trough serum voriconazole concentrations in individual patients (AII). Unlike in adults, voriconazole PO bioavailability in children is only approximately 60%, so trough levels are crucial.[27]	Aggressive surgical debulking/excision is essential for CNS lesions. These can be highly resistant infections, so strongly recommend antifungal susceptibility testing to guide therapy and consultation with a pediatric infectious diseases expert. Antifungal susceptibilities are often variable, but empiric therapy with voriconazole is the best start. Optimal voriconazole trough serum concentrations (generally thought to be 2–5 μg/mL) are important for success. It is critical to monitor trough concentrations to guide therapy due to high inter-patient variability,[28] Low voriconazole concentrations are a leading cause of clinical failure. Younger children often have lower voriconazole levels and need much higher dosing.
	Alternatives could include posaconazole (trough concentrations >0.7 μg/mL) or combination therapy with an echinocandin + azole or an echinocandin + L-AmB (BIII).	
Blastomycosis (North American)[40-46]	For moderate-severe pulmonary disease: ABLC or L-AmB 5 mg/kg IV daily for 1–2 wk or until improvement noted, followed by itraconazole oral solution 10 mg/kg/day PO div bid (max 400 mg/day) PO for a total of 6–12 mo (AIII). Itraconazole loading dose (double dose for first 2 days) is recommended in adults but has not been studied in children (but likely helpful).	Itraconazole oral solution provides greater and more reliable absorption than capsules and only the oral solution should be used (on an empty stomach); serum concentrations of itraconazole should be determined 2 wk after start of therapy to ensure adequate drug exposure. For blastomycosis, maintain trough itraconazole concentrations at >1.0 μg/mL (values for both itraconazole and hydroxyl-itraconazole are added together). If only itraconazole

For mild-moderate pulmonary disease: itraconazole oral solution 10 mg/kg/day div bid (max 400 mg/day) PO for a total of 6–12 mo (AIII). Itraconazole loading dose (double dose for first 2 days) recommended in adults but has not been studied in children (but likely helpful).

For CNS blastomycosis: ABLC/L-AmB for 4–6 wk, followed by an azole (fluconazole is preferred, at 12 mg/kg/day after a loading dose of 25 mg/kg; alternatives for CNS disease are voriconazole or itraconazole), for a total of at least 12 mo and until resolution of CSF abnormalities (AII). Some experts suggest combination therapy with L-AmB plus high-dose fluconazole as induction therapy in CNS blastomycosis until clinical improvement (BII).

capsules are available, use 20 mg/kg/d div q12h and take with cola product to increase gastric acidity and bioavailability.

Alternative to itraconazole: 12 mg/kg/day fluconazole (BII) after a loading dose of 25 mg/kg/day.

Patients with extrapulmonary blastomycosis should receive at least 12 mo of total therapy.

If induction with L-AmB alone is failing, add itraconazole or high-dose fluconazole until clinical improvement. Lifelong itraconazole if immunosuppression cannot be reversed.

Candidiasis[47-51] (See Chapter 2.)

– Cutaneous

Topical therapy (alphabetic order): ciclopirox, clotrimazole, econazole, haloprogin, ketoconazole, miconazole, oxiconazole, sertaconazole, sulconazole

Fluconazole 6 mg/kg/day PO qd for 5–7 days

Relapse common in cases of chronic mucocutaneous disease, and antifungal susceptibilities critical to drive appropriate therapy

Preferred Therapy for Specific Fungal Pathogens

8

B. SYSTEMIC INFECTIONS (continued)

Infection	Therapy (evidence grade)	Comments
– Disseminated, acute (including catheter fungemia) infection	For neutropenic patients An echinocandin is recommended as initial therapy. Caspofungin 70 mg/m² IV loading dose on day 1 (max dose 70 mg), followed by 50 mg/m² IV (max dose 70 mg) on subsequent days (AII); OR micafungin 2 mg/kg/day q24h (children weighing <40 kg), up to max dose 100 mg/day (AII).[52] ABLC or L-AmB 5 mg/kg/day IV q24h (BII) is an effective but less attractive alternative due to potential toxicity (AII). Fluconazole (12 mg/kg/day q24h, after a load of 25 mg/kg/day) is an alternative for patients who are not critically ill and have had no prior azole exposure (CII). A fluconazole loading dose is standard of care in adult patients but has only been studied in infants[53]—it is likely that the beneficial effect of a loading dose extends to children. Fluconazole can be used as step-down therapy in stable neutropenic patients with susceptible isolates and documented bloodstream clearance (CIII). For children on ECMO, 35 mg/kg load on day 1 followed by 12 mg/kg/day (BII).[54] For non-neutropenic patients An echinocandin is recommended as initial therapy. Caspofungin 70 mg/m² IV loading dose on day 1 (max dose 70 mg), followed by 50 mg/m² IV (max dose 70 mg) on subsequent days (AII); OR micafungin 2 mg/kg/day q24h (children weighing <40 kg), up to max dose 100 mg/day (AI).[52] Fluconazole (12 mg/kg/day IV or PO q24h, after a load of 25 mg/kg/day) is an acceptable alternative to an echinocandin as initial therapy in	Prompt removal of infected IV catheter or any infected devices is absolutely critical to success (AII). For infections with C krusei or C glabrata, an echinocandin is preferred; however, there are increasing reports of some C glabrata resistance to echinocandins (treatment would, therefore, be lipid formulation AmB) (BIII). Lipid formulation AmB (5 mg/kg daily) is a reasonable alternative if there is intolerance, limited availability, or resistance to other antifungal agents (AI). Transition from lipid AmB to fluconazole is recommended after 5–7 days among patients who have isolates that are susceptible to fluconazole, who are clinically stable, and in whom repeat cultures on antifungal therapy are negative (AI). Voriconazole (18 mg/kg/day div q12h load, followed by 16 mg/kg/day div q12h) is effective for candidemia but offers little advantage over fluconazole as initial therapy. Voriconazole is recommended as step-down oral therapy for selected cases of candidemia due to C krusei or if mold coverage is needed. Follow-up blood cultures should be performed every day or every other day to establish the time point at which candidemia has been cleared (AIII). Duration of therapy is for 2 wk AFTER negative cultures in pediatric patients without obvious metastatic complications and after symptom resolution (AII). In neutropenic patients, ophthalmologic findings of chorioidal and vitreal infection are minimal until recovery from neutropenia; therefore, dilated funduscopic examinations should be performed within the first week after recovery from neutropenia (AIII).

selected patients, including those who are not critically ill and who are considered unlikely to have a fluconazole-resistant Candida species (AI). For children on ECMO, use 35 mg/kg load followed by 12 mg/kg/day (BII).[54]

Transition from an echinocandin to fluconazole (usually within 5–7 days) is recommended for non-neutropenic patients who are clinically stable, have isolates that are susceptible to fluconazole (eg, C albicans), and have negative repeat blood cultures following initiation of antifungal therapy (AII).

For CNS infections

AmB-D (1 mg/kg/day) or L-AmB/ABLC (5 mg/kg/day) with or without flucytosine 100 mg/kg/day PO div q6h (AII) until initial clinical response, followed by step-down therapy with fluconazole (12 mg/kg/day q24h, after a load of 25 mg/kg/day); echinocandins do not achieve therapeutic concentrations in CSF.

All non-neutropenic patients with candidemia should have a dilated ophthalmologic examination, preferably performed by an ophthalmologist, within the first week after diagnosis (AIII).

– Disseminated, chronic (hepatosplenic) infection	Initial therapy with lipid formulation AmB (5 mg/kg daily) OR an echinocandin (caspofungin 70 mg/m² IV loading dose on day 1 [max dose 70 mg], followed by 50 mg/m² IV [max dose 70 mg] on subsequent days OR micafungin 2 mg/kg/day q24h in children weighing <40 kg [max dose 100 mg]) for several weeks, followed by oral fluconazole in patients unlikely to have a fluconazole-resistant isolate (12 mg/kg/day q24h, after a load of 25 mg/kg/day) (AIII). Therapy should continue until lesions resolve on repeat imaging, which is usually several months. Premature discontinuation of antifungal therapy can lead to relapse (AIII).	If chemotherapy or hematopoietic cell transplantation is required, it should not be delayed because of the presence of chronic disseminated candidiasis, and antifungal therapy should be continued throughout the period of high risk to prevent relapse (AIII).

Preferred Therapy for Specific Fungal Pathogens

8

B. SYSTEMIC INFECTIONS (continued)

Infection	Therapy (evidence grade)	Comments
– Neonatal[50] (See Chapter 5.)	AmB-D (1 mg/kg/day) is recommended therapy (AII). Fluconazole (12 mg/kg/day q24h, after a load of 25 mg/kg/day) is an alternative if patient has not been on fluconazole prophylaxis (AII).[53] For treatment of neonates and young infants (<120 days) on ECMO, fluconazole is loaded with 35 mg/kg on day 1, followed by 12 mg/kg/day q24h (BII). Lipid formulation AmB is an alternative but carries a theoretic risk of less urinary tract penetration compared with AmB-D (CII). Duration of therapy for candidemia without obvious metastatic complications is for 2 wk after documented clearance and resolution of symptoms. Echinocandins should be used with caution and generally limited to salvage therapy or to situations in which resistance or toxicity preclude the use of AmB-D or fluconazole (CIII). Role of flucytosine in neonates with meningitis is questionable and not routinely recommended due to toxicity concerns. The addition of flucytosine (100 mg/kg/day div q6h) may be considered as salvage therapy in patients who have not had a clinical response to initial AmB therapy, but adverse effects are frequent (CIII).	In nurseries with high rates of candidiasis (>10%), IV or oral fluconazole prophylaxis (AI) (3–6 mg/kg twice weekly for 6 wk) in high-risk neonates (birth weight <1,000 g) is recommended. Oral nystatin, 100,000 units 3 times daily for 6 wk, is an alternative to fluconazole in neonates with birth weights <1,500 g in situations in which availability or resistance precludes the use of fluconazole (CII). Lumbar puncture and dilated retinal examination recommended in neonates with cultures positive for *Candida* species from blood and/or urine (AIII). CT or ultrasound imaging of genitourinary tract, liver, and spleen should be performed if blood cultures are persistently positive (AIII). Meningoencephalitis in the neonate occurs at a higher rate than in older children/adults. Central venous catheter removal is strongly recommended. Infected CNS devices, including ventriculostomy drains and shunts, should be removed if possible.
– Oropharyngeal, esophageal[47]	Mild oropharyngeal disease: clotrimazole 10 mg troches PO 5 times daily OR nystatin 100,000 U/mL, 4–6 mL 4 times daily for 7–14 days.	For fluconazole-refractory oropharyngeal or esophageal disease: itraconazole oral solution OR posaconazole OR AmB IV OR an echinocandin for up to 28 days (AII).

	Esophageal disease always requires systemic antifungal therapy. A diagnostic trial of antifungal therapy for esophageal candidiasis is appropriate before performing an endoscopic examination (AI). Chronic suppressive therapy (3 times weekly with fluconazole is recommended for recurrent infections (AI). Alternatives also include miconazole mucoadhesive buccal 50-mg tablet to the mucosal surface over the canine fossa once daily for 7–14 days OR 1–2 nystatin pastilles (200,000 U each) 4 times daily for 7–14 days (AII). Moderate-severe oropharyngeal disease: fluconazole 6 mg/kg qd PO for 7–14 days (AII). Esophageal candidiasis: oral fluconazole (6–12 mg/kg/day), after a loading dose of 25 mg/kg/day) for 14–21 days (AI). If cannot tolerate oral therapy, use fluconazole IV OR ABLC/L-AmB/AmB-D OR an echinocandin (AI).
– Urinary tract infection	Cystitis: fluconazole 6 mg/kg qd IV or PO for 2 wk (AII). For fluconazole-resistant *C glabrata* or *C krusei*, AmB-D for 1–7 days (AIII). Pyelonephritis: fluconazole 12 mg/kg qd IV or PO for 2 wk (AIII) after a loading dose of 25 mg/kg/day. For fluconazole-resistant *C glabrata* or *C krusei*, AmB-D with or without flucytosine for 1–7 days (AIII). Treatment is NOT recommended in asymptomatic candiduria unless neutropenic, low-birth weight neonate, or patient will undergo urologic manipulation (AIII). Removing Foley catheter, if present, may lead to a spontaneous cure in the normal host; check for additional upper urinary tract disease. AmB-D bladder irrigation is not generally recommended due to high relapse rate (an exception may be in fluconazole-resistant *Candida*) (CIII). For renal collecting system fungus balls, surgical debridement may be required in non-neonates (BIII). Echinocandins have poor urinary concentrations.
– Vulvovaginal[55]	Topical vaginal cream/tablets/suppositories (alphabetic order); butoconazole, clotrimazole, econazole, fenticonazole, miconazole, sertaconazole, terconazole, or tioconazole for 3–7 days (AI) OR fluconazole 10 mg/kg (max 150 mg) as a single dose (AII) For uncomplicated vulvovaginal candidiasis, no topical agent is clearly superior. Avoid azoles during pregnancy. For recurring disease, consider 10–14 days of induction with topical agent or fluconazole, followed by fluconazole once weekly for 6 mo (AI).
Chromoblastomycosis (subcutaneous infection by dematiaceous fungi)[56–59]	Itraconazole oral solution 10 mg/kg/day PO for 12–18 mo, in combination with surgical excision or repeated cryotherapy (AII) Alternative: terbinafine plus surgery; heat and potassium iodide; posaconazole. Lesions are recalcitrant and difficult to treat.

Preferred Therapy for Specific Fungal Pathogens

Preferred Therapy for Specific Fungal Pathogens

8

B. SYSTEMIC INFECTIONS (continued)

Infection	Therapy (evidence grade)	Comments
Coccidioidomycosis[60–68]	For moderate infections: fluconazole 12 mg/kg IV PO q24h (AIII) after loading dose of 25 mg/kg/day. For severe pulmonary disease: AmB-D 1 mg/kg/day IV q24h OR ABLC/L-AmB 5 mg/kg/day IV q24h (AIII) as initial therapy for several weeks until clear improvement, followed by an oral azole for total therapy of at least 12 mo, depending on genetic or immunocompromised risk factors. For meningitis: fluconazole 12 mg/kg/day IV q24h (AII) after loading dose of 25 mg/kg/day (AII). Itraconazole has also been effective (BIII). If no response to azole, use intrathecal AmB-D (0.1–1.5 mg/dose) with or without fluconazole (AIII). Lifelong azole suppressive therapy required due to high relapse rate. For extrapulmonary (non-meningeal), particularly for osteomyelitis: itraconazole solution 10 mg/kg/day div bid for at least 12 mo appears more effective than fluconazole in bone disease (AIII), and AmB as an alternative if worsening.	Mild pulmonary disease does not require therapy in the normal host and only requires periodic reassessment. There is experience with posaconazole for disease in adults but little experience in children. Isavuconazole experience in adults is increasing. Treat until serum cocci complement fixation titers drop to 1:8 or 1:4, about 3–6 mo. Disease in immunocompromised hosts may need to be treated longer, including potentially lifelong azole secondary prophylaxis. Watch for relapse up to 1–2 y after therapy.
Cryptococcosis[69–73]	For mild-moderate pulmonary disease: fluconazole 12 mg/kg/day (max 400 mg) IV/PO q24h after loading dose of 25 mg/kg/day for 6–12 mo (AIII). Itraconazole is alternative if cannot tolerate fluconazole. For meningitis or severe pulmonary disease: induction therapy with AmB-D 1 mg/kg/day IV q24h OR ABLC/L-AmB 5 mg/kg/day q24h; AND flucytosine 100 mg/kg/day PO div q6h for a	Serum flucytosine concentrations should be obtained after 3–5 days to achieve a 2-h post-dose peak <100 µg/mL (ideally 30–80 µg/mL) to prevent neutropenia. For HIV-positive patients, continue maintenance therapy with fluconazole (6 mg/kg/day) indefinitely. Initiate HAART 2–10 wk after commencement of antifungal therapy to avoid immune reconstitution syndrome.

minimum of 2 wk and a repeat CSF culture is negative, followed by consolidation therapy with fluconazole (12 mg/kg/day with max dose 400 mg after a loading dose of 25 mg/kg/day) for a minimum of 8 more wk (AI). Then use maintenance therapy with fluconazole (6 mg/kg/day) for 6–12 mo (AI). Alternative induction therapies for meningitis or severe pulmonary disease (listed in order of preference): AmB product for 4–6 wk (AII); AmB product plus fluconazole for 2 wk, followed by fluconazole for 8 wk (BII); fluconazole plus flucytosine for 6 wk (BII).	In organ transplant recipients, continue maintenance fluconazole (6 mg/kg/day) for 6–12 mo after consolidation therapy with higher dose fluconazole. For cryptococcal relapse, restart induction therapy (this time for 4–10 wk), repeat CSF analysis every 2 wk until sterile, and determine antifungal susceptibility of relapse isolate. Successful use of voriconazole, posaconazole, and isavuconazole for cryptococcosis has been reported in adult patients.
Fusarium, Scedosporium prolificans, Pseudallescheria boydii (and its asexual form, **Scedosporium apiospermum**),[32,74–78] and other agents of **hyalohyphomycosis**	Voriconazole (AII) 18 mg/kg/day IV div q12h for a loading dose on the first day, then 16 mg/kg/day IV div q12h as a maintenance dose for children 2–12 y or 12–14 y and weighing <50 kg. In children ≥15 y or 12–14 y and weighing >50 kg, use adult dosing (load 12 mg/kg/day IV div q12h on the first day, then 8 mg/kg/day div q12h as a maintenance dose) (AII). When stable, may switch from voriconazole IV to voriconazole PO at a dose of 18 mg/kg/day div bid for children 2–12 y and at least 400 mg/day div bid for children >12 y (AII). Dosing in children <2 y is less clear, but doses are generally higher (AIII). These are only initial dosing recommendations; continued dosing in all ages is guided by close monitoring of trough serum voriconazole concentrations in individual patients (AII). Unlike in adults, voriconazole PO bioavailability in children is only approximately 60%, so trough levels are crucial at this stage.[27]	These can be highly resistant infections, so strongly recommend antifungal susceptibility testing against a wide range of agents to guide specific therapy and consultation with a pediatric infectious diseases expert. Optimal voriconazole trough serum concentrations (generally thought to be 2–5 μg/mL) are important for success. It is critical to monitor trough concentrations to guide therapy due to high inter-patient variability.[28] Low voriconazole concentrations are a leading cause of clinical failure. Younger children often have lower voriconazole levels and need much higher dosing. Often resistant to AmB in vitro. Alternatives: posaconazole (trough concentrations >0.7 μg/mL) can be active; echinocandins have been reportedly successful as salvage therapy in combination with azoles; while there are reports of promising in vitro combinations with terbinafine, terbinafine does not obtain good tissue concentrations for these disseminated infections; miltefosine (for leishmaniasis) use has been reported.

Preferred Therapy for Specific Fungal Pathogens

B. SYSTEMIC INFECTIONS (continued)

Infection	Therapy (evidence grade)	Comments
Histoplasmosis[79-81]	For severe acute pulmonary disease: ABLC/L-AmB 5 mg/kg/day q24h for 1–2 wk, followed by itraconazole 10 mg/kg/day div bid (max 400 mg daily) to complete a total of 12 wk (AIII). Add methylprednisolone (0.5–1.0 mg/kg/day) for first 1–2 wk in patients with hypoxia or significant respiratory distress. For mild-moderate acute pulmonary disease: if symptoms persist for >1 mo, itraconazole 10 mg/kg/day PO solution div bid for 6–12 wk (AIII). For progressive disseminated histoplasmosis: ABLC/L-AmB 5 mg/kg/day q24h for 4–6 wk; alternative treatment is lipid AmB for 1–2 wk followed by itraconazole 10 mg/kg/day div bid (max 400 mg daily) to complete a total of 12 wk (AIII).	Mild pulmonary disease may not require therapy and, in most cases, resolves in 1 mo. CNS histoplasmosis requires initial AmB therapy for 4–6 wk, followed by itraconazole for at least 12 mo and until CSF antigen resolution. Itraconazole oral solution provides greater and more reliable absorption than capsules and only the oral solution should be used (on an empty stomach); serum concentrations of itraconazole should be determined 2 wk after start of therapy to ensure adequate drug exposure. Maintain trough itraconazole concentrations at >1–2 µg/mL (values for both itraconazole and hydroxyl-itraconazole are added together). If only itraconazole capsules are available, use 20 mg/kg/day div q12h and take with cola product to increase gastric acidity and bioavailability. Potential lifelong suppressive itraconazole if cannot reverse immunosuppression. Corticosteroids recommended for 2 wk for pericarditis with hemodynamic compromise. Voriconazole and posaconazole use has been reported. Fluconazole is inferior to itraconazole.
Mucormycosis (previously known as zygomycosis)[82-86]	Aggressive surgical debridement combined with induction antifungal therapy: L-AmB at 5–10 mg/kg/day q24h (AIII) for 3 wk. Lipid formulations of AmB are preferred to AmB-D due to increased penetration and decreased toxicity. Many experts advocate induction combination therapy with L-AmB plus an echinocandin (although data are largely in diabetic patients with rhinocerebral disease) (CII).	Following clinical response with AmB, long-term oral step-down therapy with posaconazole (trough concentrations ideally for mucormycosis at >2 µg/mL) can be attempted for 2–6 mo. No pediatric dosing exists for isavuconazole. Voriconazole has NO activity against mucormycosis or other Zygomycetes. Return of immune function is paramount to treatment success; for children receiving corticosteroids, decreasing the corticosteroid dosage or changing to steroid-sparing protocols is also important.

8

For salvage therapy, isavuconazole (AI) or posaconazole (AIII).

Following successful induction antifungal therapy (for at least 3 wk), can continue consolidation therapy with posaconazole (or use intermittent L-AmB) (BII).

Paracoccidioidomycosis[87–90]	Itraconazole 10 mg/kg/day (max 400 mg daily) PO solution div bid for 6 mo (AIII) OR voriconazole (dosing listed under Aspergillosis) (BI)	Alternatives: fluconazole; isavuconazole; sulfadiazine or TMP/SMX for 3–5 y. AmB is another alternative and may be combined with sulfa or azole antifungals.
***Pneumocystis jiroveci (carinii)* pneumonia**[91,92]	Severe disease: preferred regimen is TMP/SMX 15–20 mg TMP component/kg/day IV div q8h (AI) OR, for TMP/SMX intolerant or TMP/SMX treatment failure, pentamidine isethionate 4 mg base/kg/day IV daily (BII), for 3 wk. Mild-moderate disease: start with IV therapy, then after acute pneumonitis is resolved, TMP/SMX 20 mg TMP component/kg/day PO div qid for 3 wk total treatment course (AII).	Alternatives: TMP AND dapsone; OR primaquine AND clindamycin; OR atovaquone. Prophylaxis: preferred regimen is TMP/SMX (5 mg TMP component/kg/day) PO div bid 3 times/wk on consecutive days; OR same dose, given qd, every day; OR atovaquone: 30 mg/kg/day for infants 1–3 mo; 45 mg/kg/day for infants/children 4–24 mo; and 30 mg/kg/day for children >24 mo; OR dapsone 2 mg/kg (max 100 mg) PO qd, OR dapsone 4 mg/kg (max 200 mg) PO once weekly. Use steroid therapy for more severe disease.
Sporotrichosis[93,94]	For cutaneous/lymphocutaneous: Itraconazole 10 mg/kg/day div bid PO solution for 2–4 wk after all lesions gone (generally total of 3–6 mo) (AII) For serious pulmonary or disseminated infection or disseminated sporotrichosis: ABLC/L-AmB at 5 mg/kg/day q24h until favorable response, then step-down therapy with itraconazole PO for at least a total of 12 mo (AIII) For less severe disease, itraconazole for 12 mo	If no response for cutaneous disease, treat with higher itraconazole dose, terbinafine, or saturated solution of potassium iodide. Fluconazole is less effective. Obtain serum concentrations of itraconazole after 2 wk of therapy; want serum trough concentration >0.5 μg/mL. For meningeal disease, initial AmB should be 4–6 wk before change to itraconazole for at least 12 mo of therapy. Surgery may be necessary in osteoarticular or pulmonary disease.

Preferred Therapy for Specific Fungal Pathogens

8

C. LOCALIZED MUCOCUTANEOUS INFECTIONS

Infection	Therapy (evidence grade)	Comments
Dermatophytoses		
– Scalp (tinea capitis, including kerion)[95-99]	Griseofulvin ultramicrosized 10–15 mg/kg/day or microsized 20–25 mg/kg/day qd PO for 6–12 wk (taken with milk or fatty foods to augment absorption). For kerion, treat concurrently with prednisone (1–2 mg/kg/day for 1–2 wk) (AIII). Terbinafine can be used for only 2–4 wk. Terbinafine dosing is 62.5 mg/day (<20 kg), 125 mg/day (20–40 kg), or 250 mg/day (>40 kg) (AII).	Griseofulvin is superior for *Microsporum* infections, but terbinafine is superior for *Trichophyton* infections. *Trichophyton tonsurans* predominates in United States. No need to routinely follow liver function tests in normal healthy children taking griseofulvin. Alternatives: itraconazole oral solution 5 mg/kg qd or fluconazole. 2.5% selenium sulfide shampoo, or 2% ketoconazole shampoo, 2–3 times/wk should be used concurrently to prevent recurrences.
– Tinea corporis (infection of trunk/limbs/face) – Tinea cruris (infection of the groin) – Tinea pedis (infection of the toes/feet)	Alphabetic order of topical agents: butenafine, ciclopirox, clotrimazole, econazole, haloprogin, ketoconazole, miconazole, naftifine, oxiconazole, sertaconazole, sulconazole, terbinafine, and tolnaftate (AII); apply daily for 4 wk.	For unresponsive tinea lesions, use griseofulvin PO in dosages provided above; fluconazole PO; itraconazole PO; OR terbinafine PO. For tinea pedis: terbinafine PO or itraconazole PO are preferred over other oral agents. Keep skin as clean and dry as possible, particularly for tinea cruris and tinea pedis.
– Tinea unguium (onychomycosis)[97,100,101]	Terbinafine 62.5 mg/day (<20 kg), 125 mg/day (20–40 kg), or 250 mg/day (>40 kg). Use for at least 6 wk (fingernails) or 12–16 wk (toenails) (AII).	Recurrence or partial response common. Alternative: itraconazole pulse therapy with 10 mg/kg/day div q12h for 1 wk per mo. Two pulses for fingernails and 3 pulses for toenails. Alternatives: fluconazole, griseofulvin.
– Tinea versicolor (also pityriasis versicolor)[97,102,103]	Apply topically: selenium sulfide 2.5% lotion or 1% shampoo daily, leave on 30 min, then rinse; for 7 days, then monthly for 6 mo (AIII); OR ciclopirox 1% cream for 4 wk (BII); OR terbinafine 1% solution (BII); OR ketoconazole 2% shampoo daily for 5 days (BII) For small lesions, topical clotrimazole, econazole, haloprogin, ketoconazole, miconazole, or naftifine	For lesions that fail to clear with topical therapy or for extensive lesions: fluconazole PO or itraconazole PO are equally effective. Recurrence common.

9. Preferred Therapy for Specific Viral Pathogens

NOTE

- **Abbreviations:** AIDS, acquired immunodeficiency syndrome; ART, antiretroviral therapy; ARV, antiretroviral; bid, twice daily; BSA, body surface area; CDC, Centers for Disease Control and Prevention; CLD, chronic lung disease; CMV, cytomegalovirus; CrCl, creatinine clearance; div, divided; EBV, Epstein-Barr virus; FDA, US Food and Drug Administration; G-CSF, granulocyte-colony stimulating factor; HAART, highly active antiretroviral therapy; HBeAg, hepatitis B e antigen; HBV, hepatitis B virus; HCV, hepatitis C virus; HHS, US Department of Health and Human Services; HIV, human immunodeficiency virus; HSV, herpes simplex virus; IFN, interferon; IG, immune globulin; IM, intramuscular; IV, intravenous; NS5A, nonstructural protein 5A; PO, orally; postmenstrual age, weeks of gestation since last menstrual period PLUS weeks of chronologic age since birth; PTLD, posttransplant lymphoprolifera-tive disorder; qd, once daily; qid, 4 times daily; RAV, resistance-associated variant; RSV, respiratory syncytial virus; SQ, subcutaneous; tid, 3 times daily; WHO, World Health Organization.

Preferred Therapy for Specific Viral Pathogens

A. OVERVIEW OF NON-HIV VIRAL PATHOGENS AND USUAL PATTERN OF SUSCEPTIBILITY TO ANTIVIRALS

Virus	Acyclovir	Adefovir	Cidofovir	Daclatasvir plus Sofosbuvir	Elbasvir/ Grazoprevir (Zepatier)	Entecavir	Famciclovir	Foscarnet	Ganciclovir
Cytomegalovirus			+					+	++
Hepatitis B virus[1]		+				++			
Hepatitis C virus[a]				++ b,c	++ d,e				
Herpes simplex virus	++						++	+	+
Influenza A and B									
Varicella-zoster virus	++						++	+	+

Virus	Interferon alfa-2b	Lamivudine	Ombitasvir/ Paritaprevir/Ritonavir Co-packaged With Dasabuvir (Viekira Pak)	Ombitasvir/ Paritaprevir/ Ritonavir plus Ribavirin	Oseltamivir	Pegylated Interferon alfa-2a	Peramivir	Ribavirin
Cytomegalovirus								
Hepatitis B virus	+	+				++		
Hepatitis C virus[a]			++ b	++ e		++ f		++ f
Herpes simplex virus								
Influenza A and B					++		+	
Varicella-zoster virus								

Virus	Simeprevir plus Sofosbuvir	Sofosbuvir/ Ledipasvir (Harvoni)	Sofosbuvir plus Ribavirin	Sofosbuvir/ Velpatasvir (Epclusa)	Telbivudine	Tenofovir	Valacyclovir	Valganciclovir	Zanamivir
Cytomegalovirus								++	
Hepatitis B virus					+	++			
Hepatitis C virus[a]	++[b]	++[b,e,g]	++[c]	+[h]					
Herpes simplex virus							++	+	
Influenza A and B									+
Varicella-zoster virus							++		

NOTE: ++ = preferred therapy(ies); + = acceptable therapy.

[a] HCV treatment guidelines from the Infectious Diseases Society of America and the American Association for the Study of Liver Diseases available at www.hcvguidelines.org (accessed September 15, 2016).

[b] Treatment-naive patients with HCV genotype 1a and 1b infection who do not have cirrhosis.

[c] Treatment-naive patients with HCV genotype 2 and 3 infection who do not have cirrhosis.

[d] Treatment-naive patients with HCV genotype 1a and 1b infection who do not have cirrhosis and in whom no baseline high fold-change NS5A RAVs for elbasvir are detected.

[e] Treatment-naive patients with HCV genotype 4 infection who do not have cirrhosis.

[f] Likely to be replaced in pediatric patients as studies of newer molecules are performed in children.

[g] Treatment-naive patients with HCV genotype 5 and 6 infection who do not have cirrhosis.

[h] Active against all genotypes of HCV; approved June 28, 2016.

Preferred Therapy for Specific Viral Pathogens

B. PREFERRED THERAPY FOR SPECIFIC VIRAL PATHOGENS

Infection	Therapy (evidence grade)	Comments
Adenovirus (pneumonia or disseminated infection in immunocompromised hosts)[2]	Cidofovir and ribavirin are active in vitro, but no prospective clinical data exist and both have significant toxicity. Two cidofovir dosing schedules have been employed in clinical settings: (1) 5 mg/kg/dose IV once weekly or (2) 1–1.5 mg/kg/dose IV 3 times/wk. If parenteral cidofovir is utilized, IV hydration and oral probenecid should be used to reduce renal toxicity.	Brincidofovir, the orally bioavailable lipophilic derivative of cidofovir also known as CMX001, is under investigation for the treatment of adenovirus in immunocompromised hosts. It is not yet commercially available.
Cytomegalovirus		
– Neonatal[3]	See Chapter 5.	
– Immunocompromised (HIV, chemotherapy, transplant-related)[4–16]	For induction: ganciclovir 10 mg/kg/day IV div q12h for 14–21 days (AII) (may be increased to 15 mg/kg/day IV div q12h). For maintenance: 5 mg/kg IV q24h for 5–7 days per week. Duration dependent on degree of immunosuppression (AII). CMV hyperimmune globulin may decrease morbidity in bone marrow transplant patients with CMV pneumonia (AII).	Use foscarnet or cidofovir for ganciclovir-resistant strains; for HIV-positive children on HAART, CMV may resolve without therapy. Also used for prevention of CMV disease posttransplant for 100–120 days. Data on valganciclovir dosing in young children for treatment of retinitis are unavailable, but consideration can be given to transitioning from IV ganciclovir to oral valganciclovir after improvement of retinitis is noted. Limited data on oral valganciclovir in infants[17,18] (32 mg/kg/day PO div bid) and children (dosing by BSA [dose (mg) = $7 \times$ BSA $\times$ CrCl]).[6]
– Prophylaxis of infection in immunocompromised hosts[5,19]	Ganciclovir 5 mg/kg IV daily (or 3 times/wk) (started at engraftment for stem cell transplant patients) (BII) Valganciclovir at total dose in milligrams = $7 \times$ BSA $\times$ CrCl (use maximum CrCl 150 mL/min/1.73 m²) orally once daily with	Neutropenia is a complication with ganciclovir prophylaxis and may be addressed with G-CSF. Prophylaxis and preemptive strategies are effective; neither has been shown clearly superior to the other.[10]

	food for children 4 mo–16 y (max dose 900 mg/day) for primary prophylaxis in HIV patients[20] who are CMV antibody positive and have severe immunosuppression (CD4 count <50 cells/mm³ in children ≥6 y; CD4 percentage <5% in children <6 y) (CIII)
Enterovirus	Supportive therapy; no antivirals currently FDA approved	Pocapavir PO is currently under investigation for enterovirus (poliovirus). Pleconaril PO is currently under consideration for approval at the FDA for treatment of neonatal enteroviral sepsis syndrome.[21]
Epstein-Barr virus		
– Mononucleosis, encephalitis[22–24]	Limited data suggest small clinical benefit of valacyclovir in adolescents for mononucleosis (3 g/day div tid for 14 days) (CIII). For EBV encephalitis: ganciclovir IV OR acyclovir IV (AIII).	No prospective data on benefits of acyclovir IV or ganciclovir IV in EBV clinical infections of normal hosts. Patients suspected to have infectious mononucleosis should not be given ampicillin or amoxicillin, which cause nonallergic morbilliform rashes in a high proportion of patients with active EBV infection (AII). Therapy with short-course corticosteroids (prednisone 1 mg/kg per day PO [maximum 20 mg/day] for 7 days with subsequent tapering) may have a beneficial effect on acute symptoms in patients with marked tonsillar inflammation with impending airway obstruction, massive splenomegaly, myocarditis, hemolytic anemia, or hemophagocytic lymphohistiocytosis (BIII).
– Posttransplant lymphoproliferative disorder[25,26]	Ganciclovir (AIII)	Decrease immune suppression if possible, as this has the most effect on control of EBV; rituximab, methotrexate have been used but without controlled data. Preemptive treatment with ganciclovir may decrease PTLD in solid organ transplants.

9

Preferred Therapy for Specific Viral Pathogens

Preferred Therapy for Specific Viral Pathogens

9

B. PREFERRED THERAPY FOR SPECIFIC VIRAL PATHOGENS (continued)

Infection	Therapy (evidence grade)	Comments
Hepatitis B virus (chronic)[27-45]	IFN-alfa 3 million U/m² BSA SQ 3 times/wk for 1 wk, followed by dose escalation to 6 million U/m² BSA (max 10 million U/dose), to complete a 24-wk course for children 1–18 y; OR lamivudine 3 mg/kg/day (max 100 mg) PO q24h for 52 wk for children ≥2 y (children coinfected with HIV and HBV should use the approved dose for HIV) (AII); OR adefovir for children ≥12 y (10 mg PO q24h for a minimum of 12 mo; optimum duration of therapy unknown) (BII); OR entecavir for children ≥2 y (optimum duration of therapy unknown) [BII] No prior nucleoside therapy: ≥16 y: 0.5 mg qd 2–15 y: 10–11 kg: 0.15 mg oral solution qd >11–14 kg: 0.2 mg oral solution qd >14–17 kg: 0.25 mg oral solution qd >17–20 kg: 0.3 mg oral solution qd >20–23 kg: 0.35 mg oral solution qd >23–26 kg: 0.4 mg oral solution qd >26–30 kg: 0.45 mg oral solution qd >30 kg: 0.5 mg oral solution or tablet qd Prior nucleoside therapy: Double the dosage in each weight bracket.	Indications for treatment of chronic HBV infection, with or without HIV coinfection, are (1) evidence of ongoing HBV viral replication, as indicated by serum HBV DNA (>20,000 without HBeAg positivity or >2,000 IU/mL with HBeAg positivity) for >6 mo and persistent elevation of serum transaminase levels for >6 mo, or (2) evidence of chronic hepatitis on liver biopsy (BII). Antiviral therapy is not warranted in children without necroinflammatory liver disease (BII). Treatment is not recommended for children with immunotolerant chronic HBV infection (ie, normal serum transaminase levels despite detectable HBV DNA) (BII). Standard IFN-alfa (IFN-2a or 2b) is recommended for treating chronic HBV infection with compensated liver disease in HIV-uninfected children aged ≥2 y who warrant treatment (AI). IFN-alfa therapy in combination with oral antiviral therapy cannot be recommended for pediatric HBV infection in HIV-uninfected children until more data are available (BII). In HIV/HBV-coinfected children who do not require ART for their HIV infection, IFN-alfa therapy is the preferred agent to treat chronic HBV (BIII), whereas adefovir can be considered in children ≥12 y (BIII). Treatment options for HIV/HBV-coinfected children who meet criteria for HBV therapy and who are already receiving lamivudine- or emtricitabine-containing HIV-suppressive ART, include the standard IFN-alfa therapy to the ARV regimen (BIII), or adefovir if the child can receive adult dosing (BIII), or use of tenofovir disoproxil fumarate in children ≥2 y (BII). HIV/HBV-coinfected children should not be given lamivudine (or emtricitabine) without additional anti-HIV drugs for treatment of chronic HBV (CIII).[20]

Alternatives

Tenofovir (adult and adolescent dose [≥12 y] 300 mg qd).

Telbivudine (adult dose 600 mg qd). There are not sufficient clinical data to identify the appropriate dose for use in children.

Lamivudine approved for children ≥2 y, but antiviral resistance develops on therapy in 30%.

Entecavir is superior to lamivudine in the treatment of chronic HBV infection and is the most potent anti-HBV agent available.

Preferred Therapy for Specific Viral Pathogens

B. PREFERRED THERAPY FOR SPECIFIC VIRAL PATHOGENS (continued)

Infection	Therapy (evidence grade)	Comments
Hepatitis C virus (chronic)[46-52]	Treatment of HCV infections in adults has been revolutionized in recent years with the licensure of numerous highly effective direct-acting antiviral drugs for use in adults. Studies of many of these drugs are underway in children, but their optimal use in children and adolescents has yet to be defined. Given the efficacy of these new treatment regimens in adults (AI),[53-68] strong consideration should be given to seeking out these studies if treatment is desired in children and adolescents. An alternative would be to not treat with the approved treatment regimen of IFN + ribavirin pending results of these pediatric studies. If treatment currently is desired and access to the studies of direct-acting antiviral agents is not available, the following treatment is the only one FDA approved for HCV infection in children 3–17 y: Pegylated IFN-alfa: 2a 180 μg/1.73 m² BSA SQ once per wk (maximum dose 180 μg) OR 2b 60 μg/m² BSA once per wk PLUS Ribavirin (oral) 7.5 mg/kg body weight bid (fixed dose by weight recommended) 25–36 kg: 200 mg in am and pm >36–49 kg: 200 mg in am and 400 mg in pm >49–61 kg: 400 mg in am and pm >61–75 kg: 400 mg in am and 600 mg in pm >75 kg: 600 mg in am and pm Treatment duration: 24–48 wk (AII)	None of the direct-acting antiviral HCV drugs currently have been approved for use in children. Treatment of children <3 y who have HCV infection usually is not recommended (BII). HCV-infected, HIV-uninfected children ≥3 y should be individualized because HCV usually causes mild disease in this population and few data exist to identify risk factors differentiating those at greater risk for progression of liver disease. Those who are chosen for treatment should receive combination therapy with IFN-alfa and ribavirin for 48 wk for genotype 1 and 24 wk for genotypes 2 or 3 (AI) (see Therapy column). Treatment should be considered for all HIV/HCV-coinfected children aged >3 y who have no contraindications to treatment (BII). A liver biopsy to stage disease is recommended before deciding whether to initiate therapy for chronic HCV genotype 1 infection (BIII). However, some specialists would treat children infected with HCV genotypes 2 or 3 without first obtaining a liver biopsy (BIII). IFN-alfa therapy is contraindicated for children with decompensated liver disease, substantial cytopenias, renal failure, severe cardiac or neuropsychiatric disorders, and non–HCV-related autoimmune disease (AII).[19]

Herpes simplex virus		
– Third trimester maternal suppressive therapy[69,70]	Acyclovir or valacyclovir maternal suppressive therapy in pregnant women reduces HSV recurrences and viral shedding at the time of delivery but does not fully prevent neonatal HSV[71] (BIII).	
– Neonatal	See Chapter 5.	
– Mucocutaneous (normal host)	Acyclovir 80 mg/kg/day PO div qid (max dose: 800 mg) for 5–7 days, or 15 mg/kg/day IV as 1–2 h infusion div q8h (AII) Suppressive therapy for frequent recurrence (no pediatric data): 20 mg/kg/dose given bid or tid (max dose: 400 mg) for 6–12 mo, then reevaluate need (AIII) Valacyclovir 20 mg/kg/dose (max dose: 1 g) PO bid[72] for 5–7 days (BII)	Foscarnet for acyclovir-resistant strains. Immunocompromised hosts may require 10–14 days of therapy. Topical acyclovir not efficacious and therefore is not recommended.
– Genital	Adult doses: acyclovir 400 mg PO tid for 7–10 days; OR valacyclovir 1 g PO bid for 10 days; OR famciclovir 250 mg PO tid for 7–10 days (AI)	All 3 drugs have been used as prophylaxis to prevent recurrence. Topical acyclovir not efficacious and therefore is not recommended.
– Encephalitis	Acyclovir 60 mg/kg/day IV as 1–2 h infusion div q8h; for 21 days for infants ≤4 mo. For older infants and children, 30–45 mg/kg/day IV as 1–2 h infusion div q8h (AIII).	Safety of high-dose acyclovir (60 mg/kg/day) not well defined beyond the neonatal period; can be used but monitor for neurotoxicity and nephrotoxicity.
– Keratoconjunctivitis	1% trifluridine or 0.15% ganciclovir ophthalmic gel (AII)	Treat in consultation with an ophthalmologist. Topical steroids may be helpful when used together with antiviral agents.

Preferred Therapy for Specific Viral Pathogens

9

B. PREFERRED THERAPY FOR SPECIFIC VIRAL PATHOGENS (continued)

Infection	Therapy (evidence grade)	Comments
Human herpesvirus 6		
– Immunocompromised children[73]	No prospective comparative data; ganciclovir 10 mg/kg/day IV div q12h used in case report (AIII)	May require high dose to control infection; safety and efficacy not defined at high doses.
Human immunodeficiency virus		
Current information on HIV treatment and opportunistic infections for children[74] is posted at http://aidsinfo.nih.gov/ContentFiles/PediatricGuidelines.pdf (accessed September 15, 2016); other information on HIV programs is available at www.cdc.gov/hiv/policies/index.html (accessed September 15, 2016). Consult with an HIV expert, if possible, for current recommendations, as treatment options are complicated and constantly evolving.		
– **Therapy of HIV infection** State-of-the-art therapy is rapidly evolving with introduction of new agents and combinations; currently there are 26 individual ARV agents approved for use by the FDA that have pediatric indications, as well as multiple combinations; guidelines for children and adolescents are continually updated on the AIDSinfo and CDC Web sites given previously.	Effective therapy (HAART) consists of ≥3 agents, including 2 nucleoside reverse transcriptase inhibitors, plus either a protease inhibitor, a non-nucleoside reverse transcriptase inhibitor, or an integrase inhibitor; many different combination regimens give similar treatment outcomes; choice of agents depends on the age of the child, viral load, consideration of potential viral resistance, and extent of immune depletion, in addition to judging the child's ability to adhere to the regimen.	Assess drug toxicity (based on the agents used) and virologic/immunologic response to therapy (quantitative plasma HIV and CD4 count) initially monthly and then every 3–6 mo during the maintenance phase.
– Children of any age	Any child with AIDS or significant HIV-related symptoms (clinical category C and most B conditions) should be treated (AI). Recent guidance from the WHO and HHS guidelines committees now recommend treatment for **all children** regardless of age, CD4 count, or clinical status, with situation-specific levels of urgency.	Adherence counseling and appropriate ARV formulations are critical for successful implementation.

– First 3 y of life	HAART with ≥3 drugs is now recommended for **all infants** ≤36 mo, regardless of clinical status or laboratory values (AI for <12 wk and for >1 y; AII for 12–52 wk).
	Preferred therapy in the first year of life is zidovudine plus lamivudine (at any age) OR abacavir plus lamivudine (>3 mo) plus lopinavir/ritonavir (toxicity concerns preclude its use until a postmenstrual age of 42 wk and a postnatal age of at least 14 days is reached). Raltegravir is equally preferred with lopinavir/ritonavir for children between 2 and 3 of age.
– HIV-infected children ≥3 y to <12 y	**Treat all** with evidence grade for the following CD4 values: 1–<6 y with CD4 <1,000 or <25% (AII) 1–<6 y with CD4 ≥1,000 or ≥25% (BI) ≥6 y with CD4 <500 (AII) ≥6 y with CD4 ≥500 (BI)
	Preferred regimens comprise zidovudine plus lamivudine (at any age) OR abacavir plus lamivudine (>3 mo) PLUS either lopinavir/ritonavir OR efavirenz OR atazanavir/ritonavir OR darunavir/ritonavir OR raltegravir.
– HIV-infected youth ≥12 y	**Treat all with evidence grades of AII–BI depending on CD4 count.**
	Preferred regimens comprise tenofovir or TAF plus emtricitabine (adolescents/Tanner stage 4 or 5) OR abacavir plus lamivudine PLUS either atazanavir/ritonavir OR darunavir/ritonavir OR dolutegravir OR elvitegravir.
– Antiretroviral-experienced child	Consult with HIV specialist.
	Consider treatment history and drug resistance testing and assess adherence.
– **HIV exposures, nonoccupational**	Therapy recommendations for exposures available on the CDC Web site at www.cdc.gov/hiv/guidelines/preventing.html (accessed September 15, 2016)
– Negligible exposure risk (urine, nasal secretions, saliva, sweat, or tears—no visible blood in secretions) OR >72 h since exposure	Prophylaxis not recommended (BIII)
	Postexposure prophylaxis remains unproven but substantial evidence supports its use; consider individually regarding risk, time from exposure, and likelihood of adherence; prophylactic regimens administered for 4 wk.

Preferred Therapy for Specific Viral Pathogens

B. PREFERRED THERAPY FOR SPECIFIC VIRAL PATHOGENS (continued)

Infection	Therapy (evidence grade)	Comments
– Significant exposure risk (blood, semen, vaginal, or rectal secretions from a known HIV-infected individual) AND <72 h since exposure	Prophylaxis recommended (BIII) Preferred regimens 4 wk–<2 y: zidovudine PLUS lamivudine PLUS either raltegravir OR lopinavir/ritonavir 2–12 y: tenofovir PLUS emtricitabine PLUS raltegravir ≥13 y: tenofovir PLUS emtricitabine PLUS either raltegravir OR dolutegravir	Consultation with a pediatric HIV specialist is advised.
– HIV exposure, occupational[75]	See guidelines on CDC Web site at www.cdc.gov/hiv/guidelines/preventing.html (accessed September 15, 2016).	

Influenza virus

Recommendations for the treatment of influenza can vary from season to season; access the American Academy of Pediatrics Web site (www.aap.org) and the CDC Web site (www.cdc.gov/flu/professionals/antivirals/summary-clinicians.htm, accessed September 15, 2016) for the most current, accurate information.

Influenza A and B

Infection	Therapy (evidence grade)	Comments
– Treatment[76–78]	Oseltamivir Preterm, <38 wk postmenstrual age: 1 mg/kg/dose PO bid[76] Preterm, 38–40 wk postmenstrual age: 1.5 mg/kg/dose PO bid[76] Preterm, >40 wk postmenstrual age: 3.0 mg/kg/dose PO bid Term, birth–8 mo: 3.0 mg/kg/dose PO bid 9–11 mo: 3.5 mg/kg/dose PO bid[77] 12–23 mo: 30 mg/dose PO bid 2–12 y: ≤15 kg: 30 mg bid; 16–23 kg: 45 mg bid; 24–40 kg: 60 mg bid; >40 kg: 75 mg bid ≥13 y: 75 mg bid OR zanamivir ≥7 y: 10 mg by inhalation bid for 5 days	Oseltamivir currently is drug of choice for treatment of influenza infections. For patients 12–23 mo, the original FDA-approved unit dose of 30 mg/dose may provide inadequate drug exposure; 3.5 mg/kg/dose PO bid has been studied,[77] but study population sizes were small. Peramivir is a third neuraminidase inhibitor that was approved for use as a parenteral drug in adults in the United States in December 2014. Pediatric studies of parenteral peramivir are underway. Studies of parenteral zanamivir have been completed in children.[79] This formulation of the drug is not yet approved in the United States, though.

	The adamantanes, amantadine and rimantadine, currently are not effective for treatment due to near-universal resistance of influenza A.
– Chemoprophylaxis	Oseltamivir 3 mo–12 y: The prophylaxis dose is one-half of the treatment dose for all ages; the same mg dose that is given bid for treatment is given qd for prophylaxis. Zanamivir ≥5 y: 10 mg by inhalation qd for as long as 28 days (community outbreaks) or 10 days (household setting)	Oseltamivir currently is drug of choice for chemoprophylaxis of influenza infection. Unless the situation is judged critical, oseltamivir chemoprophylaxis not recommended for patients <3 mo because of limited safety and efficacy data in this age group. The adamantanes, amantadine and rimantadine, currently are not effective for chemoprophylaxis of influenza A.
Measles[80]	No prospective data on antiviral therapy. Ribavirin is active against measles virus in vitro. Vitamin A is beneficial in children with measles and is recommended by WHO for all children with measles regardless of their country of residence (qd dosing for 2 days); for children ≥1 y: 200,000 IU; for infants 6–12 mo: 100,000 IU; for infants <6 mo: 50,000 IU (BII). Even in countries where measles is not usually severe, vitamin A should be given to all children with severe measles (eg, requiring hospitalization). Parenteral and oral formulations are available in the United States.	IG prophylaxis for exposed, susceptible children: 0.5 mL/kg (max 15 mL) IM
Respiratory syncytial virus[81,82]		
– Therapy (severe disease in compromised host)	Ribavirin (6-g vial to make 20 mg/mL solution in sterile water), aerosolized over 18–20 h daily for 3–5 days (BII)	Aerosol ribavirin provides a small benefit and should only be used for life-threatening infection with RSV. Airway reactivity with inhalation precludes routine use.

Preferred Therapy for Specific Viral Pathogens

9

B. PREFERRED THERAPY FOR SPECIFIC VIRAL PATHOGENS (continued)

Infection	Therapy (evidence grade)	Comments
– Prophylaxis (palivizumab, Synagis for high-risk infants) (BI)[81,82]	Prophylaxis: palivizumab (a monoclonal antibody) 15 mg/kg IM monthly (max 5 doses) for the following high-risk infants (AI): In first y of life, palivizumab prophylaxis is recommended for infants born before 29 wk 0 days' gestation. Palivizumab prophylaxis is not recommended for otherwise healthy infants born at ≥29 wk 0 days' gestation. In first y of life, palivizumab prophylaxis is recommended for preterm infants with CLD of prematurity, defined as birth at <32 wk 0 days' gestation and a requirement for >21% oxygen for at least 28 days after birth. Clinicians may administer palivizumab prophylaxis in the first y of life to certain infants with hemodynamically significant heart disease.	Palivizumab does not provide benefit in the treatment of an active RSV infection. Palivizumab prophylaxis may be considered for children <24 mo who will be profoundly immunocompromised during the RSV season. Palivizumab prophylaxis is not recommended in the second year of life except for children who required at least 28 days of supplemental oxygen after birth and who continue to require medical support (supplemental oxygen, chronic corticosteroid therapy, or diuretic therapy) during the 6-mo period before the start of the second RSV season. Monthly prophylaxis should be discontinued in any child who experiences a breakthrough RSV hospitalization. Children with pulmonary abnormality or neuromuscular disease that impairs the ability to clear secretions from the upper airways may be considered for prophylaxis in the first year of life. Insufficient data are available to recommend palivizumab prophylaxis for children with cystic fibrosis or Down syndrome. The burden of RSV disease and costs associated with transport from remote locations may result in a broader use of palivizumab for RSV prevention in Alaska Native populations and possibly in selected other American Indian populations. Palivizumab prophylaxis is not recommended for prevention of health care–associated RSV disease.

Varicella-zoster virus[83]		
– Infection in a normal host	Acyclovir 80 mg/kg/day (max single dose 800 mg) PO div qid for 5 days (AI)	The sooner antiviral therapy can be started, the greater the clinical benefit.
– Severe primary chickenpox, disseminated infection (cutaneous, pneumonia, encephalitis, hepatitis); immunocompromised host with primary chickenpox or disseminated zoster	Acyclovir 30 mg/kg/day IV as 1–2 h infusion div q8h for 10 days (acyclovir doses of 45–60 mg/kg/day in 3 div doses IV should be used for disseminated or central nervous system infection). Dosing also can be provided as 1,500 mg/m²/day IV div q8h. Duration in immunocompromised children: 7–14 days, based on clinical response (AI).	Oral valacyclovir, famciclovir, foscarnet also active

10. Preferred Therapy for Specific Parasitic Pathogens

NOTES

- For some parasitic diseases, therapy may be available only from the Centers for Disease Control and Prevention (CDC), as noted. The CDC provides up-to-date information about parasitic diseases and current treatment recommendations at www.cdc.gov/parasites. Consultation is available from the CDC for parasitic disease diagnostic services (www.cdc.gov/dpdx, accessed September 15, 2016); parasitic disease testing and experimental therapy at 404/639-3670; for malaria, 770/488-7788 or 855/856-4713 Monday through Friday, 9:00 am to 5:00 pm ET, and 770/488-7100 after hours, weekends, and holidays. Antiparasitic drugs available from the CDC can be reviewed and requested at www.cdc.gov/laboratory/drugservice/formulary.html (accessed September 15, 2016).

- Additional information about many of the organisms and diseases mentioned here, along with treatment recommendations, can be found in the appropriate sections in the American Academy of Pediatrics *Red Book*.

- **Abbreviations:** AmB, amphotericin B; A-P, atovaquone/proguanil; bid, twice daily; BP, blood pressure; CDC, Centers for Disease Control and Prevention; CNS, central nervous system; CrCl, creatinine clearance; CSF, cerebrospinal fluid; DEC, diethylcarbamazine; div, divided; DS, double strength; ECG, electrocardiogram; FDA, US Food and Drug Administration; G6PD, glucose-6-phosphate dehydrogenase; GI, gastrointestinal; h, hour; HAART, highly active antiretroviral therapy; HIV, human immunodeficiency virus; IM, intramuscular; IV, intravenous; MRI, magnetic resonance imaging; PAIR, percutaneous aspiration, injection, re-aspiration; PHMB, polyhexamethylene biguanide; PO, orally; qd, once daily; qid, 4 times daily; qod, every other day; spp, species; tab, tablet; tid, 3 times daily; TMP/SMX, trimethoprim/sulfamethoxazole.

Preferred Therapy for Specific Parasitic Pathogens

10

PREFERRED THERAPY FOR SPECIFIC PARASITIC PATHOGENS

Disease/Organism	Treatment (evidence grade)	Comments
AMEBIASIS[1–5]		
Entamoeba histolytica		
– Asymptomatic intestinal colonization	Paromomycin 25–35 mg/kg/day PO div tid for 7 days; OR iodoquinol 30–40 mg/kg/day (max 650 mg/dose) PO div tid for 20 days; OR diloxanide furoate (not commercially available in the United States) 20 mg/kg/day PO div tid (max 500 mg/dose) for 10 days (CII)	Follow-up stool examination to ensure eradication of carriage; screen/treat positive close contacts. *Entamoeba dispar* infections do not require treatment.
– Colitis	Metronidazole 35–50 mg/kg/day PO div tid for 10 days; OR tinidazole (age >3 y) 50 mg/kg/day PO (max 2 g) qd for 3 days FOLLOWED by paromomycin or iodoquinol as above to eliminate cysts (BII)	Avoid antimotility drugs, steroids. Take tinidazole with food to decrease GI side effects; if unable to take tabs, pharmacists can crush tabs and mix with syrup. Avoid alcohol ingestion with metronidazole and tinidazole. Preliminary data support use of nitazoxanide to treat clinical infection but it may not prevent parasitologic failure: age ≥12 y, 500 mg bid for 3 days; ages 4–11 y, 200 mg bid for 3 days; ages 1–3 y, 100 mg bid for 3 days.
– Liver abscess, extraintestinal disease	Metronidazole 35–50 mg/kg/day IV q8h, switch to PO when tolerated, for 10 days; OR tinidazole (age >3 y) 50 mg/kg/day PO (max 2 g) qd for 5 days FOLLOWED by paromomycin or iodoquinol as above to eliminate cysts (BII) Nitazoxanide 500 mg bid for 10 days (≥12 y)	Serologic assays >95% positive in extraintestinal amebiasis. Percutaneous or surgical drainage may be indicated for large liver abscesses or inadequate response to medical therapy. Avoid alcohol ingestion with metronidazole and tinidazole. Take tinidazole with food to decrease GI side effects; if unable to take tabs, pharmacists can crush tabs and

MENINGOENCEPHALITIS[6–10]

Naegleria	AmB 1.5 mg/kg/day IV qd ± intrathecally PLUS rifampin 10 mg/kg/day PO qd or div tid PLUS fluconazole 10 mg/kg/day IV or PO qd PLUS miltefosine <45 kg 50 mg PO bid; ≥45 kg 50 mg PO tid PLUS azithromycin 500 mg IV or PO; duration uncertain with ranges from 9–30 days; PLUS steroids to control cerebral edema	Optimal treatment regimen uncertain. Liposomal AmB is less effective in animal models. Treatment outcomes usually unsuccessful; early therapy (even before diagnostic confirmation if indicated) may improve survival.
Acanthamoeba	Combination regimens including miltefosine, fluconazole, and pentamidine favored by some experts; TMP/SMX, metronidazole, and a macrolide may be added. Other drugs that have been used alone or in combination include rifampin, azoles, pentamidine, sulfadiazine, flucytosine, and caspofungin. Keratitis: topical therapies include PHMB (0.02%) or biguanide chlorhexidine, combined with propamidine isethionate (0.1%) or hexamidine (0.1%) (topical therapies not approved in United States but available at compounding pharmacies).	Optimal treatment regimens uncertain; combination therapy favored Keratitis should be evaluated by an ophthalmologist. Prolonged treatment often needed.
Balamuthia	Combination regimens preferred. Drugs that have been used alone or in combination include pentamidine, 5-flucytosine, fluconazole, macrolides, sulfadiazine, miltefosine, thioridazine, AmB, itraconazole, and albendazole.	Optimal treatment regimen uncertain; regimens based on case reports. Surgical resection of CNS lesions may be beneficial.
Hartmannella spp		
Ancylostoma caninum	See EOSINOPHILIC COLITIS.	

10

Preferred Therapy for Specific Parasitic Pathogens

Preferred Therapy for Specific Parasitic Pathogens

10

PREFERRED THERAPY FOR SPECIFIC PARASITIC PATHOGENS (continued)

Disease/Organism	Treatment (evidence grade)	Comments
Ancylostoma duodenale	SEE HOOKWORM.	
ANGIOSTRONGYLIASIS[1-14]		
Angiostrongylus cantonensis (cerebral disease)	Supportive care	Most patients recover without antiparasitic therapy; treatment may provoke severe neurologic symptoms. Corticosteroids, analgesics, and repeat lumbar puncture may be of benefit. Prednisolone (60 mg daily for 2 wk) may shorten duration of headache and reduce need for repeat lumbar puncture. Ocular disease may require surgery or laser treatment.
Angiostrongylus costaricensis (eosinophilic enterocolitis)	Supportive care	Surgery may be pursued to exclude another diagnosis such as appendicitis.
ASCARIASIS (*Ascaris lumbricoides*)[15]	First line: albendazole 400 mg PO once OR mebendazole 500 mg once or 100 mg bid for 3 days (BII) Pregnant women: pyrantel pamoate 11 mg/kg max 1 g once Alternatives: ivermectin 150–200 µg/kg PO once (CII); nitazoxanide 7.5 mg/kg once	Follow-up stool ova and parasite examination after therapy not essential. Take albendazole with food (bioavailability increases with food, especially fatty meals). Albendazole has theoretic risk of causing seizures in patients coinfected with cysticercosis.
BABESIOSIS (*Babesia* spp)[16-18]	Clindamycin 30 mg/kg/day IV or PO div tid (max 600 mg per dose), PLUS quinine 25 mg/kg/day PO (max 650 mg/dose) div tid for 7–10 days (BII) (preferred for severe disease); OR atovaquone 40 mg/kg/day (max 750 mg/dose) div bid, PLUS azithromycin 12 mg/kg/day (max 500 mg/dose) for 7–10 days (CII) (preferred for mild disease due to more favorable adverse event profile)	Daily monitoring of hematocrit and percentage of parasitized red blood cells (until <5%) should be done. Exchange blood transfusion may be of benefit for severe disease; *Babesia divergens*. Higher doses of medications and prolonged therapy may be needed for asplenic or immunocompromised individuals.
Balantidium coli[19]	Tetracycline (patients >7 y) 40 mg/kg/day PO div qid for 10 days (max 2 g/day) (CII); OR metronidazole 35–50 mg/kg/day PO tid for 5 days	Repeated stool examination may be needed for diagnosis; prompt stool examination may increase detection of rapidly degenerating trophozoites. Follow-up stool exam if symptoms continue

Baylisascaris procyonis[20,21] (raccoon roundworm)	Albendazole 25 mg/kg/day PO div q12h for 20 days given as soon as possible after exposure (ingestion of raccoon feces, etc) might prevent clinical disease (CIII).	Therapy generally unsuccessful to prevent fatal outcome or severe neurologic sequelae once CNS disease present. Steroids may be of value in decreasing inflammation in CNS or ocular infection. Retinal worms may be killed by direct photocoagulation. If albendazole not immediately available, mebendazole, levamisole, or ivermectin may be useful in the interim. Albendazole bioavailability increased with food, especially fatty meals.
Blastocystis spp[22,23]	Metronidazole 30 mg/kg/day (max 750 mg per dose) PO div tid for 5–10 days (BII); OR tinidazole 50 mg/kg (max 2 g) once (age >3 y) (BII)	Pathogenesis debated. Asymptomatic individuals do not need treatment; diligent search for other pathogenic parasites recommended for symptomatic individuals with *B hominis*. Paromomycin, nitazoxanide, and TMP/SMX also may be effective. Metronidazole resistance may occur. Take tinidazole with food; tablets may be crushed and mixed with flavored syrup.
CHAGAS DISEASE (*Trypanosoma cruzi*)[24-26]	See TRYPANOSOMIASIS.	
Clonorchis sinensis	See FLUKES.	

10

Preferred Therapy for Specific Parasitic Pathogens

PREFERRED THERAPY FOR SPECIFIC PARASITIC PATHOGENS (continued)

Disease/Organism	Treatment (evidence grade)	Comments
CRYPTOSPORIDIOSIS (*Cryptosporidium parvum*)[27–30]	Nitazoxanide, age 12–47 mo, 5 mL (100 mg) bid for 3 days; age 4–11 y, 10 mL (200 mg) bid for 3 days; age ≥12 y, 500 mg (tab or suspension) PO bid for 3 days (BII). Paromomycin 30 mg/kg/day div bid–qid (CII); OR azithromycin 10 mg/kg/day for 5 days (CII); or paromomycin AND azithromycin given as combination therapy may yield initial response but may not result in sustained cure in immunocompromised individuals.	Recovery depends largely on the immune status of the host; treatment not required in all immunocompetent individuals. Medical therapy may have limited efficacy in HIV-infected patients not receiving HAART.
CUTANEOUS LARVA MIGRANS or CREEPING ERUPTION[31,32] (dog and cat hookworm) (*Ancylostoma caninum, Ancylostoma braziliense, Uncinaria stenocephala*)	Albendazole 15 mg/kg/day (max 400 mg) PO qd for 3 days (CII); OR ivermectin 200 µg/kg PO for 1–2 days (CII)	Albendazole bioavailability increased with food, especially fatty meals
***Cyclospora* spp**[33,34] (cyanobacterium-like agent)	TMP/SMX 10 mg TMP/kg/day (max 1 DS tablet) PO div bid for 7–10 days (BIII); OR nitazoxanide 500 mg bid for 7 days	HIV-infected patients may require higher doses/longer therapy. Ciprofloxacin 30 mg/kg/day div bid for 7 days is an alternative, although treatment failures have been reported.
CYSTICERCOSIS[35–38] (*Cysticercus cellulosae*; larva of *Taenia solium*)	Neurocysticercosis. Albendazole 15 mg/kg/day PO bid (max 800 mg/day) (CII) plus steroids (prednisone 1.0 mg/kg/day or dexamethasone 0.1 mg/kg/day) for 5–10 days followed by rapid taper to reduce inflammation associated with dying organisms; OR praziquantel 50 mg/kg/day PO div tid (CII) plus steroids (prednisone 1.0 mg/kg/day or dexamethasone 0.1 mg/kg/day) (AI) for 5–10 days followed by rapid taper.	Collaboration with a specialist with experience treating this condition recommended Management of seizures, edema, intracranial hypertension, or hydrocephalus, when present, is the focus of initial therapy. Treatment generally recommended for symptomatic patients with multiple live lesions; generally will not provide benefit when all lesions are calcified, although viable, live cysts may not be identified on MRI scans.

	Steroids may not be needed for single lesion disease, as there may be minimal CNS swelling with treatment, particularly if there are few viable parasites present at the time of treatment.[38] Intravesicular and intraocular cysts should be treated with surgical removal; antiparasitic therapy relatively contraindicated.
Combination therapy with albendazole plus praziquantel may be more effective than albendazole alone (CII). Optimal duration of therapy depends on form of disease (single enhancing lesions, 3–7 days; multiple viable parenchymal lesion, 10–14 days; subarachnoid disease, prolonged [≥28 days] therapy).	
	Treatment indicated when no other cause except *Dientamoeba* found for abdominal pain or diarrhea lasting more than a week. Take paromomycin with meals and iodoquinol after meals. Tinidazole, nitazoxanide, and doxycycline also may be effective. Albendazole and mebendazole have no activity against *Dientamoeba*.
DIENTAMOEBIASIS[39,40] (*Dientamoeba fragilis*)	Metronidazole 35–50 mg/kg/day PO div tid for 10 days (max 500–750 mg/dose); OR paromomycin 25–35 mg/kg/day PO div tid for 7 days; OR iodoquinol 30–40 mg/kg/day (max 650 mg/dose) PO div tid for 20 days (BII)
Diphyllobothrium latum	See TAPEWORMS.
ECHINOCOCCOSIS[41,42]	
	Involvement with specialist with experience treating this condition recommended. Surgery is the treatment of choice for management of complicated cysts. PAIR technique effective for appropriate cysts. Praziquantel has proto-scolicidal activity but clinical efficacy variable; may be used in combination therapy with albendazole.
Echinococcus granulosus	Albendazole 15 mg/kg/day PO bid (max 800 mg/day) for 1–6 mo alone (CIII) or as adjunctive therapy with surgery or percutaneous treatment; initiate 4–30 days before and continue for at least 1 mo after surgery.
	Surgical treatment generally the treatment of choice; postoperative albendazole 15 mg/kg/day PO bid (max 800 mg/day) should be administered to reduce relapse; duration uncertain (at least 2 y with long-term monitoring for relapse). Benefit of preoperative albendazole unknown.
Echinococcus multilocularis	

10

10

PREFERRED THERAPY FOR SPECIFIC PARASITIC PATHOGENS (continued)

Disease/Organism	Treatment (evidence grade)	Comments
Entamoeba histolytica	See AMEBIASIS.	
Enterobius vermicularis	See PINWORMS.	
Fasciola hepatica	See FLUKES.	
EOSINOPHILIC COLITIS[43] (*Ancylostoma caninum*)	Albendazole 400 mg PO once or mebendazole 100 mg bid for 3 days (BIII)	Endoscopic removal may be considered if medical treatment not successful.
EOSINOPHILIC MENINGITIS	See ANGIOSTRONGYLIASIS.	
FILARIASIS[44,45]		
– River blindness (*Onchocerca volvulus*)	Ivermectin 150 µg/kg PO once (AII); repeat q6–12mo until asymptomatic and no ongoing exposure; OR doxycycline 100–200 mg PO daily for 6 wk followed by a single dose of ivermectin	Doxycycline targets *Wolbachia*, the endosymbiotic bacteria associated with *O volvulus*.
– *Wuchereria bancrofti, Brugia malayi, Brugia timori, Mansonella streptocerca*	DEC (from CDC) 6 mg/kg/day div tid for 12 days OR 6 mg/kg/day PO as a single dose (AII). Consider adding doxycycline 200 mg daily for 4–6 wk.	Avoid DEC with *Onchocerca* and *Loa loa* coinfection; doxycycline (200 mg daily for 4–6 wk) may be used; albendazole is an alternative if doxycycline cannot be used.
Mansonella ozzardi	Ivermectin 200 µg/kg PO once may be effective.	DEC and albendazole not effective
Mansonella perstans	Albendazole 400 mg PO bid for 10 days or mebendazole 100 mg PO bid for 30 days	Relatively resistant to DEC and ivermectin; doxycycline 200 mg daily for 6 wk beneficial for clearing microfilaria in Mali
Loa loa	When no evidence of microfilaremia: DEC (from CDC) 8–10 mg/kg/day PO div tid for 21 days. When microfilaremia present: day 1: 1 mg/kg (max 50 mg); day 2: 1 mg/kg (max 50 mg) div tid; day 3: 1–2 mg/kg (max 100 mg) div tid; days 4–21: 9 mg/kg/day PO div tid	Albendazole is an alternative agent.

Tropical pulmonary eosinophilia[46]	DEC (from CDC) 6 mg/kg/day PO tid for 12–21 days; antihistamines/corticosteroids for allergic reactions (CII)
FLUKES	
Liver flukes[47] (*Clonorchis sinensis*, *Opisthorchis* spp)	Praziquantel 75 mg/kg PO div tid for 2 days (BII); OR albendazole 10 mg/kg/day PO for 7 days (CIII) OR mebendazole 30 mg/kg for 20–30 days	Take praziquantel with liquids and food.
Lung fluke[48,49] (*Paragonimus westermani* and other *Paragonimus* lung flukes)	Praziquantel 75 mg/kg PO div tid for 3 days (BII)	Triclabendazole (available from CDC) (10 mg/kg PO once or twice) may also be effective; triclabendazole should be taken with food to facilitate absorption.
Sheep liver fluke[50] (*Fasciola hepatica*)	Triclabendazole (from CDC) 10 mg/kg PO for 1–2 days (BII) OR nitazoxanide PO (take with food), age 12–47 mo, 100 mg/dose bid for 7 days; age 4–11 y, 200 mg/dose bid for 7 days; age ≥12 y, 1 tab (500 mg)/dose bid for 7 days (CII)	Responds poorly to praziquantel; albendazole and mebendazole ineffective
GIARDIASIS (*Giardia intestinalis* [formerly *lamblia*])[51-53]	Metronidazole 15–30 mg/kg/day (max 250 mg/dose) PO div tid for 5–7 days (BII); OR tinidazole 50 mg/kg/day (max 2 g) for 1 day (BII); OR nitazoxanide PO (take with food), age 1–3 y, 100 mg/dose bid for 3 days; age 4–11 y, 200 mg/dose bid for 3 days; age ≥12 y, 500 mg/dose bid for 3 days (BII)	Alternatives: albendazole 10–15 mg/kg/day (max 400 mg/dose) PO for 5 days (CII) OR mebendazole 200 mg PO tid for 5 days; OR paromomycin 30 mg/kg/day div tid for 5–10 days; furazolidone 6 mg/kg/day in 4 doses for 7–10 days (not available in United States). If therapy ineffective, may try a higher dose or longer course of the same agent, or an agent in a different class; combination therapy may be considered for refractory cases. Prolonged courses may be needed for immunocompromised patients (eg, hypogammaglobulinemia). Treatment of asymptomatic carriers not usually indicated.

10

Preferred Therapy for Specific Parasitic Pathogens

PREFERRED THERAPY FOR SPECIFIC PARASITIC PATHOGENS (continued)

Disease/Organism	Treatment (evidence grade)	Comments
HOOKWORM[54–56]		
Necator americanus, Ancylostoma duodenale	Albendazole 400 mg once (repeat dose may be necessary) (BII); OR mebendazole 100 mg PO for 3 days; OR pyrantel pamoate 11 mg/kg (max 1 g/day) (BII) PO qd for 3 days	
Hymenolepis nana	See TAPEWORMS.	
Cystoisospora belli (formerly Isospora belli)[19]	TMP/SMX 8–10 mg TMP/kg/day PO (or IV) div bid for 7–10 days (max 160 mg TMP/800 mg SMX bid); OR ciprofloxacin 500 mg PO div bid for 7 days	Infection often self-limited in immunocompetent hosts; consider treatment if symptoms do not resolve by 5–7 days or are severe. Pyrimethamine plus leucovorin and nitazoxanide are alternatives. Immunocompromised patients should be treated; longer courses or suppressive therapy may be needed for severely immunocompromised patients.
LEISHMANIASIS,[57–63] **including kala-azar**		
Leishmania spp	Visceral: liposomal AmB 3 mg/kg/day on days 1–5, day 14, and day 21 (AI); OR sodium stibogluconate (from CDC) 20 mg/kg/day IM or IV for 28 days (or longer) (BIII); OR miltefosine 2.5 mg/kg/day PO (max 150 mg/day) for 28 days (BIII); OR AmB 1 mg/kg/day IV daily for 15–20 days or qod for 4–8 wk (BIII). Uncomplicated cutaneous: combination of debridement of eschars, cryotherapy, thermotherapy, intralesional pentavalent antimony, and topical paromomycin (not available in United States). Complicated cutaneous: oral or parenteral systemic therapy with miltefosine 2.5 mg/kg/day PO (max 150 mg/day) for 28 days (BIII); OR sodium stibogluconate 20 mg/kg/day IM or IV for 10–20 days (BIII); OR	Consultation with a specialist familiar with management of leishmaniasis is advised strongly, especially when treating patients with HIV coinfection. Region where infection acquired, species of Leishmania, skill of practitioner with some local therapies, and drugs available in the United States affect therapeutic choices. For immunocompromised patients, FDA-approved dosing of liposomal amphotericin is 4 mg/kg on days 1–5, 10, 17, 24, 31, and 38, with further therapy on an individual basis.

pentamidine isethionate 2–4 mg/kg IV or IM daily or qod for 4–7 doses or until healed (BII); OR amphotericin 0.5–1 mg/kg IV qod for 20–30 days; OR azoles (fluconazole 200–600 mg PO qd for 6 wk; or ketoconazole or itraconazole; treatment failures are common).

Mucosal: sodium stibogluconate 20 mg/kg/day IM or IV for 28 days (may use with pentoxifylline for synergistic activity); OR AmB 0.5–1 mg/kg/day IV daily for 15–20 days or qod for 4–8 wk; OR miltefosine 2.5 mg/kg/day PO (max 150 mg/day) for 28 days.

LICE

Pediculosis capitis or humanus, Phthirus pubis[64]	Follow manufacturer's instructions for topical use: permethrin 1% (≥2 mo) OR pyrethrin (children aged ≥2 y) (BII); OR 0.5% ivermectin lotion (BII); OR spinosad 0.9% topical suspension (≥6 mo) (BIII); OR benzyl alcohol lotion 5% (≥6 mo) (BIII); OR malathion 0.5% (children aged ≥2 y) (BIII); OR topical or oral ivermectin 200 µg/kg PO once (400 µg/kg for ≥15 kg).	Launder bedding and clothing; for eyelash infestation, use petrolatum; for head lice, remove nits with comb designed for that purpose. Benzyl alcohol can be irritating to skin; parasite resistance unlikely to develop. Consult health care professional before re-treatment with ivermectin lotion; re-treatment with spinosad topical suspension usually not needed unless live lice seen 1 wk after treatment. Administration of 3 doses of ivermectin (1 dose/wk separately by weekly intervals) may be needed to eradicate heavy infection.

MALARIA[65–69]

Plasmodium falciparum, Plasmodium vivax, Plasmodium ovale, Plasmodium malariae	CDC Malaria Hotline 770/488-7788 or 855/856-4713 toll-free (Monday–Friday, 9:00 am–5:00 pm ET) or emergency consultation after hours 770/488-7100; online information at www.cdc.gov/malaria (accessed September 15, 2016). Consult infectious diseases or tropical medicine specialist if unfamiliar with malaria.	Consultation with a specialist familiar with management of malaria is advised, especially for severe malaria. No antimalarial drug provides absolute protection against malaria; fever after return from an endemic area should prompt an immediate evaluation. Emphasize personal protective measures (insecticides, bed nets, clothing, and avoidance of dusk–dawn mosquito exposures).

Preferred Therapy for Specific Parasitic Pathogens

PREFERRED THERAPY FOR SPECIFIC PARASITIC PATHOGENS (continued)

Disease/Organism	Treatment (evidence grade)	Comments
Prophylaxis		
For areas with chloroquine-resistant *P falciparum* or *P vivax*	A-P: 5–8 kg, ½ pediatric tab/day; ≥9–10 kg, ¾ pediatric tab/day; ≥11–20 kg, 1 pediatric tab (62.5 mg atovaquone/25 mg proguanil); ≥21–30 kg, 2 pediatric tabs; ≥31–40 kg, 3 pediatric tabs; ≥40 kg, 1 adult tab (250 mg atovaquone/100 mg proguanil) PO daily starting 1–2 days before travel and continuing 7 days after last exposure; for children <5 kg, data on A-P limited (BII); OR mefloquine: for children <5 kg, 5 mg/kg; ≥5–9 kg, ⅛ tab; ≥10–19 kg, ¼ tab; 20–30 kg, ½ tab; ≥31–45 kg, ¾ tab; ≥45 kg (adult dose), 1 tab PO once weekly starting the wk before arrival in area and continuing for 4 wk after leaving area (BII); OR doxycycline (patients >7 y): 2 mg/kg (max 100 mg) PO daily starting 1–2 days before arrival in area and continuing for 4 wk after leaving area (BII); OR primaquine (check for G6PD deficiency before administering): 0.5 mg/kg base daily starting 1 day before travel and continuing for 5 days after last exposure (BII)	Avoid mefloquine for persons with a history of seizures or psychosis, active depression, or cardiac conduction abnormalities; see black box warning. Avoid A-P in severe renal impairment (CrCl <30). *P falciparum* resistance to mefloquine exists along the borders between Thailand and Myanmar and Thailand and Cambodia, Myanmar and China, and Myanmar and Laos; isolated resistance has been reported in southern Vietnam. Take doxycycline with adequate fluids to avoid esophageal irritation and food to avoid GI side effects; use sunscreen and avoid excessive sun exposure.
For areas without chloroquine-resistant *P falciparum* or *P vivax*	Chloroquine phosphate 5 mg base/kg (max 300 mg base) PO once weekly, beginning the wk before arrival in area and continuing for 4 wk after leaving area (available in suspension outside the United States and Canada and at compounding pharmacies) (AII). For heavy or prolonged (months) exposure to mosquitoes: consider treatment with primaquine (check for G6PD deficiency before administering) 0.5 mg base/kg PO qd with final 2 wk of chloroquine for prevention of relapse with *P ovale* or *P vivax*.	

Treatment of disease

– Chloroquine-resistant *P falciparum* or *P vivax*	Oral therapy: artemether/lumefantrine 6 doses over 3 days at 0, 8, 24, 36, 48, and 60 h; <15 kg, 1 tab/dose; ≥15–25 kg, 2 tabs/dose; ≥25–35 kg, 3 tabs/dose; ≥35 kg, 4 tabs/dose (BII); A-P: for children <5 kg, data limited; ≥5–8 kg, 2 pediatric tabs (62.5 mg atovaquone/25 mg proguanil) PO qd for 3 days; ≥9–10 kg, 3 pediatric tabs qd for 3 days; ≥11–20 kg, 1 adult tab (250 mg atovaquone/100 mg proguanil) qd for 3 days; ≥21–30 kg, 2 adult tabs qd for 3 days; 31–40 kg, 3 adult tabs qd for 3 days; ≥40 kg, 4 adult tabs qd for 3 days (BII); OR quinine 30 mg/kg/day (max 2 g/day) PO div tid for 3–7 days AND doxycycline (age >7 y) 4 mg/kg/day div bid for 7 days OR clindamycin 30 mg/kg/day div tid (max 900 mg tid) for 7 days.

Parenteral therapy (check with CDC): quinidine gluconate salt 10 mg/kg (max 600 mg) IV (1 h infusion in normal saline) followed by continuous infusion of 0.02 mg/kg/min until oral therapy can be given (BII); alternative: artesunate 2.4 mg/kg/dose IV for 3 days at 0, 12, 24, 48, and 72 h (from CDC) (BI) AND a second oral agent (A-P, clindamycin, or doxycycline for aged ≥7 y).

For prevention of relapse with *P vivax, P ovale*: primaquine (check for G6PD deficiency before administering) 0.5 mg base/kg/day PO for 14 days. | Mild disease may be treated with oral antimalarial drugs; severe disease (impaired level of consciousness, convulsion, hypotension, or parasitemia >5%) should be treated parenterally.

Avoid mefloquine for treatment of malaria if possible given higher dose and increased incidence of adverse events.

Take clindamycin and doxycycline with plenty of liquids.

Do not use primaquine during pregnancy.

For relapses of primaquine-resistant *P vivax* or *P ovale*, consider retreating with primaquine 30 mg (base) for 28 days.

Continuously monitor ECG, BP, and glucose in patients receiving quinidine.

Avoid artemether/lumefantrine and mefloquine in patients with cardiac arrhythmias, and avoid concomitant use of drugs that prolong QT interval.

Take A-P and artemether/lumefantrine with food or milk.

Use artesunate for quinidine intolerance, lack of quinidine availability, or treatment failure; www.cdc.gov/malaria/resources/pdf/treatmenttable.pdf (accessed September 15, 2016); artemisinin should be used in combination with other drugs to avoid resistance. |
| – Chloroquine-susceptible *P falciparum*, chloroquine-susceptible *P vivax, P ovale, P malariae* | Oral therapy: chloroquine 10 mg/kg base (max 600 mg base) PO then 5 mg/kg 6, 24, and 48 h after initial dose.

Parenteral therapy: quinidine, as above.

See above for prevention of relapse due to *P vivax* and *P ovale*. | Alternative if chloroquine not available: hydroxychloroquine 10 mg base/kg PO immediately, followed by 5 mg base/kg PO at 6, 24, and 48 hours. |

Preferred Therapy for Specific Parasitic Pathogens

10

PREFERRED THERAPY FOR SPECIFIC PARASITIC PATHOGENS (continued)

Disease/Organism	Treatment (evidence grade)	Comments
Paragonimus westermani	See FLUKES.	
PINWORMS (*Enterobius vermicularis*)	Mebendazole 100 mg once, repeat in 2 wk; OR albendazole <20 kg, 200 mg PO once; ≥20 kg, 400 mg PO once; repeat in 2 wk (BII); OR pyrantel pamoate 11 mg/kg (max 1 g) PO once (BII); repeat in 2 wk.	Treat entire household (and if this fails, consider close child care/school contacts); re-treatment of contacts after 2 wk may be needed to prevent reinfection.
PNEUMOCYSTIS	See Chapter 8, Table 8B, *Pneumocystis jiroveci (carinii)* pneumonia.	
SCABIES (*Sarcoptes scabiei*)[70]	Permethrin 5% cream applied to entire body (including scalp in infants), left on for 8–14 h then bathe, repeat in 1 wk (BII); OR ivermectin 200 µg/kg PO once weekly for 2 doses (BII); OR crotamiton 10% applied topically overnight on days 1, 2, 3, and 8, bathe in am (BII).	Launder bedding and clothing. Reserve lindane for patients who do not respond to other therapy. Crotamiton treatment failure has been observed. Ivermectin safety not well established in children <15 kg and pregnant women. Itching may continue for weeks after successful treatment; can be managed with antihistamines.
SCHISTOSOMIASIS (*Schistosoma haematobium, Schistosoma japonicum, Schistosoma mansoni, Schistosoma mekongi, Schistosoma intercalatum*)[71–73]	Praziquantel 40 (for *S haematobium, S mansoni,* and *S intercalatum*) or 60 (for *S japonicum* and *S mekongi*) mg/kg/day PO div bid (if 40 mg/day) or tid (if 60 mg/day) for 1 day (AI)	Take praziquantel with food and liquids. Oxamniquine (not available in United States) 20 mg/kg PO div bid for 1 day (Brazil) or 40–60 mg/kg/day for 2–3 days (most of Africa) (BII).
STRONGYLOIDIASIS (*Strongyloides stercoralis*)[74,75]	Ivermectin 200 µg/kg PO qd for 1–2 days (BII); OR albendazole 400 mg PO bid for 7 days (or longer for disseminated disease) (BII)	Albendazole is less effective but may be adequate if longer courses used. For immunocompromised patients (especially with hyperinfection syndrome), parenteral veterinary formulations may be lifesaving. Ivermectin safety not well established in children <15 kg and pregnant women.

TAPEWORMS

– *Taenia saginata, Taenia solium, Hymenolepis nana, Diphyllobothrium latum, Dipylidium caninum*	Praziquantel 5–10 mg/kg PO once (25 mg/kg once then repeated 10 days later for *H nana*) (BIII); OR niclosamide 50 mg/kg (max 2 g) PO once, chewed thoroughly (not available in United States)	Nitazoxanide may be effective (published clinical data limited) 500 mg PO bid for 3 days for >11 y of age; 200 mg PO bid for 3 days for ages 4–11 y; 100 mg PO bid for 3 days for ages 1–3 y.
TOXOCARIASIS[76] (*Toxocara canis* [dog roundworm] and *Toxocara cati* [cat roundworm])	Visceral larval migrans: albendazole 400 mg PO bid for 5 days (BII) Ocular larva migrants: albendazole 400 mg PO daily (800 mg daily for adults) for 2–4 wk with prednisone (0.5–1 mg/kg/day with slow taper)	Mild disease often resolves without treatment. Corticosteroids may be used for severe symptoms in visceral larval migrans. Mebendazole (100–200 mg/day PO bid for 5 days) and DEC (available only from CDC) are alternatives.
TOXOPLASMOSIS (*Toxoplasma gondii*)[77–79]	Pyrimethamine 2 mg/kg/day PO div bid for 2 days (max 100 mg) then 1 mg/kg/day (max 25 mg/day) PO daily AND sulfadiazine 120 mg/kg/day PO div qid (max 6 g/day); with supplemental folinic acid and leucovorin 10–25 mg with each dose of pyrimethamine (AI) for 3–6 wk. See Chapter 5 for congenital infection. For treatment in pregnancy, spiramycin 50–100 mg/kg/day PO qid (available as investigational therapy through the FDA at 301/796-0563) (CII).	Experienced ophthalmologic consultation encouraged for treatment of ocular disease. Treatment continued for 2 wk after resolution of illness (approximately 3–6 wk); concurrent corticosteroids given for ocular or CNS infection. Prolonged therapy if HIV positive. Take pyrimethamine with food to decrease GI adverse effects; sulfadiazine should be taken on an empty stomach with water. Clindamycin, azithromycin, or atovaquone plus pyrimethamine may be effective for patients intolerant of sulfa-containing drugs. Consult expert advice for treatment during pregnancy and management of congenital infection.
TRAVELERS' DIARRHEA[80–82]	Azithromycin 10 mg/kg qd for 1–3 days (BII); OR rifaximin 200 mg PO tid for 3 days (ages ≥12 y) (BIII); OR ciprofloxacin (BII); OR cefixime (CII); OR rifaximin 200 mg tid for 3 days for ages ≥12 y.	Azithromycin preferable to ciprofloxacin for travelers to Southeast Asia given high prevalence of quinolone-resistant *Campylobacter*. Rifaximin may not be as efficacious for *Shigella* and other enterics in patients with bloody diarrhea and invasive infection.

10

Preferred Therapy for Specific Parasitic Pathogens

PREFERRED THERAPY FOR SPECIFIC PARASITIC PATHOGENS (continued)

Disease/Organism	Treatment (evidence grade)	Comments
TRICHINELLOSIS (*Trichinella spiralis*)[83]	Albendazole 20 mg/kg/day (max 400 mg/dose) PO div bid for 8–14 days (BII) OR mebendazole 200–400 mg PO tid for 3 days, then 400–500 mg PO tid for 10 days	Therapy ineffective for larvae already in muscles. Anti-inflammatory drugs, steroids for CNS or cardiac involvement or severe symptoms.
TRICHOMONIASIS (*Trichomonas vaginalis*)	Tinidazole 50 mg/kg (max 2 g) PO for 1 dose (BII) OR metronidazole 500 mg PO tid for 7 days (BII)	Treat sex partners simultaneously. Metronidazole resistance occurs and may be treated with higher-dose metronidazole or tinidazole.
Trichuris trichiura	See WHIPWORM (TRICHURIASIS).	
TRYPANOSOMIASIS		
– Chagas disease[24-26] (*Trypanosoma cruzi*)	Benznidazole PO (from CDC): age <12 y, 5–7.5 mg/kg/day div bid for 60 days; ≥12 y, 5–7 mg/kg/day div bid for 60 days (BIII); OR nifurtimox PO (from CDC): age 1–10 y, 15–20 mg/kg/day div tid or qid for 90 days; 11–16 y, 12.5–15 mg/kg/day div tid or qid for 90 days; ≥17 y, 8–10 mg/kg/day div tid–qid for 90–120 days (BIII)	Therapy recommended for acute and congenital infection, reactivated infection, and chronic infection in children aged <18 y; consider in those up to age 50 with chronic infection without advanced cardiomyopathy. Side effects fairly common. Both drugs contraindicated in pregnancy.
– Sleeping sickness[84-87] (*Trypanosoma brucei gambiense* [West African]; *T brucei rhodesiense* [East African]; acute [hemo-lymphatic] stage)	*Tb gambiense:* pentamidine isethionate 4 mg/kg/day (max 300 mg) IM or IV for 7–10 days (BII) *Tb rhodesiense:* suramin (from CDC) 100–200 mg test dose IV, then 20 mg/kg (max 1 g) IV on days 1, 3, 5, 14, and 21 (BII)	CSF examination required for all patients to assess CNS involvement. Consult with infectious diseases or tropical medicine specialist if unfamiliar with trypanosomiasis. Examination of the buffy coat of peripheral blood may be helpful. *Tb gambiense* may be found in lymph node aspirates.
Late (CNS) stage	*Tb gambiense:* eflornithine (from CDC) 400 mg/kg/day IV div bid for 7 days PLUS nifurtimox 5 mg/kg PO tid for 10 days (BIII); OR eflornithine 400 mg/kg/day IV div qid for 14 days (BII); OR melarsoprol (from CDC) 2.2 mg/kg/day (max 180 mg) IV for 10 days (BIII).	CSF examination needed for management (double-centrifuge technique recommended); perform repeat CSF examinations every 6 mo for 2 y to detect relapse.

10

Tb rhodesiense: melarsoprol, 2–3.6 mg/kg/day IV for 3 days; after 7 days, 3.6 mg/kg/day for 3 days; after 7 days, 3.6 mg/kg/day for 3 days; corticosteroids often given with melarsoprol to decrease risk of CNS toxicity.

WHIPWORM (TRICHURIASIS)

Trichuris trichiura	Mebendazole 100 mg PO bid for 3 days or 500 mg once; OR albendazole 400 mg PO for 3 days; OR ivermectin 200 µg/kg/day PO daily for 3 days (BII)	Treatment can be given for 5–7 days for heavy infestation.
Wuchereria bancrofti	See FILARIASIS.	
Yaws	Azithromycin 30 mg/kg max 2 g once (also treats bejel and pinta)	Alternative regimens include IM benzathine penicillin and second-line agents doxycycline, tetracycline, and erythromycin.

10

11. Alphabetic Listing of Antimicrobials

NOTES

- Higher dosages in a dose range are generally indicated for more serious infections. For pathogens with higher minimal inhibitory concentrations against beta-lactam antibiotics, a more prolonged infusion of the antibiotic will allow increased antibacterial effect (see Chapter 3).

- Maximum dosages for adult-sized children (eg, >40 kg) are based on US Food and Drug Administration (FDA)-approved product labeling or post-marketing data.

- For information on dosing in children who are obese, see Chapter 12.

- Antiretroviral medications are not listed. See Chapter 9.

- Drugs with FDA-approved dosage, or dosages based on randomized clinical trials, are given a Level of Evidence I. Dosages for which data are collected from non-comparative trials or small comparative trials are given a Level of Evidence II. Dosages based on expert or consensus opinion or case reports are given a Level of Evidence III.

- If no oral liquid form is available, round the child's dose to a combination of available solid dosage forms. Consult a pediatric pharmacist for recommendations on mixing with food (crushing tablets, emptying capsule contents) and the availability of extemporaneously compounded liquid formulations.

- Cost estimates are in US dollars per course, or per month for continual regimens. Estimates are based on prices at the editor's institution. These may differ from that of the reader due to contractual differences, regional market forces, and supply fluctuations. Legend: $ = <$100, $$ = $100–$400, $$$ = $401–$1,000, $$$$ = >$1,000, $$$$$ = >$10,000.

- There are some agents that we do not recommend even though they may be available. We believe they are significantly inferior to those we do recommend (see chapters 5–10) and could possibly lead to poor outcomes if used. Such agents are not listed.

- **Abbreviations:** AOM, acute otitis media; bid, twice daily; BSA, body surface area; CABP, community-acquired bacterial pneumonia; CA-MRSA, community-associated methicillin-resistant *Staphylococcus aureus;* cap, capsule or caplet; CDC, Centers for Disease Control and Prevention; CF, cystic fibrosis; CMV, cytomegalovirus; CNS, central nervous system; CrCl, creatinine clearance; DI, drug interactions; div, divided; DR, delayed release; EC, enteric coated; ER, extended release; FDA, US Food and Drug Administration; hs, bedtime; HSV, herpes simplex virus; IBW, ideal body weight; IM, intramuscular; IV, intravenous; IVPB, IV piggyback (premixed bag); LD, loading dose; MAC, *Mycobacterium avium* complex; MRSA, methicillin-resistant *S aureus;* NS, normal saline; oint, ointment; OPC, oropharyngeal candidiasis; ophth, ophthalmic; PCP, *Pneumocystis* pneumonia; PIP, piperacillin; PMA, post-menstrual age; PO, oral;

pwd, powder; qd, once daily; qhs, every bedtime; qid, 4 times daily; RSV, respiratory syncytial virus; SIADH, syndrome of inappropriate antidiuretic hormone; SMX, sulfamethoxazole; soln, solution; SPAG-2, small particle aerosol generator model-2; SQ, subcutaneous; supp, suppository; susp, suspension; tab, tablet; TB, tuberculosis; TBW, total body weight; tid, 3 times daily; TMP, trimethoprim; top, topical; UTI, urinary tract infection; vag, vaginal; VZV, varicella-zoster virus.

A. SYSTEMIC ANTIMICROBIALS WITH DOSAGE FORMS AND USUAL DOSAGES

Generic and Trade Names	Dosage Form (cost estimate)	Route	Dose (evidence level)	Interval
Acyclovir,[a] Zovirax	500-, 1,000-mg vial ($)	IV	15–45 mg/kg/day (I) (See Chapter 9.) Max 1,500 mg/m²/day (II) (See Chapter 12.)	q8h
	200-mg/5-mL susp ($$) 200-mg cap ($) 400-, 800-mg tab ($)	PO	900 mg/m²/day (I) 60–80 mg/kg/day, max 4 g/day (I) (See chapters 5 and 9.)	q8h q6–8h
Albendazole, Albenza	200-mg tab ($$$$)	PO	15 mg/kg/day, max 800 mg/day (I) See Chapter 10 for other dosages	q12h
Amikacin,[a] Amikin	250-mg/mL in 2 or 4 mL vials ($-$$)	IV, IM	15–22.5 mg/kg/day[c] (I) (See Chapter 1.) 30–35 mg/kg/day[c] for CF (II)	q8–24h q24h
		Intravesical	50–100 mL of 0.5 mg/mL in NS (III)	q12h
Amoxicillin,[a] Amoxil	125-, 200-, 250-, 400-mg/5-mL susp ($) 125-, 250-mg chew tab ($) 250-, 500-mg cap ($) 500-, 875-mg tab ($)	PO	Standard dose: 40–45 mg/kg/day (I) High dose: 80–90 mg/kg/day (I) 150 mg/kg/day for penicillin-resistant *S pneumoniae* otitis media (III) Max 4 g/day (III)	q8–12h q12h q8h
Amoxicillin extended release,[a] Moxatag	775-mg tab ($$)	PO	≥12 y and adults 775 mg/day	q24h

11

Alphabetic Listing of Antimicrobials

Alphabetic Listing of Antimicrobials

11

A. SYSTEMIC ANTIMICROBIALS WITH DOSAGE FORMS AND USUAL DOSAGES (continued)

Generic and Trade Names	Dosage Form (cost estimate)	Route	Dose (evidence level)	Interval
Amoxicillin/ clavulanate,[a] Augmentin	16:1 Augmentin XR: 1,000/62.5-mg tab ($–$$)	PO	16:1 formulation: ≥40 kg and adults 4,000 mg amoxicillin component/day (I)	q12h
	14:1 Augmentin ES: 600/42.9-mg/5-mL susp ($)	PO	14:1 formulation: 90-mg amoxicillin component/kg/ day (I), max 4 g/day (III)	q12h
	7:1 Augmentin ($): 875/125-mg tab 200/28.5-, 400/57-mg chew tab 200/28.5-, 400/57-mg/5-mL susp	PO	7:1 formulation: 25- to 45-mg amoxicillin component/kg/day, max 1,750 mg/day (I)	q12h
	4:1 Augmentin: 500/125-mg tab ($) 125/31.25-mg/5-mL susp ($$$) 250/62.5-mg/5-mL susp ($)	PO	20- to 40-mg amoxicillin component/kg/day (max 1,500 mg/day) (I)	q8h
Amphotericin B deoxycholate,[a] Fungizone	50-mg vial ($$)	IV	1–1.5 mg/kg pediatric and adults (I), no max 0.5 mg/kg for Candida esophagitis or cystitis (II)	q24h
		Intravesical	50–100 µg/mL in sterile water × 50–100 mL (III)	q8h
Amphotericin B, lipid complex, Abelcet	100-mg/20-mL vial ($$$$)	IV	5 mg/kg pediatric and adult dose (I) No max	q24h
Amphotericin B, liposomal, AmBisome	50-mg vial ($$$$)	IV	5 mg/kg pediatric and adult dose (I) No max	q24h
Ampicillin/ampicillin trihydrate[a]	250-, 500-mg cap ($) 125-, 250-mg/5-mL susp ($)	PO	50–100 mg/kg/day if <20 kg (I) ≥20 kg and adults 1–2 g/day (I)	q6h

Drug	Form	Route	Dosage	Interval
Ampicillin sodium[a]	250-, 500-mg vial ($) 1-, 2-, 10-g vial ($)	IV, IM	50–200 mg/kg/day, max 8 g/day (I)	q6h
			300–400 mg/kg/day, max 12 g/day endocarditis/meningitis (III)	q4–6h
Ampicillin/sulbactam,[a] Unasyn	1/0.5-, 2/1-, 10/5-g vial ($)	IV, IM	200-mg ampicillin component/kg/day (I) ≥40 kg and adults 4–max 8 g/day (I)	q6h
Anidulafungin, Eraxis	50-, 100-mg vial ($$)	IV	1.5–3 mg/kg LD, then 0.75–1.5 mg/kg (II) Max 200-mg LD, then 100 mg (I)	q24h
Atovaquone,[a] Mepron	750-mg/5-mL susp ($$$)	PO	30 mg/kg/day if 1–3 mo or >24 mo (I) 45 mg/kg/day if >3 mo–24 mo (I) Max 1,500 mg/day (I)	q12h q24h for prophylaxis
Atovaquone and proguanil,[a] Malarone	62.5/25-mg pediatric tab ($–$$) 250/100-mg adult tab ($$)	PO	Prophylaxis for malaria: 11–20 kg: 1 pediatric tab, 21–30 kg: 2 pediatric tabs, 31–40 kg: 3 pediatric tabs, >40 kg: 1 adult tab (I) Treatment: 5–8 kg: 2 pediatric tabs, 9–10 kg: 3 pediatric tabs, 11–20 kg: 1 adult tab, 21–30 kg: 2 adult tabs, 31–40 kg: 3 adult tabs, >40 kg: 4 adult tabs (I)	q24h
Azithromycin,[a] Zithromax	250-, 500-, 600-mg tab ($) 100-, 200-mg/5-mL susp ($)	PO	Otitis: 10 mg/kg/day for 1 day, then 5 mg/kg for 4 days; or 10 mg/kg/day for 3 days; or 30 mg/kg once (I). Pharyngitis: 12 mg/kg/day for 5 days (I). Sinusitis: 10 mg/kg/day for 3 days (I). CABP: 10 mg/kg for 1 day, then 5 mg/kg/day for 4 days or 60 mg/kg once of ER (Zmax) susp, max 2 g (I). Total cumulative dose max 2.5 g (I). MAC prophylaxis: 5 mg/kg/day, max 250 mg (I), or 20 mg/kg, max 1.2 g qwk. See Chapter 6 for other specific disease dosing recommendations.	q24h
Azithromycin, Zmax	2-g/60-mL ER susp (Zmax) ($$)			
	500-mg vial[a] ($)	IV	10 mg/kg, max 500 mg (II)	q24h

11

Alphabetic Listing of Antimicrobials

A. SYSTEMIC ANTIMICROBIALS WITH DOSAGE FORMS AND USUAL DOSAGES (continued)

Generic and Trade Names	Dosage Form (cost estimate)	Route	Dose (evidence level)	Interval
Aztreonam,[a] Azactam	1-, 2-g vial ($$–$$$)	IV, IM	90–120 mg/kg/day, max 8 g/day (I)	q6–8h
Capreomycin, Capastat	1-g vial ($$$$)	IV, IM	15–30 mg/kg/day (III), max 1 g (I)	q24h
Caspofungin, Cancidas	50-, 70-mg vial ($$$$)	IV	Load with 70 mg/m² once, then 50 mg/m², max 70 mg (I)	q24h
Cefaclor,[a] Ceclor	125-, 250-, 375-mg/5-mL susp ($$) 250-, 500-mg cap ($) 500-mg ER tab ($)	PO	20–40 mg/kg/day, max 1 g/day (I)	q12h
Cefadroxil,[a] Duricef	250-, 500-mg/5-mL susp ($) 500-mg cap ($) 1-g tab ($)	PO	30 mg/kg/day, max 2 g/day (I)	q12–24h
Cefazolin,[a] Ancef	0.5-, 1-, 10-, 20-g vial ($)	IV, IM	25–100 mg/kg/day (I) 100–150 mg/kg/day for serious infections (III), max 12 g/day	q8h q6h
Cefdinir,[a] Omnicef	125-, 250-mg/5-mL susp ($) 300-mg cap ($)	PO	14 mg/kg/day, max 600 mg/day (I)	q24h
Cefditoren, Spectracef	200-, 400-mg tab ($$)	PO	≥12 y and adults 400–800 mg/day (I)	q12h
Cefepime,[a] Maxipime	1-, 2-g vial ($$) 1-, 2-g IVPB ($$$)	IV, IM	100 mg/kg/day, max 4 g/day (I) 150 mg/kg/day empiric therapy of fever with neutropenia, max 6 g/day (I)	q12h q8h
Cefixime, Suprax	100-, 200-mg/5-mL susp[a] ($$) 100-, 200-mg chew tab ($$) 400-mg cap ($$)	PO	8 mg/kg/day, max 400 mg/day (I) For convalescent oral therapy of serious infections, up to 20 mg/kg/day (III)	q24h q12h

Cefotaxime,[a] Claforan	0.5-, 1-, 2-, 10-g vial (\$) 1-, 2-g IVPB (\$\$)	IV, IM	150–180 mg/kg/day, max 8 g/day (I)	q8h
			200–225 mg/kg/day for meningitis, max 12 g/day (I)	q6h
Cefotetan,[a] Cefotan	1-, 2-, 10-g vial (\$\$) 1-, 2-g IVPB (\$\$)	IV, IM	60–100 mg/kg/day (II), max 6 g/day (I)	q12h
Cefoxitin,[a] Mefoxin	1-, 2-, 10-g vial (\$) 1-, 2-g IVPB (\$)	IV, IM	80–160 mg/kg/day, max 12 g/day (I)	q6–8h
Cefpodoxime,[a] Vantin	50-, 100-mg/5-mL susp (\$) 100-, 200-mg tab (\$)	PO	10 mg/kg/day, max 400 mg/day (I)	q12h
Cefprozil,[a] Cefzil	125-, 250-mg/5-mL susp (\$) 250-, 500-mg tab (\$)	PO	15–30 mg/kg/day, max 1 g/d (I)	q12h
Ceftaroline, Teflaro	400-, 600-mg vial (\$\$\$\$)	IV	For skin or CABP (I): ≥2 mo–<2 y: 24 mg/kg/day ≥2 y: 36 mg/kg/day, max 1,200 mg/day For complicated pneumonia (see Chapter 6): ≥2 mo–<6 mo: 30 mg/kg/day ≥6 mo: 45 mg/kg/day, max 1,800 mg/day	q8h
Ceftazidime,[a] Tazicef, Fortaz	0.5-, 1-, 2-, 6-g vial (\$) 1-, 2-g IVPB (\$\$)	IV, IM	90–150 mg/kg/day, max 6 g/day (I)	q8h
		IV	200–300 mg/kg/day for serious *Pseudomonas* infection, max 12 g/day (II)	q8h
Ceftazidime/ avibactam, Avycaz	2 g/0.5 g vial (\$\$\$\$)	IV	Adults 7.5 g (6 g/1.5 g)/day (I)	q8h
Ceftibuten,[a] Cedax	180-mg/5-mL susp (\$\$\$) 400-mg cap (\$\$\$)	PO	9 mg/kg/day, max 400 mg/day (I)	q24h
Ceftolozane/ tazobactam, Zerbaxa	1.5-g (1-g/0.5-g) vial (\$\$\$\$)	IV	Adults 4.5 g (3 g/1.5 g)/day (I)	q8h

11

Alphabetic Listing of Antimicrobials

Alphabetic Listing of Antimicrobials

11

A. SYSTEMIC ANTIMICROBIALS WITH DOSAGE FORMS AND USUAL DOSAGES (continued)

Generic and Trade Names	Dosage Form (cost estimate)	Route	Dose (evidence level)	Interval
Ceftriaxone,[a] Rocephin	0.25-, 0.5-, 1-, 2-, 10-g vial ($) 1-, 2-g IVPB ($)	IV, IM	50 mg/kg, max 1 g, 1–3 doses for AOM (II) 50–75 mg/kg/day, max 2 g/day (I) Meningitis: 100 mg/kg/day, max 4 g/day (I)	q24h q24h q12h
Cefuroxime axetil, Ceftin	125-, 250-mg/5-mL susp ($$) 250-, 500-mg tab[a] ($)	PO	20–30 mg/kg/day, max 1 g/day (I) For bone and joint infections, up to 100 mg/kg/day, max 3 g/day (III)	q12h q8h
Cefuroxime sodium,[a] Zinacef	0.75-, 1.5-, 7.5-g vial ($)	IV, IM	100–150 mg/kg/day, max 6 g/day (I)	q8h
Cephalexin,[a] Keflex	125-, 250-mg/5-mL susp ($) 250-, 500-mg cap ($) 250-, 500-mg tab ($)	PO	25–50 mg/kg/day (I) 75–100 mg/kg/day for bone and joint, or severe infections (II), max 4 g/day (I)	q12h q6–8h
Chloroquine phosphate,[a] Aralen	250-, 500-mg (150-, 300-mg base) tabs ($$)	PO	See Chapter 10.	
Cidofovir,[a] Vistide	375-mg/5-mL vial ($$$)	IV	5 mg/kg (III); see also Chapter 9.	Weekly
Ciprofloxacin,[a] Cipro	250-, 500-mg/5-mL susp ($) 250-, 500-, 750-mg tab ($)	PO	20–40 mg/kg/day, max 1.5 g/day (I)	q12h
	200-, 400-mg vial ($) 200-, 400-mg IVPB ($)	IV	20–30 mg/kg/day, max 1.2 g/day (I)	q12h
Ciprofloxacin extended release,[a] Cipro XR	500-, 1,000-mg ER tab ($)	PO	Adults 500–1,000 mg (I)	q24h
Clarithromycin,[a] Biaxin	125-, 250-mg/5-mL susp ($) 250-, 500-mg tab ($)	PO	15 mg/kg/day, max 1 g/day (I)	q12h
Clarithromycin extended release,[a] Biaxin XL	500-mg ER tab ($)	PO	Adults 1,000 mg (I)	q24h

Clindamycin,[a] Cleocin	75 mg/5-mL soln ($–$$) 75-, 150-, 300-mg cap ($)	PO	10–25 mg/kg/day, max 1.8 g/day (I) 30–40 mg/kg/day for CA-MRSA, intra-abdominal infection, or AOM (III)	q8h
	0.3-, 0.6-, 0.9-g vial ($) 0.3-, 0.6-, 0.9-g IVPB ($$)	IV, IM	20–40 mg/kg/day, max 2.7 g/day (I)	q8h
Clotrimazole,[a] Mycelex	10-mg lozenge ($)	PO	≥3 y and adults, dissolve lozenge in mouth (I).	5 times daily
Colistimethate,[a] Coly-Mycin M	150-mg (colistin base) vial ($) 1-mg base = 2.7-mg colistimethate	IV, IM	2.5- to 5-mg base/kg/day based on IBW (I) Up to 5- to 7-mg base/kg/day (III)	q8h
Cycloserine, Seromycin	250-mg cap ($$$)	PO	10–20 mg/kg/day (III) Adults max 1 g/day (I)	q12h
Dalbavancin, Dalvance	500-mg vial ($$$$)	IV	Adults 1 g one time then 500 mg in 1 wk	Once weekly
Daclatasvir, Daklinza	30-, 60-, 90-mg tab ($$$$$)	PO	Adults 30–90 mg + sofosbuvir (I)	q24h
Dapsone[a]	25-, 100-mg tab ($)	PO	2 mg/kg, max 100 mg (I)	q24h
			4 mg/kg, max 200 mg (I)	Once weekly
Daptomycin, Cubicin (investigational in children <12 y)	500-mg vial ($$$$)	IV	2–5 y: 10 mg/kg (III) ≥6–11 y: 7 mg/kg (II) ≥12 y and adults: 4–6 mg/kg TBW (I)	q24h
Dasabuvir co-packaged with ombitasvir, paritaprevir, ritonavir (Viekira Pak)	Ombitasvir/paritaprevir/ ritonavir (12.5-/75-/50-mg) tab + dasabuvir 250-mg tab ($$$$$)	PO	Adults 2 ombitasvir, paritaprevir, ritonavir tabs + 1 dasabuvir 250-mg tab	qam q12h
Demeclocycline,[a] Declomycin	150-, 300-mg tab ($)	PO	≥8 y: 7–13 mg/kg/day, max 600 mg/day (I) Dosage differs for SIADH.	q6h
Dicloxacillin,[a] Dynapen	250-, 500-mg cap ($)	PO	12–25 mg/kg/day (adults 0.5–1 g/day) (I) For bone and joint infections, up to 100 mg/kg/day, max 2 g/day (III)	q6h

11

Alphabetic Listing of Antimicrobials

Alphabetic Listing of Antimicrobials

11

A. SYSTEMIC ANTIMICROBIALS WITH DOSAGE FORMS AND USUAL DOSAGES (continued)

Generic and Trade Names	Dosage Form (cost estimate)	Route	Dose (evidence level)	Interval
Doxycycline,[a] Vibramycin	25-mg/5-mL susp ($) 50-mg/5-mL syrup ($) 20-, 50-, 75-, 100-mg tab/cap ($)	PO	≥8 y: 4 mg/kg/day loading dose on day 1, then 2–4 mg/kg/day, max 200 mg/day (I)	q12h 12–24h
	100-mg vial ($$)	IV		
Elbasvir/Grazoprevir, Zepatier	50-mg/100-mg tab ($$$$$)	PO	Adults 1 tab	q24h
Entecavir, Baraclude	0.05-mg/mL soln ($$$) 0.5-, 1-mg tab ($$$)	PO	≥2 y and ≥10 kg: 0.015 mg/kg to nearest mL, max 0.5 mg; double dose if 3TC exposed (I) Adults 0.5–1 mg (I)	q24h
Ertapenem, Invanz	1-g vial ($$$)	IV, IM	30 mg/kg/day, max 1 g/day (I) ≥13 y and adults: 1 g/day (I)	q12h q24h
Erythromycin base	250-, 500-mg tab ($$–$$$) 250-mg cap EC pellets[a] ($$) 333-, 500-mg EC particle tab (PCE) ($$) 250-, 333-, 500-mg DR tab (EryTab) ($$)	PO	50 mg/kg/day, max 4 g/day (I)	q6–8h
Erythromycin ethylsuccinate, EES, EryPed	200-, 400-mg/5-mL susp ($$$) 400-mg tab ($$)	PO	50 mg/kg/day, max 4 g/day (I)	q6–8h
Erythromycin lactobionate, Erythrocin	0.5-g vial ($$$)	IV	20 mg/kg/day, max 4 g/day (I)	q6h
Erythromycin stearate	250-mg tab ($$)	PO	50 mg/kg/day, max 4 g/day (I)	q6–8h
Ethambutol,[a] Myambutol	100-, 400-mg tab ($)	PO	15–25 mg/kg, max 2.5 g (I)	q24h

Drug	Form	Route	Dosage	Interval
Ethionamide, Trecator	250-mg tab ($$)	PO	15–20 mg/kg/day, max 1 g/day (I)	q12–24h
Famciclovir,[a] Famvir	125-, 250-, 500-mg tab (S)	PO	Adults 0.5–1.5 g/day (I)	q8–12h
Fluconazole,[a] Diflucan	50-, 100-, 150-, 200-mg tab (S); 50-, 200-mg/5-mL susp (S)	PO	6–12 mg/kg/day, max 800 mg/day (I). 800–1,000 mg/day may be used for some CNS fungal infections. See Chapter 8.	q24h
	200-, 400-mg vial, IVPB (S)	IV		
Flucytosine,[a] Ancobon	250-, 500-mg cap ($$$$)	PO	100 mg/kg/day (I)[b]	q6h
Foscarnet, Foscavir	6-g vial ($$$$)	IV	CMV/VZV: 180 mg/kg/day (I)	q8h
			CMV suppression: 90–120 mg/kg/day (I)	q24h
			HSV: 120 mg/kg/day (I)	q8–12h
Ganciclovir,[a] Cytovene	500-mg vial ($$)	IV	CMV treatment: 10 mg/kg/day (I)	q12h
			CMV suppression: 5 mg/kg (I)	q24h
			VZV: 10 mg/kg/day (III)	q12h
Gentamicin[a,b]	20-mg/2-mL (S); 40-mg/mL in 2-mL and 20-mL (S)	IV, IM	3–7.5 mg/kg/day, CF 7–10 mg/kg/day See Chapter 1 for q24h dosing.	q8–24h
		Intravesical	0.5 mg/mL in NS x 50–100 mL (III)	q12h
Griseofulvin microsized,[a] Grifulvin V	125-mg/5-mL susp (S); 500-mg tab ($$)	PO	20–25 mg/kg/day (II), max 1 g (I)	q24h
Griseofulvin ultra-microsized,[a] Gris-PEG	125-, 250-mg tab (S)	PO	10–15 mg/kg (II), max 750 mg (I)	q24h
Imipenem/cilastatin,[a] Primaxin	250/250-, 500/500-mg vial ($$)	IV, IM	60–100 mg/kg/day, max 4 g/day (I). IM form not approved for <12 y	q6h
Interferon-PEG Alfa-2a, Pegasys Alfa-2b, PegIntron Alfa-2b, Sylatron	Vials, prefilled syringes: 135-, 180-µg ($$$$); 50-, 80-, 120-, 150-µg ($$$$); 200-, 300-, 600-µg ($$$$)	SQ	See Chapter 9, Hepatitis C virus.	Weekly

11

Alphabetic Listing of Antimicrobials

Alphabetic Listing of Antimicrobials

11

A. SYSTEMIC ANTIMICROBIALS WITH DOSAGE FORMS AND USUAL DOSAGES (continued)

Generic and Trade Names	Dosage Form (cost estimate)	Route	Dose (evidence level)	Interval
Isavuconazonium (isavuconazole), Cresemba	186-mg cap (100-mg base) ($$$$) 372-mg vial (200-mg base) ($$$$)	PO IV	Adults 200 mg base per dose PO/IV (base = isavuconazole)	q8h x 6 doses then q24h
Isoniazid,[a] Nydrazid	50-mg/5-mL syrup ($$) 100-, 300-mg tab ($) 1,000-mg vial ($$)	PO IV, IM	10–15 mg/kg/day, max 300 mg/day (I) With directly observed biweekly therapy, dosage is 20–30 mg/kg, max 900 mg/dose (I).	q12–24h Twice weekly
Itraconazole, Sporanox	50-mg/5-mL soln ($$$) 100-mg cap[a] ($$) 200-mg tab ($$$)	PO	10 mg/kg/day (III), max 200 mg/day 5 mg/kg/day for chronic mucocutaneous *Candida* (III)	q12h q24h
Ivermectin,[a] Stromectol	3-mg tab ($)	PO	0.15–0.2 mg/kg, no max (I)	1 dose
Ketoconazole,[a] Nizoral	200-mg tab ($)	PO	≥2 y: 3.3–6.6 mg/kg, max 400 mg (I)	q24h
Levofloxacin,[a] Levaquin	125-mg/5-mL soln ($) 250-, 500-, 750-mg tab ($) 500-, 750-mg vial ($) 250-, 500-, 750-mg IVPB ($)	PO, IV	For postexposure anthrax prophylaxis (I): <50 kg: 16 mg/kg/day, max 500 mg/day ≥50 kg: 500 mg For respiratory infections: <5 y: 20 mg/kg/day (II) ≥5 y: 10 mg/kg/day, max 500 mg/day (II)	q12h q24h q12h q24h
Linezolid,[a] Zyvox	100-mg/5-mL susp ($$$) 600-mg tab ($$) 200-mg IVPB ($$) 600-mg IVPB ($$)	PO, IV	Pneumonia, complicated skin infections, vancomycin-resistant enterococci: Birth–11 y: 30 mg/kg/day (I) >11 y: 1,200 mg/day (I) Uncomplicated skin infections: Birth–5 y: 30 mg/kg/day (I) 5–11 y: 20 mg/kg/day (I) >11–18 y: 1,200 mg/day (I)	q8h q12h q8h q12h q12h

Mebendazole, Emverm	100-mg chew tab ($$$)	PO	100 mg (not per kg)	q12h x3d
			100 mg x1 for *Enterobius*. See Chapter 10.	
Mefloquine,[a] Lariam	250-mg tab ($)	PO	See Chapter 10, Malaria.	
Meropenem,[a] Merrem	0.5-, 1-g vial ($$)	IV	60 mg/kg/day, max 3 g/day (I)	q8h
			120 mg/kg/day meningitis, max 6 g/day (I)	q8h
Methenamine hippurate,[a] Hiprex	1-g tab ($)	PO	6–12 y: 1–2 g/day (I)	q12h
			>12 y: 2 g/day (I)	
Methenamine mandelate[a]	0.5-, 1-g tab ($)		<6 y: 75 mg/kg/day (I)	q6h
			6–12 y: 2 g/day (I)	
			>12 y: 4 g/day (I)	
Metronidazole,[a] Flagyl	250-, 500-mg tab ($)	PO	30–50 mg/kg/day, max 2,250 mg/day (I)	q8h
	375-mg cap ($$)			
	500-mg vial ($)	IV	22.5–40 mg/kg/day (III), max 4 g/day (I)	q6–8h
	500-mg IVPB ($)			
Micafungin, Mycamine	50-, 100-mg vial ($$$)	IV	2–4 mg/kg, max 150 mg (I)	q24h
Miltefosine, Impavido	50-mg cap	PO	2.5 mg/kg/day (II). See Chapter 10.	
	Available from CDC		≥12 y (I):	
			30–44 kg: 100 mg/day	bid
			≥45 kg: 150 mg/day	tid
Minocycline, Minocin	50-, 75-, 100-mg cap[a] ($)	PO, IV	≥8 y: 4 mg/kg/day, max 200 mg/day (I)	q12h
	50-, 75-, 100-mg tab[a] ($$)			
	100-mg vial ($$$$)			
Minocycline, Solodyn	55-, 65-, 80-, 105-, 115-mg ER tabs ($$$)	PO	≥8 y: 1 mg/kg/day for acne	q24h
Moxifloxacin,[a] Avelox	400-mg tab ($), IVPB ($$$)	PO, IV	Adults 400 mg/day (I)	q24h
Nafcillin,[a] Nallpen	1-, 2-, 10-g vial ($$)	IV, IM	150–200 mg/kg/day (II)	q6h
			Max 12 g/day div q4h (I)	

11

Alphabetic Listing of Antimicrobials

Alphabetic Listing of Antimicrobials

A. SYSTEMIC ANTIMICROBIALS WITH DOSAGE FORMS AND USUAL DOSAGES (continued)

Generic and Trade Names	Dosage Form (cost estimate)	Route	Dose (evidence level)	Interval
Neomycin sulfate[a]	500-mg tab ($)	PO	50–100 mg/kg/day (III), max 12 g/day (I)	q6–8h
Nitazoxanide, Alinia	100-mg/5-mL susp ($$) 500-mg tab ($$$)	PO	1–3 y: 200 mg/day (I) 4–11 y: 400 mg/day (I) ≥12 y: 1 g/day (I)	q12h
Nitrofurantoin,[a] Furadantin	25-mg/5-mL susp ($$)	PO	5–7 mg/kg/day, max 400 mg/day (I)	q6h
			1–2 mg/kg for UTI prophylaxis (I)	q24h
Nitrofurantoin, macrocrystalline,[a] Macrodantin	25-, 50-, 100-mg cap ($)	PO	Same as susp	
Nitrofurantoin monohydrate and macrocrystalline,[a] Macrobid	100-mg cap ($)	PO	>12 y: 200 mg/day (I)	q12h
Nystatin,[a] Mycostatin	500,000-U/5-mL susp ($) 500,000-U tabs ($)	PO	Infants 2 mL/dose, children 4–6 mL/dose, to coat oral mucosa	q6h
			Tabs: 3–6 tabs/day	tid–qid
Oritavancin, Orbactiv	400-mg vial ($$$$)	IV	Adults 1,200 mg/day (I)	One time
Oseltamivir, Tamiflu (See Chapter 9, Influenza virus.)	30-mg/5-mL susp ($$) 30-, 45-, 75-mg cap ($$)	PO	Preterm, <38 wk PMA (II): 1 mg/kg/dose PO bid Preterm, 38–40 wk PMA (II): 1.5 mg/kg/dose PO bid Preterm, >40 wk PMA (II), and term, birth–8 mo (I): 3 mg/kg/dose PO bid 9–11 mo (II): 3.5 mg/kg/dose PO bid ≥12 mo (I): ≤15 kg: 60 mg/day	q12h

11

	Form (cost)	Route	Dosage	Interval
			>15–23 kg: 90 mg/day >23–40 kg: 120 mg/day >40 kg: 150 mg/day	q24h
			Prophylaxis: Give at the same mg/kg dose but qd rather than bid. Not recommended for infants <3 mo.	
Oxacillin,[a] Bactocill	1-, 2-, 10-g vial ($$)	IV, IM	100 mg/kg/day, max 12 g/day (I) 150–200 mg/kg/day for meningitis (III)	q4-6h
Palivizumab, Synagis	50-, 100-mg vial ($$$$)	IM	15 mg/kg (I)	Monthly
Paromomycin,[a] Humatin	250-mg cap ($)	PO	25–35 mg/kg/day, max 4 g/day (I)	q8h
Penicillin G intramuscular				
– Penicillin G benzathine, Bicillin L-A	600,000 U/mL in 1-, 2-, 4-mL prefilled syringes ($–$$)	IM	50,000 U/kg for newborns and infants, children <60 lb: 300,000–600,000 units, children ≥60 lb: 900,000 units (FDA approved in 1952 for dosing by lbs) Adults: 1.2–2.4 million units	1 dose
– Penicillin G benzathine/procaine, Bicillin C-R, Bicillin C-R pediatric	1,200,000 IU per 2 mL pre-filled syringe as 600,000 IU benzathine + 600,000 IU procaine per mL ($). Pediatric has a 1-inch needle.	IM	<30 lb: 600,000 U 30–60 lb: 900,000–1,200,000 U >60 lb: 2,400,000 U (I)	1 dose (may need repeat injections q2–3d)
– Penicillin G procaine[a]	600,000 U/mL in 1-, 2-mL pre-filled syringes ($$)	IM	50,000 U/kg/day, max 1,200,000 U per dose (I)	q12-24h
Penicillin G intravenous				
– Penicillin G K,[a] Pfizerpen	5-, 20-million unit vial ($)	IV, IM	100,000–300,000 units/kg/day (I). Max daily dose is 24 million units.	q4-6h
– Penicillin G sodium[a]	5-million unit vial ($$)	IV, IM	100,000–300,000 unit/kg/day (I). Max daily dose is 24 million units.	q4-6h

11

Alphabetic Listing of Antimicrobials

Alphabetic Listing of Antimicrobials

11

A. SYSTEMIC ANTIMICROBIALS WITH DOSAGE FORMS AND USUAL DOSAGES (continued)

Generic and Trade Names	Dosage Form (cost estimate)	Route	Dose (evidence level)	Interval
Penicillin V oral				
– Penicillin V K[a]	125-, 250-mg/5-mL soln ($) 250-, 500-mg tab ($)	PO	25–50 mg/kg/day, max 2 g/day (I)	q6h
Pentamidine Pentam, Nebupent	300-mg vial ($$$)	IV, IM	4 mg/kg/day (I), max 300 mg	q24h
	300-mg vial ($)	Inhaled	300 mg monthly for prophylaxis (I)	Monthly
Peramivir, Rapivab	200-mg vial ($$-$$$)	IV	10 mg/kg (II), max 600 mg (I)	One time
Piperacillin/tazobactam,[a] Zosyn	2/0.25-, 3/0.375-, 4/0.5-, 36/4.5-g vial ($-$$)	IV	≤40 kg: 240–300 mg PIP/kg/day, max 16 g PIP/day (I)	q8h
Polymyxin B[a]	500,000 U vial ($) 1 mg = 10,000 U	IV	2.5 mg/kg/day (I) Adults 2 mg/kg LD, then 2.5–3 mg/kg/day, dose based on TBW, no max (II)	q12h
Posaconazole, Noxafil (See Chapter 8.)	200-mg/5-mL susp ($$$$)	PO	<13 y: under investigation, 18 mg/kg/day with serum trough monitoring	q8h
			≥13 y and adults (I):	
			Candida or *Aspergillus* prophylaxis: 600 mg/day	q8h
			OPC treatment: 100 mg q12h for 1 day, then 100 mg	q24h
			Refractory OPC: 800 mg/day	q12h
	100-mg DR tab ($$$$) 300-mg/16.7-mL vial ($$$$)	PO, IV	≥13 y and adults (I): *Candida* or *Aspergillus* prophylaxis: 300 mg q12h for 1 day, then 300 mg/day	q24h

Drug	Formulation	Dose	Route	Interval
Praziquantel, Biltricide	600-mg tri-scored tab ($$)	20–25 mg/kg, no max (I)	PO	q4–6h for 3 doses
Primaquine phosphate[a]	15-mg base tab ($) (26.3-mg primaquine phosphate)	0.3 mg base/kg, max 30 mg (III) (See Chapter 10.)	PO	q24h
Pyrantel pamoate,[a]	250-mg base/5-mL susp ($) 250-mg base chew tab ($)	11 mg (base)/kg, max 1 g (I) (144-mg pyrantel pamoate = 50-mg base)	PO	Once
Pyrazinamide[a]	500-mg tab ($)	30 mg/kg/day, max 2 g/day (I) Directly observed biweekly therapy, 50 mg/kg (I) use IBW, no max.	PO	q24h Twice weekly
Quinupristin/ dalfopristin, Synercid	150/350-mg vial (500 mg total) ($$$$)	22.5 mg/kg/day (II) Adults 15–22.5 mg/kg/day, no max (I)	IV	q8h q8–12h
Raxibacumab	1,700-mg/35-mL vial Available from CDC	≤15 kg: 80 mg/kg 15–50 kg: 60 mg/kg >50 kg: 40 mg/kg (I)	IV	Once
Ribavirin, Rebetol (See Chapter 9.)	200-mg/5-mL soln ($$) 200-mg cap/tab ($) 400-, 600-mg tab ($$$$) 600-, 800-, 1,000-, 1,200-mg dose paks[a] ($$$–$$$$)	15 mg/kg/day (with interferon) (I)	PO	q12h
Ribavirin, Virazole	6-g vial ($$$$$)	1 vial by SPAG-2; see Chapter 9, RSV.	Inhaled	
Rifabutin,[a] Mycobutin	150-mg cap ($$$)	5 mg/kg for MAC prophylaxis (II) 10–20 mg/kg for MAC or TB treatment (I) Max 300 mg/day	PO	q24h

11

Alphabetic Listing of Antimicrobials

Alphabetic Listing of Antimicrobials

11

A. SYSTEMIC ANTIMICROBIALS WITH DOSAGE FORMS AND USUAL DOSAGES (continued)

Generic and Trade Names	Dosage Form (cost estimate)	Route	Dose (evidence level)	Interval
Rifampin,[a] Rifadin	150-, 300-mg cap ($) 600-mg vial ($$-$$$)	PO, IV	10–20 mg/kg, max 600 mg for TB (I)	q24h
			With directly observed biweekly therapy, dosage is still 10–20 mg/kg/dose (max 600 mg).	Twice weekly
			20 mg/kg/day for 2 days for meningococcus prophylaxis, max 1.2 g/day (I)	q12h
Rifampin/isoniazid/ pyrazinamide, Rifater	120-/50-/300-mg tab ($$$)	PO	≥15 y and adults: ≤44 kg: 4 tab 45–54 kg: 5 tab ≥55 kg: 6 tab	q24h
Rifapentine, Priftin	150-mg tab ($$)	PO	≥12 y and adults: 600 mg/dose (I)	Twice weekly
Rifaximin, Xifaxan	200-mg tab ($$)	PO	≥12 y and adults: 600 mg/day (I) 20–30 mg/kg/day, max 1,600 mg/day (III)	q8h
Simeprevir, Olysio	150-mg cap ($$$$$)	PO	Adults 150 mg[c] (I)	q24h
Sofosbuvir, Sovaldi	400-mg tab ($$$$$)	PO	Adults 400 mg[c] (I)	q24h
Sofosbuvir/ Ledipasvir, Harvoni	400-/90-mg tab ($$$$$)	PO	Adults 1 tab (I)	q24h
Sofosbuvir/ Velpatasvir, Epclusa	400-/100-mg tab ($$$$$)	PO	Adults 1 tab (I)	q12h
Streptomycin[a]	1-g vial ($$)	IM, IV	20–40 mg/kg/day, max 1 g/day[b] (I)	q12–24h
Sulfadiazine[a]	500-mg tab ($$)	PO	120–150 mg/kg/day, max 4–6 g/day (I)	q6h
			Rheumatic fever secondary prophylaxis 500 mg once daily if ≤27 kg, 1,000 mg once daily if >27 kg (II)	q24h
			See also Chapter 10.	

Tedizolid, Sivextro	200-mg tab ($$$$) 200-mg vial ($$$$)	PO, IV	Adults 200 mg (I)	q24h
Telavancin, Vibativ	250-, 750-mg vial ($$$$)	IV	Adults 10 mg/kg	q24h
Telbivudine, Tyzeka	600-mg tab ($$$$)	PO	≥16 y and adults: 600 mg/day (I)	q24h
Terbinafine, Lamisil	125-, 187.5-mg granules ($$$) 250-mg tab[a] ($)	PO	>4 y: <25 kg: 125 mg/day 25–35 kg: 187.5 mg/day >35 kg: 250 mg/day (I)	q24h
Tetracycline[a]	250-, 500-mg cap ($$)	PO	≥8 y: 25–50 mg/kg/day (I)	q6h
Tinidazole,[a] Tindamax	250-, 500-mg tab ($)	PO	50 mg/kg, max 2 g (I) See also Chapter 10.	q24h
Tobramycin,[a] Nebcin	20-mg/2-mL vial ($) 40-mg/mL 2-, 30-, 50-mL vial ($) 1.2-g vial ($)	IV, IM	3–7.5 mg/kg/day (CF 7–10)[b]; see Chapter 1 regarding q24h dosing.	q8–24h
Tobramycin inhalation,[a] Tobi	300-mg ampule ($$$$)	Inhaled	≥6 y: 600 mg/day (I)	q12h
Tobi Podhaler	28-mg cap for inhalation ($$$$)	Inhaled	≥6 y: 224 mg/day via Podhaler device (I)	q12h
Trimethoprim/ sulfamethoxazole,[a] Bactrim, Septra	80-mg TMP/400-mg SMX tab (single strength) ($) 160-mg TMP/800-mg SMX tab (double strength) ($) 40-mg TMP/200-mg SMX per 5-mL oral susp ($) 16-mg TMP/80-mg SMX per mL inj soln in 5-, 10-, 30-mL vial ($$)	PO, IV	8–10 mg TMP/kg/day (I)	q12h
			2 mg TMP/kg/day for UTI prophylaxis (I)	q24h
			15–20 mg TMP/kg/day for PCP treatment (I), no max	q6–8h
			150 mg TMP/m²/day, OR 5 mg TMP/kg/day for PCP prophylaxis (I), max 160 mg TMP/day	q12h 3 times a wk OR q24h

11

Alphabetic Listing of Antimicrobials

Alphabetic Listing of Antimicrobials

11

A. SYSTEMIC ANTIMICROBIALS WITH DOSAGE FORMS AND USUAL DOSAGES (continued)

Generic and Trade Names	Dosage Form (cost estimate)	Route	Dose (evidence level)	Interval
Valacyclovir,[a] Valtrex	500-mg, 1-g tab ($)	PO	VZV: ≥3 mo: 60 mg/kg/day (I, II) HSV: ≥3 mo: 40 mg/kg/day (I, II) Max single dose 1 g (I)	q8h q12h
Valganciclovir, Valcyte	250-mg/5-mL soln ($$$) 450-mg tab[a] ($$$)	PO	Congenital CMV treatment: 32 mg/kg/day (II). CMV prophylaxis: 7 × BSA × CrCl (using the modified Schwartz formula for CrCl), max 900 mg (I). See also Chapter 9.	q12h q24h
Vancomycin,[a] Vancocin	125-, 250-mg/5-mL susp ($) 125-, 250-mg cap ($)	PO	40 mg/kg/day (I), max 500 mg/day (III)	q6h
	0.5-, 0.75-, 1-, 5-, 10-g vial ($–$$)	IV	30–40 mg/kg/day[a] (I) For life-threatening invasive MRSA infection, 60–70 mg/kg/day adjusted to achieve an AUC:MIC of >400 mg/L × h (II)	q6–8h
Voriconazole,[a] Vfend (See Chapter 8.)	200-mg/5-mL susp ($$$) 50-, 200-mg tab ($$)	PO	2–12 y: 18 mg/kg/day (II) >12 y: 400 mg/day (I)	q12h
	200-mg vial ($$$)	IV	2–12 y: 18 mg/kg/day LD for 1 day, then 16 mg/kg/day (II) >12 y: 12 mg/kg/day LD for 1 day, then 8 mg/kg/day (max 600 mg/day) (I)	q12h
Zanamivir, Relenza	5-mg blister cap for inhalation ($)	Inhaled	Prophylaxis: ≥5 y: 10 mg/day (I)	q24h
			Treatment: ≥7 y: 20 mg/day (I)	q12h

[a] Available in a generic formulation.
[b] Monitor serum concentrations.
[c] Given as a cocktail with ribavirin ± interferon-PEG.

B. TOPICAL ANTIMICROBIALS (SKIN, EYE, EAR)

Generic and Trade Names	Dosage Form	Route	Dose	Interval
Acyclovir, Sitavig	50-mg tab	Buccal	Adults 50 mg, for herpes labialis	One time
Azithromycin, AzaSite	1% ophth soln	Ophth	1 drop	bid for 2 days then qd for 5 days
Bacitracin[a]	Ophth oint	Ophth	Apply to affected eye.	q3–4h
	Oint[b]	Top	Apply to affected area.	bid–qid
Benzyl alcohol, Ulesfia	5% lotion	Top	Apply to scalp and hair.	Once; repeat in 7 days.
Besifloxacin, Besivance	0.6% ophth susp	Ophth	≥1 y: 1 drop to affected eye	tid
Butenafine, Mentax, Lotrimin-Ultra	1% cream	Top	≥12 y: apply to affected area.	qd
Butoconazole, Gynazole-1	2% prefilled cream	Vag	Adults 1 applicatorful	One time
Ciclopirox,[a] Loprox, Penlac	0.77% cream, gel, lotion	Top	≥10 y: apply to affected area.	bid
	1% shampoo		≥16 y: apply to scalp.	Twice weekly
	8% nail lacquer		≥12 y: apply to infected nail.	qd
Ciprofloxacin,[a] Cetraxal	0.2% otic soln	Otic	≥1 y: apply 3 drops to affected ear.	bid for 7 days
Ciprofloxacin, Ciloxan	0.3% ophth soln[a]	Ophth	≥12 y: apply to affected eye.	q2h for 2 days then q4h for 5 days
	0.3% ophth oint			q8h for 2 days then q12h for 5 days
Ciprofloxacin + dexamethasone, Ciprodex	0.3% + 0.1% otic soln	Otic	≥6 mo: apply 4 drops to affected ear.	bid for 7 days
Ciprofloxacin + hydrocortisone, Cipro HC	0.2% + 1% otic soln	Otic	≥1 y: apply 3 drops to affected ear.	bid for 7 days

11

Alphabetic Listing of Antimicrobials

Alphabetic Listing of Antimicrobials

B. TOPICAL ANTIMICROBIALS (SKIN, EYE, EAR) (continued)

Generic and Trade Names	Dosage Form	Route	Dose	Interval
Clindamycin				
Clindesse	2% cream	Vag	Adolescents and adults 1 applicatorful	One time
Cleocin	100-mg ovule		1 ovule	qhs for 3 days
	2% vaginal cream[a]		1 applicatorful	qhs for 3–7 days
Cleocin-T[a]	1% soln, gel, lotion	Top	Apply to affected area.	qd–bid
Evoclin[a]	1% foam			qd
Clindamycin + benzoyl peroxide, BenzaClin	1% gel[a]	Top	≥12 y: apply to affected area.	bid
Acanya	1.2% gel	Top	Apply small amount to face.	q24h
Clindamycin + tretinoin, Ziana, Veltin	1.2% gel	Top	Apply small amount to face.	hs
Clotrimazole,[a,b] Lotrimin	1% cream, lotion, soln	Top	Apply to affected area.	bid
Gyne-Lotrimin-7[a,b]	1% cream	Vag	≥12 y: 1 applicatorful	qhs for 7–14 days
Gyne-Lotrimin-3[a,b]	2% cream		≥12 y: apply to affected area.	qhs for 3 days
Clotrimazole + betamethasone,[a] Lotrisone	1% + 0.05% cream, lotion	Top	≥12 y: apply to affected area.	bid
Colistin + neomycin + hydrocortisone, Coly-Mycin S, Cortisporin TC otic	0.3% otic susp	Otic	Apply 3–4 drops to affected ear canal; may use with wick.	q6–8h
Cortisporin; bacitracin + neomycin + polymyxin B + hydrocortisone	Oint	Top	Apply to affected area.	bid–qid
Cortisporin; neomycin + polymyxin B + hydrocortisone	Otic soln[a]	Otic	3 drops to affected ear	bid–qid
	Cream	Top	Apply to affected area.	bid–qid

Dapsone, Aczone	5% gel 7.5% gel	Top	Apply to affected area.	bid qd
Econazole,[a] Spectazole	1% cream	Top	Apply to affected area.	qd–bid
Efinaconazole, Jublia	10% soln	Top	Apply to toenail.	qd for 48 wk
Erythromycin[a]	0.5% ophth oint	Ophth	Apply to affected eye.	q4h
Eryderm,[a] Erygel[a]	2% soln, gel	Top	Apply to affected area.	bid
Ery Pads	2% pledgets[a]			
Akne-Mycin	2% oint			
Erythromycin + benzoyl peroxide,[a] Benzamycin	3% gel	Top	≥12 y: apply to affected area.	qd–bid
Ganciclovir, Zirgan	0.15% ophth gel	Ophth	≥2 y: 1 drop in affected eye	q3h while awake (5 times/day) until healed then tid for 7 days
Gatifloxacin,[a] Zymaxid	0.5% ophth soln	Ophth	Apply to affected eye.	q2h for 1 day then q6h
Gentamicin,[a] Garamycin	0.1% cream, oint	Top	Apply to affected area.	tid–qid
	0.3% ophth soln, oint	Ophth	Apply to affected eye.	q1–4h (soln) q4–8h (oint)
Gentamicin + prednisolone, Pred-G	0.3% ophth soln, oint	Ophth	Adults: apply to affected eye.	q1–4h (soln) qd–tid (oint)
Ivermectin, Sklice	0.5% lotion	Top	≥6 mo: thoroughly coat hair and scalp, rinse after 10 minutes.	Once
Ivermectin, Soolantra	1% cream	Top	Adults: apply to face	qd

11

Alphabetic Listing of Antimicrobials

Alphabetic Listing of Antimicrobials

11

B. TOPICAL ANTIMICROBIALS (SKIN, EYE, EAR) (continued)

Generic and Trade Names	Dosage Form	Route	Dose	Interval
Ketoconazole		Top	≥12 y: apply to affected area.	
Nizoral	2% shampoo[a]			qd
	2% cream[a]			qd–bid
Nizoral A-D[a]	1% shampoo			bid
Extina, Xolegel	2% foam,[a] gel			bid
Levofloxacin,[a] Quixin	0.5% ophth soln	Ophth	Apply to affected eye.	q1–4h
Luliconazole, Luzu	1% cream	Top	Adults: apply to affected area.	q24h for 1–2 wk
Mafenide, Sulfamylon	8.5% cream	Top	Apply to burn.	qd–bid
	5-g pwd for reconstitution		To keep burn dressing wet	q4–8h as needed
Malathion,[a] Ovide	0.5% soln	Top	≥6 y: apply to hair and scalp.	Once
Maxitrol[a], neomycin + polymyxin + dexamethasone	Susp, oint	Ophth	Apply to affected eye.	q4h (oint) q1–4h (susp)
Metronidazole[a]	0.75% cream, gel, lotion	Top	Adults: apply to affected area.	bid
	0.75% vag gel	Vag	Adults 1 applicatorful	qd–bid
	1% gel	Top	Adults: apply to affected area.	qd
Noritate	1% cream	Top	Adults: apply to affected area.	qd
Miconazole				
· Micatin[a,b] and others	2% cream, pwd, oint, spray, lotion, gel	Top	Apply to affected area.	qd–bid
Fungoid[a,b]	2% tincture	Top	Apply to affected area.	bid

			To diaper dermatitis	Each diaper change for 7 days
Vusion	0.25% oint	Top		
Monistat-1[a,b]	1.2-g ovule + 2% cream	Vag	≥12 y: insert one ovule (plus cream to external vulva bid as needed).	Once
Monistat-3[a,b]	200-mg ovule, 4% cream			qhs for 3 days
Monistat-7[a,b]	100-mg ovule, 2% cream			qhs for 7 days
Moxifloxacin, Vigamox	0.5% ophth soln	Ophth	Apply to affected eye.	tid
Mupirocin, Bactroban	2% oint,[a] cream,[a] nasal oint	Top	Apply to infected skin or nasal mucosa.	tid
Naftifine, Naftin	1%, 2% cream[a] 2% gel	Top	Adults: apply to affected area.	qd
Natamycin, Natacyn	5% ophth soln	Ophth	Adults: apply to affected eye.	q1–4h
Neosporin[a]				
bacitracin + neomycin + polymyxin B	Ophth oint	Ophth	Apply to affected eye.	q4h
	Oint[a,b]	Top	Apply to affected area.	bid–qid
gramicidin + neomycin + polymyxin B	Ophth soln	Ophth	Apply to affected eye.	q4h
Nystatin,[a] Mycostatin	100,000 U/g cream, oint, pwd	Top	Apply to affected area.	bid–qid
Nystatin + triamcinolone,[a] Mycolog II	100,000 U/g + 0.1% cream, oint	Top	Apply to affected area.	bid
Ofloxacin,[a] Floxin Otic, Ocuflox	0.3% otic soln	Otic	5–10 drops to affected ear	qd–bid
	0.3% ophth soln	Ophth	Apply to affected eye.	q1–6h
Oxiconazole, Oxistat	1% cream,[a] lotion	Top	Apply to affected area.	qd–bid

Alphabetic Listing of Antimicrobials

11

B. TOPICAL ANTIMICROBIALS (SKIN, EYE, EAR) (continued)

Generic and Trade Names	Dosage Form	Route	Dose	Interval
Permethrin, Nix[a,b]	1% cream	Top	Apply to hair/scalp.	Once for 10 min
Elimite[a]	5% cream		Apply to all skin surfaces.	Once for 8–14 h
Piperonyl butoxide + pyrethrins,[a,b] Rid	4% + 0.3% shampoo, gel	Top	Apply to affected area.	Once for 10 min
Polysporin,[a] polymyxin B + bacitracin	Ophth oint	Ophth	Apply to affected eye.	qd–tid
	Oint[b]	Top	Apply to affected area.	qd–tid
Polytrim,[a] polymyxin B + trimethoprim	Ophth soln	Ophth	Apply to affected eye.	q3–4h
Retapamulin, Altabax	1% oint	Top	Apply thin layer to affected area.	bid for 5 days
Selenium sulfide,[a] Selsun	2.5% lotion 2.25% shampoo	Top	Lather into scalp or affected area.	Twice weekly then every 1–2 wk
Selsun Blue[a,b]	1% shampoo	Top		qd
Sertaconazole, Ertaczo	2% cream	Top	≥12 y: apply to affected area.	bid
Silver sulfadiazine,[a] Silvadene	1% cream	Top	Apply to affected area.	qd–bid
Spinosad,[a] Natroba	0.9% susp	Top	Apply to scalp and hair.	Once; may repeat in 7 days.
Sulconazole, Exelderm	1% soln, cream	Top	Adults: apply to affected area.	qd–bid
Sulfacetamide sodium[a]	10% soln	Ophth	Apply to affected eye.	q1–3h
	10% ophth oint			q4–6h
	10% lotion, wash, cream	Top	≥12 y: apply to affected area.	bid–qid
Sulfacetamide sodium + prednisolone,[a] Blephamide	10% ophth oint, soln	Ophth	Apply to affected eye.	tid–qid
Tavaborole, Kerydin	5% soln	Top	Adults: apply to toenail.	qd for 48 wk

Terbinafine,[b] Lamisil-AT	1% cream,[a] spray, gel	Top	Apply to affected area.	qd–bid
Terconazole[a] Terazol	0.4% cream	Vag	Adults 1 applicatorful or 1 suppository	qhs for 7 days
	0.8% cream 80-mg suppository			qhs for 3 days
Tioconazole[a,b]	6.5% ointment	Vag	≥12 y: 1 applicatorful	One time
Tobramycin, Tobrex	0.3% soln,[a] oint	Ophth	Apply to affected eye.	q1–4h (soln) q4–8h (oint)
Tobramycin + dexamethasone, Tobradex	0.3% soln,[a] oint	Ophth	Apply to affected eye.	q2–6h (soln) q6–8h (oint)
Tolnaftate,[a,b] Tinactin	1% cream, soln, pwd, spray	Top	Apply to affected area.	bid
Trifluridine,[a] Viroptic	1% ophth soln	Ophth	1 drop (max 9 drops/day)	q2h

[a] Generic available.
[b] Over the counter.

11

Alphabetic Listing of Antimicrobials

12. Antibiotic Therapy for Children Who Are Obese

When prescribing an antimicrobial for a child who is obese, selecting a dose based on mg per kg of total body weight (TBW) may expose the child to supratherapeutic plasma concentrations if the drug doesn't freely distribute into fat tissue. The aminoglycosides are an example of such potentially problematic antibiotics; they are hydrophilic molecules with distribution volumes that correlate with extracellular fluid. This likely explains why their weight-adjusted distribution volumes are lower in obese compared to nonobese children.

For **aminoglycosides** in obese adults and children, a 40% adjustment in dosing weight has been recommended. When performing this empiric dosing strategy with aminoglycosides in children who are obese, we recommend closely following serum concentrations.

Vancomycin is traditionally dosed based on TBW in obese adults due to increases in kidney size and glomerular filtration rate. In children who are obese, weight-adjusted distribution volume and clearance area are lower, and TBW-based dosing may result in supratherapeutic concentrations. Dosing adjustments using body surface area may be more appropriate. We recommend closely following serum concentrations.

In the setting of **cephalosporins** for surgical prophylaxis (see Chapter 14), adult studies of obese patients have generally found that distribution to the subcutaneous fat tissue target is subtherapeutic when standard doses are used. Given the wide safety margin of these agents in the short-term setting of surgical prophylaxis, maximum single doses are recommended in obese adults (eg, cefazolin 2–3 g instead of the standard 1 g) with re-dosing at 4-hour intervals for longer cases. Based on the adult data, we recommend dosing cephalosporins for surgical prophylaxis based on TBW up to the adult maximum.

In critically ill obese adults, extended infusion times have been shown to increase the likelihood of achieving therapeutic serum concentrations with **carbapenems** and **piperacillin/tazobactam**.

Monitor creatine kinase when using **daptomycin** in a child who is obese.

Listed in the Table are the major classes of antimicrobials and our suggestion on how to calculate the most appropriate dose. The levels of evidence to support these recommendations are Level II–III (pharmacokinetic studies in children, extrapolations from adult studies, and expert opinion). Whenever a dose is used that is greater than one prospectively investigated for efficacy and safety, the clinician must weigh the benefits with potential risks. Data are not available on all agents.

DRUG CLASS	DOSING RECOMMENDATIONS		
	BY EBW[a]	INTERMEDIATE DOSING	BY TBW[b]
ANTIBACTERIALS			
Beta-lactams	EBW + 0.5 (TBW-EBW)		
Penicillins		X	
Cephalosporins		X	X (surgical prophylaxis)
Carbapenems		X	
Macrolides			
Erythromycin	X		
Azithromycin	X (for gastrointestinal infections)		X
Clarithromycin	X		
Lincosamides			
Clindamycin			X
Glycopeptides			
Vancomycin		1,500–2,000 mg/m²/d	X
Aminoglycosides	EBW + 0.4 (TBW-EBW)		
Gentamicin		X	
Tobramycin		X	
Amikacin		X	
Fluoroquinolones	EBW + 0.45 (TBW-EBW)		
Ciprofloxacin		X	
Levofloxacin		X	
Rifamycins			
Rifampin	X		
Miscellaneous			
TMP/SMX			X
Metronidazole	X		
Linezolid	X		
Daptomycin			X

	DOSING RECOMMENDATIONS		
DRUG CLASS	**BY EBW**[a]	**INTERMEDIATE DOSING**	**BY TBW**[b]
ANTIFUNGALS			
Polyenes			
Amphotericin B (conventional and lipid formulations)			X
Azoles			
Fluconazole			X (max 1,200 mg/day)
Posaconazole	X		
Voriconazole	X		
Pyrimidine Analogues			
Flucytosine	X		
Echinocandins			
Anidulafungin	X		
Caspofungin			X (max 150 mg/day)
Micafungin			
ANTIVIRALS (NON-HIV)			
Nucleoside analogues (acyclovir, ganciclovir)	X		
Oseltamivir	X		
ANTIMYCOBACTERIALS			
Isoniazid	X		
Rifampin			X (max 1,200 mg/day)
Pyrazinamide			X (max 2,000 mg/day)
Ethambutol			X (max 1,600 mg/day)

Abbreviations: BMI, body mass index; EBW, expected body weight; HIV, human immunodeficiency virus; TBW, total body weight; TMP/SMX, trimethoprim/sulfamethoxazole.

[a] EBW (kg) = BMI 50th percentile for age $\times$ actual height (m)^2; from Le Grange D, et al. *Pediatrics*. 2012;129:e438–e446.

[b] Actual measured body weight.

Bibliography

Camaione L, et al. *Pharmacotherapy.* 2013;33(12):1278–1287

Hall RG. *Curr Pharm Des.* 2015;21(32):4748–4751

Harskamp-van Ginkel MW, et al. *JAMA Pediatr.* 2015;169(7):678–685

Heble DE Jr, et al. *Pharmacotherapy.* 2013;33(12):1273–1277

Le J, et al. *Clin Ther.* 2015;37(6):1340–1351

Pai MP, et al. *Antimicrob Agents Chemother.* 2011;55(12):5640–5645

Payne KD, et al. *Expert Rev Anti Infect Ther.* 2014;12(7):829–854

Payne KD, et al. *Expert Rev Anti Infect Ther.* 2016;14(2):257–267

Sampson M, et al. *GaBi J.* 2013;2(2):76–81

Smith M, et al. *E-PAS.* 2015:4194.689

13. Sequential Parenteral-Oral Antibiotic Therapy (Oral Step-down Therapy) for Serious Infections

Bone and joint infections,[1-3] complicated bacterial pneumonia with empyema,[4] deep-tissue abscesses, and appendicitis,[5,6] as well as cellulitis or pyelonephritis,[7] may require initial parenteral therapy to control the growth and spread of pathogens and minimize injury to tissues. For abscesses in soft tissues, joints, bones, and empyema, most organisms are removed by surgical drainage and, presumably, killed by the initial parenteral therapy. When the signs and symptoms of infection begin to resolve, often within 2 to 4 days, continuing intravenous (IV) therapy may not be required, as a normal host neutrophil response begins to assist in clearing the infection.[8] In addition to following the clinical response prior to oral switch, following objective laboratory markers, such as C-reactive protein (CRP) or procalcitonin (PCT), during the hospitalization may also help the clinician better assess the response to antibacterial therapy, particularly in the infant or child who is difficult to examine.[9,10]

For the beta-lactam class of antibiotics, absorption of orally administered antibiotics in *standard* dosages provides peak serum concentrations that are routinely only 5% to 20% of those achieved with IV or intramuscular administration. However, *high-dose* oral beta-lactam therapy provides the tissue antibiotic exposure thought to be required to eradicate the remaining pathogens at the infection site as the tissue perfusion improves. For beta-lactams, begin with a dosage 2 to 3 times the normal dosage (eg, 75–100 mg/kg/day of amoxicillin or 100 mg/kg/day of cephalexin). High-dose oral beta-lactam antibiotic therapy of osteoarticular infections has been associated with treatment success since 1978.[4] It is reassuring that high-quality retrospective cohort data have recently confirmed similar outcomes achieved in those treated with oral step-down therapy compared with those treated with IV.[8] High-dose prolonged oral beta-lactam therapy may be associated with reversible neutropenia; checking for hematologic toxicity every few weeks during therapy is recommended.[11]

Clindamycin and many antibiotics of the fluoroquinolone class (ciprofloxacin, levofloxacin)[4] and oxazolidinone class (linezolid, tedizolid) have excellent absorption of their oral formulations and provide virtually the same tissue antibiotic exposure at a particular mg/kg dose, compared with that dose given intravenously. Trimethoprim/sulfamethoxazole and metronidazole are also very well absorbed.

One must also assume that the parent and child are compliant with the administration of each oral antibiotic dose, that the oral antibiotic will be absorbed from the gastrointestinal tract into the systemic circulation (no vomiting or diarrhea), and that the parents will seek medical care if the clinical course does not continue to improve for their child.

Monitor the child clinically for a continued response on oral therapy; follow CRP or PCT after the switch to oral therapy, if there are concerns about continued response, to make sure the antibiotic and dosage you selected are appropriate and the family is compliant. From the first published cases of oral step-down therapy, failures caused by noncompliance have occurred.[12]

13

14. Antimicrobial Prophylaxis/Prevention of Symptomatic Infection

This chapter provides a summary of recommendations for prophylaxis of infections, defined as providing therapy prior to the onset of clinical signs or symptoms of infection. Prophylaxis can be considered in several clinical scenarios.

A. Postexposure Short-term Antimicrobial Prophylaxis

Given for a short, specified period after exposure to specific pathogens/organisms, where the risks of acquiring the infection are felt to justify antimicrobial treatment to eradicate the pathogen or prevent symptomatic infection in situations in which the child (healthy or with increased susceptibility to infection) is likely to have been inoculated (eg, asymptomatic child closely exposed to meningococcus; a neonate born to a mother with active genital herpes simplex virus).

B. Long-term Antimicrobial Prophylaxis to Prevent Symptomatic Disease

Given to a particular, defined population of children who are of relatively high risk of acquiring a severe infection (eg, a child postsplenectomy; a child with documented rheumatic heart disease to prevent subsequent streptococcal infection), with prophylaxis provided during the period of risk, potentially months or years.

C. Preemptive Treatment/Latent Infection Treatment ("Prophylaxis of Symptomatic Disease in Children Who Have Asymptomatic Infection")

Where a child has a documented but asymptomatic infection and targeted antimicrobials are given to prevent the development of symptomatic disease (eg, latent tuberculosis infection or therapy of a stem cell transplant patient with documented cytomegalovirus viremia but no symptoms of infection or rejection). Treatment period is usually defined, but certain circumstances, such as reactivation of a herpesvirus, may require re-treatment.

D. Surgical/Procedure Prophylaxis

A child receives a surgical/invasive catheter procedure, planned or unplanned, where the risk of infection postoperatively or post-procedure may justify prophylaxis to prevent an infection from occurring (eg, prophylaxis to prevent infection following spinal rod placement). Treatment is usually short-term, beginning just prior to the procedure and ending at the conclusion of the procedure, or within 24 to 48 hours.

E. Travel-Related Exposure Prophylaxis

Not discussed in this chapter; please refer to information on specific disease entities (eg, traveler's diarrhea, Chapter 6) or pathogens (eg, malaria, Chapter 10). Constantly updated, current information for travelers about prophylaxis and current worldwide infection risks can be found on the Centers for Disease Control and Prevention Web site at www.cdc.gov/travel (accessed September 19, 2016).

NOTE

- **Abbreviations:** AHA, American Heart Association; ALT, alanine aminotransferase; amox/clav, amoxicillin/clavulanate; ARF, acute rheumatic fever; bid, twice daily; CDC, Centers for Disease Control and Prevention; CSF, cerebrospinal fluid; div, divided; DOT, directly observed therapy; GI, gastrointestinal; HSV, herpes simplex virus; IGRA, interferon-gamma release assay; IM, intramuscular; INH, isoniazid; IV, intravenous; MRSA, methicillin-resistant *Staphylococcus aureus;* N/A, not applicable; PCR, polymerase chain reaction; PO, orally; PPD, purified protein derivative; qd, once daily; qid, 4 times daily; spp, species; TB, tuberculosis; tid, 3 times daily; TIG, tetanus immune globulin; TMP/SMX, trimethoprim/sulfamethoxazole; UTI, urinary tract infection.

A. POSTEXPOSURE SHORT-TERM ANTIMICROBIAL PROPHYLAXIS

Prophylaxis Category	Therapy (evidence grade)	Comments
Bacterial		
Bites, animal and human[1-5] (*Pasteurella multocida* [animal], *Eikenella corrodens* [human], *Staphylococcus* spp, and *Streptococcus* spp)	Amox/clav 45 mg/kg/day PO div tid (amox/clav 7:1; see Chapter 1 for amox/clav description) for 3–5 days (AII) OR ampicillin and clindamycin (BII). For penicillin allergy, consider ciprofloxacin (for *Pasteurella*) plus clindamycin (BII).	Recommended for children who are (1) immunocompromised; (2) asplenic; (3) have moderate to severe injuries, especially to the hand or face; or (4) have injuries that may have penetrated the periosteum or joint capsule (AII).[3] Consider rabies prophylaxis for animal bites (AI)[6]; consider tetanus prophylaxis.[7] Human bites have a very high rate of infection (do not close open wounds routinely). Cat bites have a higher rate of infection than dog bites. *Staphylococcus aureus* coverage is only fair with amox/clav and provides no coverage for MRSA.
Endocarditis Prophylaxis[8]: Given that (1) endocarditis is rarely caused by dental/GI procedures and (2) prophylaxis for procedures prevents an exceedingly small number of cases, the risks of antibiotics most often outweigh benefits. However, some "highest risk" conditions are currently recommended for prophylaxis: (1) prosthetic heart valve (or prosthetic material used to repair a valve); (2) previous endocarditis; (3) cyanotic congenital heart disease that is unrepaired (or palliatively repaired with shunts and conduits); (4) congenital heart disease that is repaired but with defects at the site of repair adjacent to prosthetic material; (5) completely repaired congenital heart disease using prosthetic material, for the first 6 months after repair; or (6) cardiac transplant patients with valvulopathy. Routine prophylaxis no longer is required for children with native valve abnormalities. Follow-up data in children suggest that following these new guidelines, no increase in endocarditis has been detected,[9] but in adults in the United States[10] and in the United Kingdom,[11] some concern for increase in the number of cases of endocarditis has been documented since widespread prophylaxis was stopped.		
– In highest-risk patients: dental procedures that involve manipulation of the gingival or periodontal region of teeth	Amoxicillin 50 mg/kg PO 1 h before procedure OR ampicillin or ceftriaxone or cefazolin, all at 50 mg/kg IM/IV 30–60 min before procedure	If penicillin allergy: clindamycin 20 mg/kg PO (60 min before) or IV (30 min before) OR azithromycin 15 mg/kg or clarithromycin 15 mg/kg (1 h before)
– Genitourinary and gastrointestinal procedures	None	No longer recommended

Antimicrobial Prophylaxis/Prevention of Symptomatic Infection

A. POSTEXPOSURE SHORT-TERM ANTIMICROBIAL PROPHYLAXIS (continued)

Prophylaxis Category	Therapy (evidence grade)	Comments
Bacterial (continued)		
Meningococcus (*Neisseria meningitidis*)[12]	For prophylaxis of close contacts, including household members, child care center contacts, and anyone directly exposed to the patient's oral secretions (eg, through kissing, mouth-to-mouth resuscitation, endotracheal intubation, endotracheal tube management) in the 7 days before symptom onset Rifampin Infants <1 mo: 5 mg/kg PO q12h for 4 doses Children ≥1 mo: 10 mg/kg PO q12h for 4 doses (max 600 mg/dose) OR Ceftriaxone Children <15 y: 125 mg IM once Children ≥16 y: 250 mg IM once OR Ciprofloxacin 500 mg PO once (adolescents and adults)	A single dose of ciprofloxacin should not present a significant risk of cartilage damage, but no prospective data exist in children for prophylaxis of meningococcal disease. For a child, an equivalent exposure for ciprofloxacin to that in adults would be 15–20 mg/kg as a single dose (max 500 mg). A few ciprofloxacin-resistant strains have now been reported. Insufficient data to recommend azithromycin at this time. Meningococcal vaccines may also be recommended in case of an outbreak.
Pertussis[13,14]	Same regimen as for treatment: azithromycin 10 mg/kg/day qd for 5 days OR clarithromycin (for infants >1 mo) 15 mg/kg/day bid for 7 days OR erythromycin (estolate preferable) 40 mg/kg/day PO div qid for 14 days (AII) Alternative: TMP/SMX 8 mg/kg/day div bid for 14 days (BII)	Prophylaxis to family members; contacts defined by CDC: persons within 21 days of exposure to an infectious pertussis case, who are at high risk of severe illness or who will have close contact with a person at high risk of severe illness (including infants, pregnant women in their third trimester, immunocompromised persons, contacts who have close contact with infants <12 mo). Close contact can be considered as face-to-face exposure within 3 feet of a symptomatic person; direct contact with respiratory, nasal, or oral secretions; or sharing the same confined space in close proximity to an infected person for ≥1 h. Community-wide prophylaxis is not currently recommended.

14

Azithromycin and clarithromycin are better tolerated than erythromycin (see Chapter 5); azithromycin is preferred in exposed young infants to reduce pyloric stenosis risk.

Tetanus
(*Clostridium tetani*)[15,16]

NEED FOR TETANUS VACCINE OR TIG[a]				
	Clean Wound		Contaminated Wound	
Number of past tetanus vaccine doses	Need for tetanus vaccine	Need for TIG 250 U IM[a]	Need for tetanus vaccine	Need for TIG 250 U IM[a]
<3 doses	Yes	No	Yes	Yes
≥3 doses	No (if <10 y[b]) Yes (if ≥10 y[b])	No	No (if <5 y[b]) Yes (if ≥5 y[b])	No

[a] IV immune globulin should be used when TIG is not available.
[b] Years since last tetanus-containing vaccine dose.

For deep, contaminated wounds, wound debridement is essential. For wounds that cannot be fully debrided, consider metronidazole 30 mg/kg/day PO div q8h until wound healing is underway and anaerobic conditions no longer exist, as short as 3–5 days (BIII).

Antimicrobial Prophylaxis/Prevention of Symptomatic Infection

14

A. POSTEXPOSURE SHORT-TERM ANTIMICROBIAL PROPHYLAXIS (continued)

Prophylaxis Category	Therapy (evidence grade)	Comments
Bacterial (continued)		
Tuberculosis (*Mycobacterium tuberculosis*) Exposed children <4 y, or immunocompromised patient (high risk of dissemination)[17,18] For treatment of latent TB infection, see Table 14C.	Scenario 1: Previously uninfected child becomes exposed to a person with active disease. Exposed children <4 y, or immunocompromised patient (high risk of dissemination): INH 10–15 mg/kg PO daily for at least 2–3 mo (AIII). For older children, may also begin prophylaxis postexposure, but if exposure is questionable, can wait 2–3 mo after exposure; if PPD/IGRA at 2–3 mo is positive at that time, start INH for 9–12 mo.	If PPD or IGRA remains negative at 2–3 mo and child remains well, consider stopping empiric therapy. However, tests at 2–3 mo may not be reliable in immunocompromised patients. This regimen is to prevent infection in a compromised host after exposure, rather than to treat latent asymptomatic infection.
	Scenario 2: Asymptomatic child is found to have a positive skin test/IGRA test for TB, documenting latent TB infection. INH 10–15 mg/kg PO daily for 9 mo (≥12 mo for an immunocompromised child) OR INH 20–30 mg/kg PO directly observed therapy twice weekly for 9 mo.	Other options For INH intolerance or INH resistance if a direct contact can be tested: rifampin 10 mg/kg PO daily for 4 mo For children ≥12 y, can use once-weekly DOT with INH AND rifapentine for 12 wk; much less data for children 2–12 y[19]
Viral		
Herpes Simplex Virus		
During pregnancy	For women with recurrent genital herpes: acyclovir 400 mg PO bid; valacyclovir 500 mg PO qd OR 1 g PO qd from 36-wk gestation until delivery (CII)[20]	Development of neonatal HSV disease after maternal suppression has been documented.
Neonatal: Primary or nonprimary maternal infection, infant exposed at delivery[21]	Asymptomatic, exposed infant: at 24 h of life, culture mucosal sites (see Comments), obtain CSF and whole-blood PCR for HSV DNA, obtain ALT, and start preemptive acyclovir IV (60 mg/kg/day div q8h) for 10 days (AII).	Reference 18 provides a management algorithm that determines the type of maternal infection and, thus, the appropriate evaluation and preemptive therapy of the neonate. Mucosal sites for culture: conjunctivae, mouth, nasopharynx, rectum.

	Some experts would evaluate at birth for exposure following presumed maternal primary infection and start preemptive therapy rather than wait 24 h.	Any symptomatic baby, at any time, requires a full evaluation for invasive infection and IV acyclovir therapy for 14–21 days.
Neonatal: Recurrent maternal infection, infant exposed at delivery[21]	Asymptomatic, exposed infant: at 24 h of life, culture mucosal sites, obtain whole-blood PCR for HSV DNA. Hold on therapy unless cultures or PCR are positive, at which time the diagnostic evaluation should be completed (CSF PCR for HSV DNA, serum ALT) and preemptive IV acyclovir (60 mg/kg/day div q8h) should be administered for 10 days (AIII).	Reference 18 provides a management algorithm that determines the type of maternal infection and, thus, the appropriate evaluation and preemptive therapy of the neonate. Any symptomatic baby, at any time, requires a full evaluation for invasive infection and IV acyclovir therapy. Risk of neonatal HSV infection following inoculation (even if not documented by newborn evaluation) lasts 6–8 wk.
Neonatal: Following symptomatic HSV disease, to prevent recurrence during first year of life[21]	300 mg/m²/dose PO tid for 6 mo following cessation of IV acyclovir treatment of acute disease (AI)	Follow absolute neutrophil counts at 2 and 4 wk, then monthly during prophylactic/suppressive therapy.
Keratitis (ocular) in otherwise healthy children	Suppressive therapy for frequent recurrence (no pediatric data): 20 mg/kg/dose bid (up to 400 mg) for ≥1 y (AIII)	Based on data from adults. Anecdotally, some children may require tid dosing to prevent recurrences. Check for acyclovir resistance for those who relapse while on appropriate therapy. Watch for severe recurrence at conclusion of suppression.
Influenza virus (A or B)[22]	Oseltamivir prophylaxis (AI) 3–≤8 mo: 3.0 mg/kg/dose qd for 10 days 9–11 mo: 3.5 mg/kg/dose PO bid qd for 10 days[23] Based on body weight for children ≥12 mo ≤15 kg: 30 mg qd for 10 days >15–23 kg: 45 mg qd for 10 days >23–40 kg: 60 mg qd for 10 days >40 kg: 75 mg qd for 10 days Zanamivir prophylaxis (AI) Children ≥5 y: 10 mg (two 5-mg inhalations) qd for as long as 28 days (community outbreaks) or 10 days (household settings)	Not recommended for infants 0 to ≤3 mo unless situation judged critical because of limited data on use in this age group.

Antimicrobial Prophylaxis/Prevention of Symptomatic Infection

A. POSTEXPOSURE SHORT-TERM ANTIMICROBIAL PROPHYLAXIS (continued)

Prophylaxis Category	Therapy (evidence grade)	Comments
Viral (continued)		
Rabies virus[24]	Rabies immune globulin, 20 IU/kg, infiltrate around wound, with remaining volume injected IM (AII). Rabies immunization should be provided postexposure (AII).	For dog, cat, or ferret bite from symptomatic animal, immediate rabies immune globulin and immunization; otherwise, can wait 10 days for observation of animal, if possible, prior to rabies immune globulin or vaccine. Bites of squirrels, hamsters, guinea pigs, gerbils, chipmunks, rats, mice and other rodents, rabbits, hares, and pikas almost never require antirabies prophylaxis. For bites of bats, skunks, raccoons, foxes, most other carnivores, and woodchucks, immediate rabies immune globulin and immunization (regard as rabid unless geographic area is known to be free of rabies or until animal proven negative by laboratory tests).
Fungal		
Pneumocystis jiroveci (previously *Pneumocystis carinii*)[25,26]	TMP/SMX as 5 mg TMP/kg/day PO, div 2 doses, q12h, either daily or 3 times/wk on consecutive days (AI); OR TMP/SMX 5 mg TMP/kg/day PO as a *single dose*, qd, given 3 times/wk on consecutive days (AI) (once-weekly regimens have also been successful); OR dapsone 2 mg/kg (max 100 mg) PO qd, or 4 mg/kg (max 200 mg) once weekly; OR atovaquone 30 mg/kg/day for infants 1–3 mo; 45 mg/kg/day for infants 4–24 mo; and 30 mg/kg/day for infants >24 mo until no longer immunocompromised, based on oncology or transplant treatment regimen	Prophylaxis in specific populations based on degree of immunosuppression

B. LONG-TERM ANTIMICROBIAL PROPHYLAXIS TO PREVENT SYMPTOMATIC DISEASE

Prophylaxis Category	Therapy (evidence grade)	Comments
Bacterial otitis media[27,28]	Amoxicillin or other antibiotics can be used in half the therapeutic dose qd or bid to prevent infections if the benefits outweigh the risks of (1) development of resistant organisms for that child and (2) the risk of antibiotic side effects.	To prevent recurrent infections, also consider the risks and benefits of placing tympanostomy tubes to improve middle ear ventilation. Studies have demonstrated that amoxicillin, sulfisoxazole, and TMP/SMX are effective. However, antimicrobial prophylaxis may alter the nasopharyngeal flora and foster colonization with resistant organisms, compromising long-term efficacy of the prophylactic drug. Continuous PO-administered antimicrobial prophylaxis should be reserved for control of recurrent acute otitis media, only when defined as ≥3 distinct and well-documented episodes during a period of 6 mo or ≥4 episodes during a period of 12 mo. Although prophylactic administration of an antimicrobial agent limited to a period when a person is at high risk of otitis media has been suggested (eg, during acute viral respiratory tract infection), this method has not been evaluated critically.
Acute rheumatic fever	For >27.3 kg (>60 lb): 1.2 million U penicillin G benzathine, q4wk (q3wk for high-risk children) For <27.3 kg: 600,000 U penicillin G benzathine, q4wk (q3wk for high-risk children) OR Penicillin V (phenoxymethyl) oral, 250 mg PO bid	AHA policy statement at http://circ.ahajournals.org/content/119/11/1541.full.pdf (accessed September 19, 2016). Doses studied many years ago, with no new data; ARF an uncommon disease currently in the United States. Alternatives to penicillin include sulfisoxazole or macrolides, including erythromycin, azithromycin, and clarithromycin.
Urinary tract infection, recurrent[29–32]	TMP/SMX 3 mg/kg/dose TMP PO qd OR nitrofurantoin 1–2 mg/kg PO qd at bedtime; more rapid resistance may develop using beta-lactams (BII).	Only for those with grade III–V reflux or with recurrent febrile UTI: prophylaxis no longer recommended for patients with grade I–II (some also exclude grade III) reflux and no evidence of renal damage. Prophylaxis prevents infection but may not prevent scarring. Early treatment of new infections is recommended for these children. Resistance eventually develops to every antibiotic; follow resistance patterns for each patient.

14

C. PREEMPTIVE TREATMENT/LATENT INFECTION TREATMENT ("PROPHYLAXIS OF SYMPTOMATIC DISEASE IN CHILDREN WHO HAVE ASYMPTOMATIC INFECTION")

Tuberculosis[17,18] (latent TB infection [asymptomatic infection], defined by a positive skin test or IGRA, with no clinical or x-ray evidence of active disease)	INH 10–15 mg/kg/day (max 300 mg) PO daily for 9 mo (12 mo for immunocompromised patients) (AII); treatment with INH at 20–30 mg twice weekly for 9 mo is also effective (AII).	Single drug therapy if no clinical or radiographic evidence of active disease. For exposure to known INH-resistant but rifampin-susceptible strains, use rifampin 10 mg/kg PO daily for 6 mo (AII). For children ≥12 y, can use once weekly DOT with INH AND rifapentine for 12 wk; much less data for children 2–12 y.[19] For exposure to multidrug-resistant strains, consult with TB specialist.

D. SURGICAL/PROCEDURE PROPHYLAXIS[33-41]

The CDC and National Healthcare Safety Network use a classification of surgical procedure-related wound infections based on an estimation of the load of bacterial contamination: Class I, clean; Class II, clean-contaminated; Class III, contaminated; and Class IV, dirty/infected.[34,37] Other major factors creating risk for postoperative surgical site infection include the duration of surgery (a longer-duration operation, defined as one that exceeded the 75th percentile for a given procedure) and the medical comorbidities of the patient, as determined by an American Society of Anesthesiologists score of III, IV, or V (presence of severe systemic disease that results in functional limitations, is life-threatening, or is expected to preclude survival from the operation). The virulence/pathogenicity of bacteria inoculated and the presence of foreign debris/devitalized tissue/surgical material in the wound are also considered risk factors for infection.

For all categories of surgical prophylaxis, dosing recommendations are derived from (1) choosing agents based on the organisms likely to be responsible for inoculation of the surgical site; (2) giving the agents shortly before starting the operation to achieve appropriate serum and tissue exposures at the time of incision through the end of the procedure; (3) providing additional doses during the procedure at times based on the standard dosing guideline for that agent; and (4) stopping the agents at the end of the procedure but no longer than 24 to 48 h after the procedure.[35-38,40,41]

Procedure/Operation	Recommended Agents	Preoperative Dose	Re-dosing Interval (h) for Prolonged Surgery
Cardiovascular			
Cardiothoracic *Staphylococcus epidermidis,* *Staphylococcus aureus,* *Corynebacterium* spp	Cefazolin, OR	30 mg/kg	4
	Vancomycin, if MRSA likely[38]	15 mg/kg	8
	Ampicillin/sulbactam if enteric gram-negative bacilli a concern	50 mg/kg of ampicillin	3
Vascular *S epidermidis, S aureus,* *Corynebacterium* spp, gram-negative enteric bacilli, particularly for procedures in the groin	Cefazolin, OR	30 mg/kg	4
	Vancomycin, if MRSA likely[38]	15 mg/kg	8
Gastrointestinal			
Gastroduodenal Enteric gram-negative bacilli, respiratory tract gram-positive cocci	Cefazolin	30 mg/kg	4
Biliary Procedure, Open Enteric gram-negative bacilli, enterococci, *Clostridia*	Cefazolin, OR	30 mg/kg	4
	Cefoxitin	40 mg/kg	2
Appendectomy, non-perforated	Cefoxitin, OR	40 mg/kg	2
	Cefazolin and metronidazole	30 mg/kg cefazolin and 10 mg/kg metronidazole	4 for cefazolin 8 for metronidazole

Antimicrobial Prophylaxis/Prevention of Symptomatic Infection

D. SURGICAL/PROCEDURE PROPHYLAXIS[33–41] (continued)

Antimicrobial Prophylaxis/Prevention of Symptomatic Infection

Procedure/Operation	Recommended Agents	Preoperative Dose	Re-dosing Interval (h) for Prolonged Surgery
Gastrointestinal (continued)			
Complicated appendicitis or other ruptured viscus Enteric gram-negative bacilli, enterococci, anaerobes. For complicated appendicitis, antibiotics provided to treat ongoing infection, rather than prophylaxis.	Cefazolin and metronidazole, OR	30 mg/kg cefazolin and 10 mg/kg metronidazole	4 for cefazolin 8 for metronidazole
	Cefoxitin, OR	40 mg/kg	2
	Ceftriaxone and metronidazole, OR	50 mg/kg ceftriaxone and 10 mg/kg metronidazole	12 for ceftriaxone 8 for metronidazole
	Ertapenem, OR	30 mg/kg	8
	Meropenem, OR	20 mg/kg	4
	Imipenem	20 mg/kg	4
Genitourinary			
Cystoscopy (only requires prophylaxis for children with suspected active UTI or those having foreign material placed) Enteric gram-negative bacilli, enterococci	Cefazolin, OR	30 mg/kg	4
	TMP/SMX (if low local resistance), OR Select a 3rd-generation cephalosporin (cefotaxime) or fluoroquinolone (ciprofloxacin) if the child is colonized with cefazolin-resistant, TMP/SMX-resistant strains.	4–5 mg/kg	N/A
Open or laparoscopic surgery Enteric gram-negative bacilli, enterococci	Cefazolin	30 mg/kg	4

Head and Neck Surgery			
Assuming incision through respiratory tract mucosa Anaerobes, enteric gram-negative bacilli, S aureus	Clindamycin, OR	10 mg/kg	6
	Cefazolin and metronidazole 30 mg/kg cefazolin and 10 mg/kg metronidazole	4 for cefazolin	8 for metronidazole
	Ampicillin/sulbactam if enteric gram-negative bacilli a concern	50 mg/kg of ampicillin	3
Neurosurgery			
Craniotomy, ventricular shunt placement S epidermidis, S aureus	Cefazolin, OR	30 mg/kg	4
	Vancomycin, if MRSA likely	15 mg/kg	8
Orthopedic			
Internal fixation of fractures, spinal rod placement,[39] prosthetic joints S epidermidis, S aureus	Cefazolin, OR	30 mg/kg	4
	Vancomycin, if MRSA likely[38]	15 mg/kg	8

Antimicrobial Prophylaxis/Prevention of Symptomatic Infection

D. SURGICAL/PROCEDURE PROPHYLAXIS[33-41] (continued)

Procedure/Operation	Recommended Agents	Preoperative Dose	Re-dosing Interval (h) for Prolonged Surgery
Trauma			
Exceptionally varied; agents should focus on skin flora (S epidermidis, S aureus) as well as the flora inoculated into the wound, based on the trauma exposure, that may include enteric gram-negative bacilli, anaerobes (including Clostridia spp), and fungi. Cultures at time of wound exploration are critical to focus therapy.	Cefazolin (for skin), OR	30 mg/kg	4
	Vancomycin (for skin), if MRSA likely, OR	15 mg/kg	8
	Meropenem OR imipenem (for anaerobes, including Clostridia spp. and non-fermenting gram-negative bacilli), OR	20 mg/kg for either	4
	Gentamicin and metronidazole (for anaerobes, including Clostridia spp. and non-fermenting gram-negative bacilli), OR	2.5 mg/kg gentamicin and 10 mg/kg metronidazole	6 for gentamicin 8 for metronidazole
	Piperacillin/tazobactam	100 mg/kg piperacillin component	2

14

15. Adverse Reactions to Antimicrobial Agents

A good rule of clinical practice is to be suspicious of an adverse drug reaction when a patient's clinical course deviates from the expected. This section focuses on reactions that may require close observation or laboratory monitoring because of their frequency or severity. For more detailed listings of reactions, review the US Food and Drug Administration (FDA)-approved package labels available at the National Library of Medicine (NLM) (http://dailymed.nlm.nih.gov, accessed September 19, 2016), with more recently approved agents actually having adverse events listed for the new agent and the comparator agent from the phase 3 prospective clinical trials. This allows one to assign drug-attributable side effects for specific drugs, such as oseltamivir, used for influenza, when influenza and the antiviral may cause nausea. The NLM also provides an online drug information service for patients (MedlinePlus) at www.nlm.nih.gov/medlineplus/druginformation.html.

Antibacterial Drugs

Aminoglycosides. Any of the aminoglycosides can cause serious nephrotoxicity and ototoxicity. Monitor all patients receiving aminoglycoside therapy for more than a few days for renal function with periodic determinations of blood urea nitrogen and creatinine to assess potential problems of drug accumulation with deteriorating renal function. Common practice has been to measure the peak serum concentration 0.5 to 1 hour after a dose to make sure one is in a safe and therapeutic range and to measure a trough serum concentration immediately preceding a dose to assess for drug accumulation and pending toxicity. Monitoring is especially important in patients with any degree of renal insufficiency. Elevated trough concentrations (>2 mg/mL for gentamicin and tobramycin; >10 mg/mL for amikacin) suggest drug accumulation and should be a warning to decrease the dose, even if the peak is not yet elevated. Renal toxicity may be related to the total exposure of the kidney to the aminoglycoside over time. With once-daily administration regimens, peak values are 2 to 3 times greater, and trough values are usually very low. Nephrotoxicity seems to be less common in adults with once-daily (as opposed to 3 times daily) dosing regimens, but data are generally lacking in children.[1,2] In patients with cystic fibrosis with pulmonary exacerbations, once-daily aminoglycosides appear less toxic and equally effective.[3]

The "loop" diuretics (furosemide and bumetanide) and other nephrotoxic drugs may potentiate the ototoxicity of the aminoglycosides. Aminoglycosides potentiate botulinum toxin neuromuscular junction dysfunction and are to be avoided in young infants with infant botulism.

Minor side effects, such as allergies, rashes, and drug fever, are rare.

Beta-lactam Antibiotics. The most feared reaction to penicillins, anaphylactic shock, is extremely rare, and no absolutely reliable means of predicting its occurrence exists. For most infections, alternative therapy to penicillin or beta-lactams exists. However, in certain situations, the benefits of penicillin or a beta-lactam may outweigh the risk of anaphylaxis, requiring that skin testing and desensitization be performed in a medically supervised environment. The commercially available skin testing material, benzylpenicilloyl polylysine (Pre-Pen, AllerQuest), contains the major determinants thought to be primarily responsible for urticarial reactions but does not contain the minor determinants that are more often associated with anaphylaxis. No commercially available minor determinant mixture is available. For adults, the Centers for Disease Control and Prevention (CDC) suggests using a dilute solution of freshly prepared benzyl penicillin G as the skin test material in place of a standardized mixture of minor determinants.[4] Testing should be performed on children with a credible history of a possible reaction to a penicillin before these drugs are used in oral or parenteral formulations. Anaphylaxis has been reported in adults receiving penicillin skin testing. Recent reviews provide more in-depth discussion,[5,6] with additional information on desensitization available in the CDC "Sexually Transmitted Diseases Treatment Guidelines, 2015."[4] Cross-reactions between classes of beta-lactam antibiotics (penicillins, cephalosporins, carbapenems, and monobactams) occur at a rate of less than 5% to 20%, with the rate of reaction to cephalosporins in patients with a *history* of penicillin allergy of about 0.1%.[7] No commercially available skin-testing reagent has been developed for beta-lactam antibiotics other than penicillin.

Amoxicillin and other aminopenicillins are associated with minor adverse effects. Diarrhea, oral or diaper-area candidiasis, morbilliform, and blotchy rashes are not uncommon. The kinds of non-urticarial rashes that may occur while a child is receiving amoxicillin are not known to predispose to anaphylaxis and may not actually be caused by amoxicillin itself; they do not represent a routine contraindication to subsequent use of amoxicillin or any other penicillins. Rarely, beta-lactams cause serious, life-threatening pseudomembranous enterocolitis due to suppression of normal bowel flora and overgrowth of toxin-producing strains of *Clostridium difficile*. Drug-related fever may occur; serum sickness is uncommon. Reversible neutropenia and thrombocytopenia may occur with any of the beta-lactams and seems to be related to dose and duration of therapy, but the neutropenia does not appear to carry the same risk of bacterial superinfection that is present with neutropenia in oncology patients.

The cephalosporins have been a remarkably safe series of antibiotics. Third-generation cephalosporins cause profound alteration of normal flora on mucosal surfaces, and all have caused pseudomembranous colitis on occasion. Ceftriaxone commonly causes loose stools, but it is rarely severe enough to require stopping therapy. Ceftriaxone in high dosages may cause fine "sand" (a calcium complex of ceftriaxone) to develop in the gallbladder. In adults, and rarely in children, these deposits may cause biliary tract symptoms; these are not gallstones, and the deposits are reversible after stopping the drug. In neonates receiving calcium-containing hyperalimentation concurrent with intravenous (IV) ceftriaxone, precipitation of ceftriaxone-calcium in the bloodstream resulting in death has been reported,[8] leading to an FDA warning against the concurrent use of ceftriaxone and parenteral calcium in neonates younger than 28 days. As ceftriaxone may also displace bilirubin from albumin-binding sites and increase free bilirubin in serum, the antibiotic is not routinely used in neonatal infections until the normal physiologic jaundice is resolving after the first few weeks of life. Cefotaxime is the preferred IV third-generation cephalosporin for neonates.

Imipenem/cilastatin, meropenem, and ertapenem have rates of adverse effects on hematopoietic, hepatic, and renal systems that are similar to other beta-lactams. However, children treated with imipenem for bacterial meningitis were noted to have an increase in probable drug-related seizures not seen with meropenem therapy in controlled studies.[9] For children requiring carbapenem therapy, meropenem is preferred for those with any underlying central nervous system inflammatory condition.

Fluoroquinolones (FQs). All quinolone antibiotics (nalidixic acid, ciprofloxacin, levofloxacin, gatifloxacin, and moxifloxacin) cause cartilage damage to weight-bearing joints in toxicity studies in various immature animals; however, no conclusive data indicate similar toxicity in young children.[10] Studies to evaluate cartilage toxicity and failure to achieve predicted growth have not consistently found statistically significant differences between those children treated with FQs and controls, although in an FDA-requested, blinded, prospective study of complicated urinary tract infections, the number of muscular/joint/tendon events was greater in the ciprofloxacin-treated group than in the comparator (www.fda.gov/downloads/Drugs/DevelopmentApprovalProcess/DevelopmentResources/UCM162536.pdf, accessed September 19, 2016). This continues to be an area of active investigation by the pediatric infectious disease community as well as the FDA. Fluoroquinolone toxicities in adults, which vary in incidence considerably between individual agents, include cardiac dysrhythmias, hepatotoxicity, and photodermatitis; other reported side effects include gastrointestinal symptoms, dizziness, headaches, tremors, confusion, seizures, and alterations of glucose metabolism producing hyperglycemia and hypoglycemia. The American Academy of Pediatrics published a clinical report on the use of fluoroquinolones and, based on the best available evidence, concluded that IV fluoroquinolones should be used when safer IV antibiotic alternatives were not available and that oral fluoroquinolones should be used if no other safe and effective oral therapy existed, even if effective alternative IV therapy existed.[11]

Lincosamides. Clindamycin can cause nausea, vomiting, and diarrhea. Pseudomembranous colitis due to suppression of normal flora and overgrowth of *C difficile* is uncommon, especially in children, but potentially serious. Urticaria, glossitis, pruritus, and skin rashes occur occasionally. Serum sickness, anaphylaxis, and photosensitivity are rare, as are hematologic and hepatic abnormalities. Extensive use of clindamycin since 2000 for treatment of community-associated methicillin-resistant *Staphylococcus aureus* infections has not been accompanied by reports of significantly increasing rates of *C difficile*–mediated colitis in children.

Macrolides. Erythromycin is one of the safest antimicrobial agents but has largely been replaced by azithromycin because of substantially decreased epigastric distress and nausea. Intravenous erythromycin lactobionate causes phlebitis and should be administered slowly (1–2 hours); the gastrointestinal side effects seen with oral administration also accompany IV use. However, IV azithromycin is better tolerated than IV erythromycin and has been evaluated for pharmacokinetics in limited numbers of children.[12]

Erythromycin therapy has been associated with pyloric stenosis in newborns and young infants; due to this toxicity and with limited data on safety of azithromycin in the first months of life, azithromycin is now the preferred macrolide for treatment of pertussis in neonates and young infants.[13]

Oxazolidinones. Linezolid represents the first oxazolidinone antibiotic approved for all children, including neonates, by the FDA. Toxicity is primarily hematologic, with thrombocytopenia and neutropenia that is dependent on dosage and duration of therapy, occurring most often with treatment courses of 2 weeks or longer. Routine monitoring for bone marrow toxicity every 1 to 2 weeks is recommended for children on long-term therapy. Peripheral neuropathy and optic neuritis may also occur with long-term therapy.[14] Tedizolid, approved for adults but not yet investigated in children, appears to have a better safety profile compared with linezolid.

Sulfonamides and Trimethoprim. The most common adverse reaction to sulfonamides is a hypersensitivity rash. Stevens-Johnson syndrome, a life-threatening systemic reaction characterized by immune-mediated injury to the skin and mucous membranes, occurs in approximately 3 of 100,000 exposed people. Neutropenia, anemia, and thrombocytopenia occur occasionally. Sulfa drugs can precipitate hemolysis in patients with glucose-6-phosphate dehydrogenase deficiency. Drug fever and serum sickness are infrequent hypersensitivity reactions. Hepatitis with focal or diffuse necrosis is rare. A rare idiosyncratic reaction to sulfa drugs is acute aseptic meningitis.

Tetracyclines. Tetracyclines are used infrequently in pediatric patients because the major indications are uncommon diseases (rickettsial infections, brucellosis, Lyme disease), with the exception of acne. Tetracyclines are deposited in growing bones and teeth, with depression of linear bone growth, dental staining, and defects in enamel formation in deciduous and permanent teeth. This effect is dose related, and the risk extends up to 8 years of age. A single treatment course of tetracyclines has not been found to cause dental staining, leading to the recommendation for tetracyclines as the drugs of choice in children for a number of uncommon pathogens. Doxycycline is likely to produce less dental staining than tetracycline. A parenteral tetracycline approved for adults in 2005, tigecycline, produces the same "staining" of bones in experimental animals as seen with other tetracyclines.

Side effects include minor gastrointestinal disturbances, photosensitization, angioedema, glossitis, pruritus ani, and exfoliative dermatitis. Potential adverse drug reactions from tetracyclines involve virtually every organ system. Hepatic and pancreatic injuries have occurred with accidental overdosage and in patients with renal failure. (Pregnant women are particularly at risk for hepatic injury.)

Vancomycin. Vancomycin can cause phlebitis if the drug is injected rapidly or in concentrated form. Vancomycin has the potential for ototoxicity and nephrotoxicity, and serum concentrations should be monitored for children on more than a few days of therapy. Hepatic toxicity is rare. Neutropenia has been reported. If the drug is infused too rapidly, a transient rash of the upper body with itching may occur from histamine release (red man syndrome). It is not a contraindication to continued use and the rash is less likely to occur if the infusion period is increased to 60 to 120 minutes and the children are pretreated with oral or IV antihistamines.

Daptomycin. This antibiotic is still undergoing investigation in children; therefore, the full adverse event profile is not yet available, but data presented at national/international meetings do not indicate adverse events that occur in children that have not been reported in adults. Specifically, no significant drug-attributable muscle toxicity or elevated creatine kinase concentrations have been reported. Of concern, prior to clinical studies in infants younger than 1 year, neonatal puppy studies indicated the possibility of the development of neurotoxicity in the first days of life; therefore, studies in infants younger than 1 year are not being performed. These concerns are presented in the current FDA-approved package label. Daptomycin should be used with caution in infants younger than 1 year.

Antituberculous Drugs

Isoniazid (INH) is generally well tolerated and hypersensitivity reactions are rare. Peripheral neuritis (preventable or reversed by pyridoxine administration) and mental aberrations from euphoria to psychosis occur more often in adults than in children. Mild elevations of alanine transaminase in the first weeks of therapy, which disappear or remain stable with continued administration, are common. Rarely, hepatitis develops but is reversible if INH is stopped; if INH is not stopped, liver failure may develop in these children. Monitoring of liver functions is not routinely required in children receiving INH single drug therapy for latent tuberculosis as long as the children can be followed closely and liver functions can be drawn if the children develop symptoms of hepatitis.

Rifampin can also cause hepatitis; it is more common in patients with preexisting liver disease or in those taking large dosages. The risk of hepatic damage increases when rifampin and INH are taken together in dosages of more than 15 mg/kg/day of each. Gastrointestinal, hematologic, and neurologic side effects of various types have been observed on occasion. Hypersensitivity reactions are rare.

Pyrazinamide also can cause hepatic damage, which again seems to be dosage related. Ethambutol has the potential for optic neuritis, but this toxicity seems to be rare in children at currently prescribed dosages. Young children who cannot comment to examiners about color blindness or other signs of optic neuritis should be considered for an ophthalmologic examination every few months on therapy. Optic neuritis is usually reversible.

Antifungal Drugs

Amphotericin B (deoxycholate) causes chills, fever, flushing, and headaches, the most common of the many adverse reactions. Some degree of decreased renal function occurs in virtually all patients given amphotericin B. Anemia is common and, rarely, hepatic toxicity and neutropenia occur. Patients should be monitored for hyponatremia, hypomagnesemia, and hypokalemia. However, much better tolerated (but more costly) lipid formulations of amphotericin B are now commonly used (see Chapter 2). For reasons of safety and tolerability, the lipid formulations should be used whenever possible, except in neonates who appear to tolerate amphotericin better than older children.

Fluconazole is usually very well tolerated from clinical and laboratory standpoints. Gastrointestinal symptoms, rash, and headache occur occasionally. Transient, asymptomatic elevations of hepatic enzymes have been reported but are rare.

Voriconazole may interfere with metabolism of other drugs the child may be receiving due to hepatic P450 metabolism. However, a poorly understood visual field abnormality has been described, usually at the beginning of a course of therapy and uniformly self-resolving, in which objects appear to the child to glow. There is no pain and no known anatomic or biochemical correlate of this side effect; lasting effects on vision have been sought, but none have yet been reported. Hepatic toxicity has also been reported but is not so common as to preclude the use of voriconazole for serious fungal infections. Phototoxic skin reaction with chronic use that has been reported to develop into carcinoma is another common reason for discontinuation.[15,16]

Caspofungin, micafungin, and anidulafungin (echinocandins) are very well tolerated as a class. Fever, rash, headache, and phlebitis at the site of infection have been reported in adults. Uncommon hepatic side effects have also been reported.

Flucytosine (5-FC) is seldom used due to the availability of safer, equally effective therapy. The major toxicity is bone marrow depression, which is dosage related, especially in patients treated concomitantly with amphotericin B. Flucytosine serum concentrations and renal function should be monitored.

Antiviral Drugs

After extensive clinical use, acyclovir has proved to be an extremely safe drug with only rare serious adverse effects. Renal dysfunction with IV acyclovir has occurred mainly with too rapid infusion of the drug. Neutropenia has been associated with administration of parenteral and oral acyclovir but is responsive to granulocyte colony-stimulating factor use and resolves spontaneously when the drug is stopped. At very high doses, parenteral acyclovir can cause neurologic irritation, including seizures. Rash, headache, and gastrointestinal side effects are uncommon. There has been little controlled experience in children with famciclovir and valacyclovir.

Ganciclovir causes hematologic toxicity that is dependent on the dosage and duration of therapy. Gastrointestinal disturbances and neurologic damage are rarely encountered. Oral valganciclovir can have these same toxicities as parenteral ganciclovir, but neutropenia is seen much less frequently following oral valganciclovir compared with IV ganciclovir. In preclinical test systems, ganciclovir is mutagenic, carcinogenic, and teratogenic. Additionally, it causes irreversible reproductive toxicity in animals.

Oseltamivir is well tolerated except for nausea with or without vomiting, which may be more likely to occur with the first few doses but usually resolves within a few days while still on therapy. Neuropsychiatric events have been reported, primarily from Japan, in patients with influenza treated with oseltamivir (a rate of approximately 1:50,000) but also are seen in patients on all of the other influenza antivirals and in patients with influenza receiving no antiviral therapy. It seems that these spontaneously reported side effects may be a function of influenza itself, oseltamivir itself, possibly a genetic predisposition to this clinical event, or a combination of all 3 factors.

Foscarnet can cause renal dysfunction, anemia, and cardiac rhythm disturbances. Alterations in plasma minerals and electrolytes occur, and any clinically significant metabolic changes should be corrected. Patients who experience mild (eg, perioral numbness or paresthesia) or severe (eg, seizures) symptoms of electrolyte abnormalities should have serum electrolyte and mineral levels assessed as close in time to the event as possible.

The primary adverse event with cidofovir is nephrotoxicity. Cidofovir concentrates in renal cells in amounts 100 times greater than in other tissues, producing severe nephrotoxicity involving the proximal convoluted tubule when concomitant hydration and administration of probenecid are not employed. Renal toxicity manifests as proteinuria and glycosuria. To decrease the potential for nephrotoxicity, aggressive IV prehydration and coadministration of probenecid are required with each cidofovir dose. In animal studies, cidofovir has been shown to be carcinogenic and teratogenic and to cause hypospermia. Intravitreal administration has been associated with ocular hypotony.

Adverse Reactions to Antimicrobial Agents

15

Appendix

Nomogram for Determing Body Surface Area

Based on the nomogram shown below, a straight line joining the patient's height and weight will intersect the center column at the calculated body surface area (BSA). For children of normal height and weight, the child's weight in pounds is used, and then the examiner reads across to the corresponding BSA in meters. Alternatively, Mosteller's formula can be used.

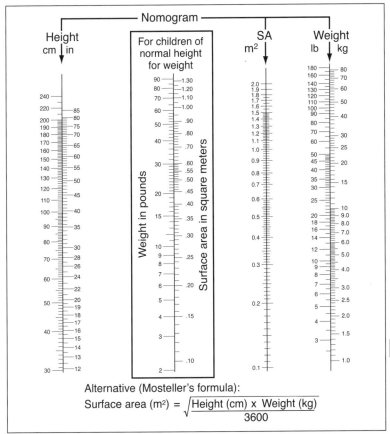

Alternative (Mosteller's formula):

$$\text{Surface area (m}^2) = \sqrt{\frac{\text{Height (cm) x Weight (kg)}}{3600}}$$

Nomogram and equation to determine body surface area. (From Engorn B, Flerlage J, eds. *The Harriet Lane Handbook*. 20th ed. Philadelphia, PA: Elsevier Mosby; 2015. Reprinted with permission from Elsevier.)

Appendix: Nomogram for Determining Body Surface Area

References

Chapter 1

1. Cannavino CR, et al. *Pediatr Infect Dis J.* 2016;35(7):752–759 PMID: 27093162
2. Blumer JL, et al. *Pediatr Infect Dis J.* 2016;35(7):760–766 PMID: 27078119
3. Korczowski B, et al. *Pediatr Infect Dis J.* 2016;35(8):e239–e247 PMID: 27164462
4. Bradley JS, et al. *Pediatrics.* 2011;128(4):e1034–e1045 PMID: 21949152
5. Bradley JS, et al. *Pediatrics.* 2014;134(1):e146–e153 PMID: 24918220

Chapter 2

1. Cornely OA, et al. *Clin Infect Dis.* 2007;44(10):1289–1297 PMID: 17443465
2. Ascher SB, et al. *Pediatr Infect Dis J.* 2012;31(5):439–443 PMID: 22189522
3. Piper L, et al. *Pediatr Infect Dis J.* 2011;30(5):375–378 PMID: 21085048
4. Friberg LE, et al. *Antimicrob Agents Chemother.* 2012;56(6):3032–3042 PMID: 22430956
5. Smith PB, et al. *Pediatr Infect Dis J.* 2009;28(5):412–415 PMID: 19319022
6. Hope WW, et al. *Antimicrob Agents Chemother.* 2010;54(6):2633–2637 PMID: 20308367
7. Benjamin DK Jr, et al. *Clin Pharmacol Ther.* 2010;87(1):93–99 PMID: 19890251
8. Cohen-Wolkowiez M, et al. *Clin Pharmacol Ther.* 2011;89(5):702–707 PMID: 21412233

Chapter 4

1. Liu C, et al. *Clin Infect Dis.* 2011;52(3):e18–e55 PMID: 21208910
2. Le J, et al. *Pediatr Infect Dis J.* 2013;32(4):e155–e163 PMID: 23340565
3. Depardieu F, et al. *Clin Microbiol Rev.* 2007;20(1):79–114 PMID: 17223624
4. Miller LG, et al. *N Engl J Med.* 2015;372(12):1093–1103 PMID: 25785967
5. Korczowski B, et al. *Pediatr Infect Dis J.* 2016;35(8):e239–e247 PMID: 27164462
6. Cannavino CR, et al. *Pediatr Infect Dis J.* 2016;35(7):752–759 PMID: 27093162
7. Blumer JL, et al. *Pediatr Infect Dis J.* 2016;35(7):760–766 PMID: 27078119
8. Huang JT, et al. *Pediatrics.* 2009;123(5):e808–e814 PMID: 19403473
9. Finnell SM, et al. *Clin Pediatr (Phila).* 2015;54(5):445–450 PMID: 25385929

Chapter 5

1. Fox E, et al. Drug therapy in neonates and pediatric patients. In: Atkinson AJ, et al, eds. *Principles of Clinical Pharmacology.* 2007:359–373
2. Wagner CL, et al. *J Perinatol.* 2000;20(6):346–350 PMID: 11002871
3. Intravenous ceftriaxone (marketed as Rocephin and generics) and calcium drug-drug interaction: potential risk for cardiovascular adverse events in neonates. US Food and Drug Administration. http://www.fda.gov/Drugs/DrugSafety/DrugSafetyNewsletter/ucm199806.htm#IntravenousCeftriaxone MarketedasRocephinandGenericsandCalciumDrug-DrugInteraction:PotentialRiskforCardiovascular AdverseEventsinNeonates. Accessed September 19, 2016
4. Martin E, et al. *Eur J Pediatr.* 1993;152(5):530–534 PMID: 8335024
5. Rours IG, et al. *Pediatrics.* 2008;121(2):e321–e326 PMID: 18245405
6. American Academy of Pediatrics. Chlamydial infections. In: Kimberlin DW, et al, eds. *Red Book: 2015 Report of the Committee on Infectious Diseases.* 2015:284–294
7. Hammerschlag MR, et al. *Pediatr Infect Dis J.* 1998;17(11):1049–1050 PMID: 9849993
8. Zar HJ. *Paediatr Drugs.* 2005;7(2):103–110 PMID: 15871630
9. Honein MA, et al. *Lancet.* 1999;354(9196):2101–2105 PMID: 10609814
10. Laga M, et al. *N Engl J Med.* 1986;315(22):1382–1385 PMID: 3095641
11. Workowski KA, et al. *MMWR Recomm Rep.* 2015;64(RR-3):1–137 PMID: 26042815
12. Newman LM, et al. *Clin Infect Dis.* 2007;44(S3):S84–S101 PMID: 17342672
13. MacDonald N, et al. *Adv Exp Med Biol.* 2008;609:108–130 PMID: 18193661
14. American Academy of Pediatrics. Gonococcal infections. In: Kimberlin DW, et al, eds. *Red Book: 2015 Report of the Committee on Infectious Diseases.* 2015:356–367
15. Cimolai N. *Am J Ophthalmol.* 2006;142(1):183–184 PMID: 16815280
16. Marangon FB, et al. *Am J Ophthalmol.* 2004;137(3):453–458 PMID: 15013867

17. American Academy of Pediatrics. Staphylococcal infections. In: Kimberlin DW, et al, eds. *Red Book: 2015 Report of the Committee on Infectious Diseases.* 2015:715–732

18. Brito DV, et al. *Braz J Infect Dis.* 2003;7(4):234–235 PMID: 14533982

19. Chen CJ, et al. *Am J Ophthalmol.* 2008;145(6):966–970 PMID: 18378213

20. Shah SS, et al. *J Perinatol.* 1999;19(6pt1):462–465 PMID: 10685281

21. Kimberlin DW, et al. *J Pediatr.* 2003;143(1):16–25 PMID: 12915819

22. Kimberlin DW, et al. *J Infect Dis.* 2008;197(6):836–845 PMID: 18279073

23. American Academy of Pediatrics. Cytomegalovirus infection. In: Kimberlin DW, et al, eds. *Red Book: 2015 Report of the Committee on Infectious Diseases.* 2015:317–322

24. Kimberlin DW, et al. *N Engl J Med.* 2015;372(10):933–943 PMID: 25738669

25. Kimberlin DW, et al. *N Engl J Med.* 2015;372(25):2463 PMID: 26083215

26. American Academy of Pediatrics. Candidiasis. In: Kimberlin DW, et al, eds. *Red Book: 2015 Report of the Committee on Infectious Diseases.* 2015:275–280

27. Hundalani S, et al. *Expert Rev Anti Infect Ther.* 2013;11(7):709–721 PMID: 23829639

28. Saez-Llorens X, et al. *Antimicrob Agents Chemother.* 2009;53(3):869–875 PMID: 19075070

29. Ericson JE, et al. *Clin Infect Dis.* 2016;63(5):604–610 PMID: 27298330

30. Smith PB, et al. *Pediatr Infect Dis J.* 2009;28(5):412–415 PMID: 19319022

31. Wurthwein G, et al. *Antimicrob Agents Chemother.* 2005;49(12):5092–5098 PMID: 16304177

32. Heresi GP, et al. *Pediatr Infect Dis J.* 2006;25(12):1110–1115 PMID: 17133155

33. Kawaguchi C, et al. *Pediatr Int.* 2009;51(2):220–224 PMID: 19405920

34. Hsieh E, et al. *Early Hum Dev.* 2012;88(S2):S6–S10 PMID: 22633516

35. Swanson JR, et al. *Pediatr Infect Dis J.* 2016;35(5):519–523 PMID: 26835970

36. Santos RP, et al. *Pediatr Infect Dis J.* 2007;26(4):364–366 PMID: 17414408

37. Frankenbusch K, et al. *J Perinatol.* 2006;26(8):511–514 PMID: 16871222

38. Thomas L, et al. *Expert Rev Anti Infect Ther.* 2009;7(4):461–472 PMID: 19400765

39. Verweij PE, et al. *Drug Resist Updat.* 2015;21–22:30–40 PMID: 26282594

40. Shah D, et al. *Cochrane Database Syst Rev.* 2012;8:CD007448 PMID: 22895960

41. Brook I. *Am J Perinatol.* 2008;25(2):111–118 PMID: 18236362

42. Denkel LA, et al. *PLoS One.* 2016;11(6):e0158136 PMID: 27332554

43. Cohen-Wolkowiez M, et al. *Clin Infect Dis.* 2012;55(11):1495–1502 PMID: 22955430

44. Jost T, et al. *PLoS One.* 2012;7(8):e44595 PMID: 22957008

45. Dilli D, et al. *J Pediatr.* 2015;166(3):545–551 PMID: 25596096

46. American Academy of Pediatrics. *Salmonella* infections. In: Kimberlin DW, et al, eds. *Red Book: 2015 Report of the Committee on Infectious Diseases.* 2015:695–702

47. Pinninti SG, et al. *Pediatr Clin North Am.* 2013;60(2):351–365 PMID: 23481105

48. American Academy of Pediatrics. Herpes simplex. In: Kimberlin DW, et al, eds. *Red Book: 2015 Report of the Committee on Infectious Diseases.* 2015:432–445

49. Jones CA, et al. *Cochrane Database Syst Rev.* 2009;(3):CD004206 PMID: 19588350

50. Kimberlin DW, et al. *N Engl J Med.* 2011;365(14):1284–1292 PMID: 21991950

51. Sampson MR, et al. *Pediatr Infect Dis J.* 2014;33(1):42–49 PMID: 24346595

52. Panel on Antiretroviral Therapy and Medical Management of HIV-Infected Children. Guidelines for the use of antiretroviral agents in pediatric HIV infection. http://aidsinfo.nih.gov/ContentFiles/PediatricGuidelines.pdf. Updated March 1, 2016. Accessed September 19, 2016

53. Panel on Treatment of HIV-Infected Pregnant Women and Prevention of Perinatal Transmission. Recommendations for use of antiretroviral drugs in pregnant HIV-1-infected women for maternal health and interventions to reduce perinatal HIV transmission in the United States. http://aidsinfo.nih.gov/guidelines/html/3/perinatal-guidelines/0. Updated June 7, 2016. Accessed September 19, 2016

54. Luzuriaga K, et al. *N Engl J Med.* 2015;372(8):786–788 PMID: 25693029

55. Nielsen-Saines K, et al. *N Engl J Med.* 2012;366(25):2368–2379 PMID: 22716975

56. American Academy of Academy Committee on Infectious Diseases. *Pediatrics.* 2015;136(4):792–808 PMID: 26347430

57. Acosta EP, et al. *J Infect Dis.* 2010;202(4):563–566 PMID: 20594104

58. McPherson C, et al. *J Infect Dis.* 2012;206(6):847–850 PMID: 22807525

59. Kamal MA, et al. *Clin Pharmacol Ther.* 2014;96(3):380–389 PMID: 24865390

60. Kimberlin DW, et al. *J Infect Dis*. 2013;207(5):709–720 PMID: 23230059

61. Blumer J, et al. Safety, tolerability and pharmacokinetics (PK) of intravenous zanamivir (IVZ) treatment in hospitalized pediatric and adolescent patients with influenza: a phase II open-label, multicenter, single-arm study. Presented at: IDWeek 2016; October 26–30, 2016; New Orleans, LA

62. Fraser N, et al. *Acta Paediatr*.2006;95(5):519–522 PMID: 16825129

63. Ulloa-Gutierrez R, et al. *Pediatr Emerg Care*. 2005;21(9):600–602 PMID: 16160666

64. Sawardekar KP. *Pediatr Infect Dis J*. 2004;23(1):22–26 PMID: 14743041

65. Bingol-Kologlu M, et al. *J Pediatr Surg*. 2007;42(11):1892–1897 PMID: 18022442

66. Brook I. *J Perinat Med*. 2002;30(3):197–208 PMID: 12122901

67. Kaplan SL. *Adv Exp Med Biol*. 2009;634:111–120 PMID: 19280853

68. Korakaki E, et al. *Jpn J Infect Dis*. 2007;60(2-3):129–131 PMID: 17515648

69. Dessi A, et al. *J Chemother*. 2008;20(5):542–550 PMID: 19028615

70. Berkun Y, et al. *Arch Dis Child*. 2008;93(8):690–694 PMID: 18337275

71. Greenberg D, et al. *Paediatr Drugs*. 2008;10(2):75–83 PMID: 18345717

72. Ismail EA, et al. *Pediatr Int*. 2013;55(1):60–64 PMID: 23039834

73. Engle WD, et al. *J Perinatol*. 2000;20(7):421–426 PMID: 11076325

74. Brook I. *Microbes Infect*. 2002;4(12):1271–1280 PMID: 12467770

75. Darville T. *Semin Pediatr Infect Dis*. 2005;16(4):235–244 PMID: 16210104

76. Eberly MD, et al. *Pediatrics*. 2015;135(3):483–488 PMID: 25687145

77. Waites KB, et al. *Semin Fetal Neonatal Med*. 2009;14(4):190–199 PMID: 19109084

78. Morrison W. *Pediatr Infect Dis J*. 2007;26(2):186–188 PMID: 17259889

79. American Academy of Pediatrics. Pertussis (whooping cough). In: Kimberlin DW, et al, eds. *Red Book: 2015 Report of the Committee on Infectious Diseases*. 2015:608–621

80. Foca MD. *Semin Perinatol*. 2002;26(5):332–339 PMID: 12452505

81. American Academy of Pediatrics Committee on Infectious Diseases and Bronchiolitis Guidelines Committee. *Pediatrics*. 2014;134(2):e620–e638 PMID: 25070304

82. Vergnano S, et al. *Pediatr Infect Dis J*. 2011;30(10):850–854 PMID: 21654546

83. Nelson MU, et al. *Semin Perinatol*. 2012;36(6):424–430 PMID: 23177801

84. Lyseng-Williamson KA, et al. *Paediatr Drugs*. 2003;5(6):419–431 PMID: 12765493

85. American Academy of Pediatrics. Group B streptococcal infections. In: Kimberlin DW, et al, eds. *Red Book: 2015 Report of the Committee on Infectious Diseases*. 2015:745–750

86. Schrag S, et al. *MMWR Recomm Rep*. 2002;51(RR-11):1–22 PMID: 12211284

87. American Academy of Pediatrics. *Ureaplasma urealyticum* and *Ureaplasma parvum* infections. In: Kimberlin DW, et al, eds. *Red Book: 2015 Report of the Committee on Infectious Diseases*. 2015:845–846

88. American Academy of Pediatrics. *Escherichia coli* and other gram-negative bacilli. In: Kimberlin DW, et al, eds. *Red Book: 2015 Report of the Committee on Infectious Diseases*. 2015:340–343

89. Venkatesh MP, et al. *Expert Rev Anti Infect Ther*. 2008;6(6):929–938 PMID: 19053905

90. Abzug MJ, et al. and the National Institute of Allergy and Infectious Diseases Collaborative Antiviral Study Group. *J. Pediatr. Infect. Dis. Soc*. 2016;5(1):53-62 PMID: 26407253

91. American Academy of Pediatrics. *Listeria monocytogenes* infections. In: Kimberlin DW, et al, eds. *Red Book: 2015 Report of the Committee on Infectious Diseases*. 2015:513–516

92. Fortunov RM, et al. *Pediatrics*. 2006;118(3):874–881 PMID: 16950976

93. Fortunov RM, et al. *Pediatrics*. 2007;120(5):937–945 PMID: 17974729

94. van der Lugt NM, et al. *BMC Pediatr*. 2010;10:84 PMID: 21092087

95. Stauffer WM, et al. *Pediatr Emerg Care*. 2003;19(3):165–166 PMID: 12813301

96. Coggins S, et al. EPAS2016:2720A.8

97. Dehority W, et al. *Pediatr Infect Dis J*. 2006;25(11):1080–1081 PMID: 17072137

98. American Academy of Pediatrics. Syphilis. In: Kimberlin DW, et al, eds. *Red Book: 2015 Report of the Committee on Infectious Diseases*. 2015:755–768

99. American Academy of Pediatrics. Tetanus. In: Kimberlin DW, et al, eds. Red Book: 2015 Report of the Committee on Infectious Diseases. 2015:773–778

100. American Academy of Pediatrics. *Toxoplasma gondii* infections. In: Kimberlin DW, et al, eds. *Red Book: 2015 Report of the Committee on Infectious Diseases*. 2015:787–796

101. Petersen E. Toxoplasmosis. *Semin Fetal Neonatal Med.* 2007;12(3):214–223 PMID: 17321812
102. Beetz R. *Curr Opin Pediatr.* 2012;24(2):205–211 PMID: 22227782
103. RIVUR Trial Investigators, et al. *N Engl J Med.* 2014;370(25):2367–2376 PMID: 24795142
104. Roberts SW, et al. Placental transmission of antibiotics. In: *Glob Libr Women's Med.* DOI 10.3843/GLOWM.10174
105. Nanovskaya TN, et al. *J Matern Fetal Neonatal Med.* 2012;25(11):2312–2315 PMID: 22590979
106. Nanovskaya T, et al. *Am J Obstet Gynecol.* 2012;207(4):331.e1–331.e6 PMID: 22867688
107. Sachs HC, et al. *Pediatrics.* 2013;132(3):e796–e809 PMID: 23979084
108. Hale TW. *Medication and Mothers' Milk: A Manual of Lactational Pharmacology.* 16th ed. 2014

Chapter 6

1. Stevens DL, et al. *Clin Infect Dis.* 2014;59(2):147–159 PMID: 24947530
2. Liu C, et al. *Clin Infect Dis.* 2011;52(3):e18–e55 PMID: 21208910
3. Elliott DJ, et al. *Pediatrics.* 2009;123(6):e959–e966 PMID: 19470525
4. Inman JC, et al. *Laryngoscope.* 2008;118(12):2111–2114 PMID: 18948832
5. Martinez-Aguilar G, et al. *Pediatr Infect Dis J.* 2003;22(7):593–598 PMID: 12867833
6. American Academy of Pediatrics. Staphylococcal infections. In: Kimberlin DW, et al, eds. *Red Book: 2015 Report of the Committee on Infectious Diseases.* 2015:715–732
7. American Academy of Pediatrics. Group A streptococcal infections. In: Kimberlin DW, et al, eds. *Red Book: 2015 Report of the Committee on Infectious Diseases.* 2015:732–744
8. Bass JW, et al. *Pediatr Infect Dis J.* 1998;17(6):447–452 PMID: 9655532
9. Hatzenbuehler LA, et al. *Pediatr Infect Dis J.* 2014;33(1):89–91 PMID: 24346597
10. Lindeboom JA. *J Oral Maxillofac Surg.* 2012;70(2):345–348 PMID: 21741739
11. Wallace RJ Jr, et al. *Chest.* 2014;146(2):276–282 PMID: 24457542
12. Lindeboom JA. *Clin Infect Dis.* 2011;52(2):180–184 PMID: 21288841
13. American Thoracic Society, et al. *MMWR Recomm Rep.* 2003;52(RR-11):1–77 PMID: 12836625
14. American Academy of Pediatrics. Tuberculosis. In: Kimberlin DW, et al, eds. *Red Book: 2015 Report of the Committee on Infectious Diseases.* 2015:805–831
15. Bradley JS, et al. *Pediatrics.* 2014;133(5):e1411–e1436 PMID: 24777226
16. Oehler RL, et al. *Lancet Infect Dis.* 2009;9(7):439–447 PMID: 19555903
17. Thomas N, et al. *Expert Rev Anti Infect Ther.* 2011;9(2):215–226 PMID: 21342069
18. Lion C, et al. *Int J Antimicrob Agents.* 2006;27(4):290–293 PMID: 16564680
19. Aziz H, et al. *J Trauma Acute Care Surg.* 2015;78(3):641–648 PMID: 25710440
20. Talan DA, et al. *N Engl J Med.* 1999;340(2):85–92 PMID: 9887159
21. Goldstein EJ, et al. *Antimicrob Agents Chemother.* 2012;56(12):6319–6323 PMID: 23027193
22. American Academy of Pediatrics. Rabies. In: Kimberlin DW, et al, eds. *Red Book: 2015 Report of the Committee on Infectious Diseases.* 2015:658–666
23. Talan DA, et al. *Clin Infect Dis.* 2003;37(11):1481–1489 PMID: 14614671
24. Miller LG, et al. *N Engl J Med.* 2015;372(12):1093–1103 PMID: 25785967
25. Talan DA, et al. *N Engl J Med.* 2016;374(9):823–832 PMID: 26962903
26. American Academy of Pediatrics. *Haemophilus influenzae* infections. In: Kimberlin DW, et al, eds. *Red Book: 2015 Report of the Committee on Infectious Diseases.* 2015:368–376
27. Yang LP, et al. *Am J Clin Dermatol.* 2008;9(6):411–413 PMID: 18973410
28. Bass JW, et al. *Pediatr Infect Dis J.* 1997;16(7):708–710 PMID: 9239775
29. Lin HW, et al. *Clin Pediatr (Phila).* 2009;48(6):583–587 PMID: 19286617
30. Pannaraj PS, et al. *Clin Infect Dis.* 2006;43(8):953–960 PMID: 16983604
31. Smith-Slatas CL, et al. *Pediatrics.* 2006;117(4):e796–e805 PMID: 16567392
32. Jamal N, et al. *Pediatr Emerg Care.* 2011;27(12):1195–1199 PMID: 22158285
33. Stevens DL. *Annu Rev Med.* 2000;51:271–288 PMID: 10774464
34. Abuhammour W, et al. *Pediatr Emerg Care.* 2006;22(1):48–51 PMID: 16418613
35. Daum RS. *N Engl J Med.* 2007;357(4):380–390 PMID: 17652653
36. Lee MC, et al. *Pediatr Infect Dis J.* 2004;23(2):123–127 PMID: 14872177
37. Karamatsu ML, et al. *Pediatr Emerg Care.* 2012;28(2):131–135 PMID: 22270497
38. Elliott SP. *Clin Microbiol Rev.* 2007;20(1):13–22 PMID: 17223620

39. Berk DR, et al. *Pediatr Ann.* 2010;39(10):627–633 PMID: 20954609
40. Braunstein I, et al. *Pediatr Dermatol.* 2014;31(3):305–308 PMID: 24033633
41. Kaplan SL. *Adv Exp Med Biol.* 2009;634:111–120 PMID: 19280853
42. Peltola H, et al. *Clin Infect Dis.* 2009;48(9):1201–1210 PMID: 19323633
43. Bradley JS. *Clin Infect Dis.* 2009;48(9):1211–1212 PMID: 19323629
44. Saphyakhajon P, et al. *Pediatr Infect Dis J.* 2008;27(8):765–767 PMID: 18600193
45. Pääkkönen M, et al. *Expert Rev Anti Infect Ther.* 2011;9(12):1125–1131 PMID: 22114963
46. Section J, et al. *J Bone Joint Surg Am.* 2015;97(6):441–449 PMID: 25788299
47. Arnold JC, et al. *Pediatrics.* 2012;130(4):e821–e828 PMID: 22966033
48. Fogel I, et al. *Pediatrics.* 2015;136(4):e776–e782 PMID: 26347429
49. Farrow L. *BMC Musculoskelet Disord.* 2015;16:241 PMID: 26342736
50. Workowski KA, et al. *MMWR Recomm Rep.* 2015;64(RR-03):1–137 PMID: 26042815
51. American Academy of Pediatrics. Gonococcal infections. In: Kimberlin DW, et al, eds. *Red Book: 2015 Report of the Committee on Infectious Diseases.* 2015:356–367
52. Pääkkönen M, et al. *N Engl J Med.* 2014;370(14):1365–1366 PMID: 24693913
53. Martinez-Aguilar G, et al. *Pediatr Infect Dis J.* 2004;23(8):701–706 PMID: 15295218
54. Messina AF, et al. *Pediatr Infect Dis J.* 2011;30(12):1019–1021 PMID: 21817950
55. Howard-Jones AR, et al. *J Paediatr Child Health.* 2013;49(9):760–768 PMID: 23745943
56. Jacqueline C, et al. *J Antimicrob Chemother.* 2014;69(Suppl1):i37–i40 PMID: 25135088
57. Ceroni D, et al. *J Pediatr Orthop.* 2010;30(3):301–304 PMID: 20357599
58. Keren R, et al. *JAMA Pediatr.* 2015;169(2):120–128 PMID: 25506733
59. Chen CJ, et al. *Pediatr Infect Dis J.* 2007;26(11):985–988 PMID: 17984803
60. Chachad S, et al. *Clin Pediatr (Phila).* 2004;43(3):213–216 PMID: 15094944
61. Bradley JS, et al. *Pediatrics.* 2011;128(4):e1034–e1045 PMID: 21949152
62. Vaska VL, et al. *Pediatr Infect Dis J.* 2011;30(11):1003–1006 PMID: 21681121
63. Seltz LB, et al. *Pediatrics.* 2011;127(3):e566–e572 PMID: 21321025
64. Peña MT, et al. *JAMA Otolaryngol Head Neck Surg.* 2013;139(3):223–227 PMID: 23429877
65. Smith JM, et al. *Am J Ophthalmol.* 2014;158(2):387–394 PMID: 24794092
66. Wald ER. *Pediatr Rev.* 2004;25(9):312–320 PMID: 15342822
67. Sheikh A, et al. *Cochrane Database Syst Rev.* 2012;9:CD001211 PMID: 22972049
68. Williams L, et al. *J Pediatr.* 2013;162(4):857–861 PMID: 23092529
69. Pichichero ME. *Clin Pediatr (Phila).* 2011;50(1):7–13 PMID: 20724317
70. Wilhelmus KR. *Cochrane Database Syst Rev.* 2015;1:CD002898 PMID: 25879115
71. Liu S, et al. *Ophthalmology.* 2012;119(10):2003–2008 PMID: 22796308
72. Young RC, et al. *Arch Ophthalmol.* 2010;128(9):1178–1183 PMID: 20837803
73. Khan S, et al. *J Pediatr Ophthalmol Strabismus.* 2014;51(3):140–153 PMID: 24877526
74. Soheilian M, et al. *Arch Ophthalmol.* 2007;125(4):460–465 PMID: 17420365
75. Riddell J 4th, et al. *Clin Infect Dis.* 2011;52(5):648–653 PMID: 21239843
76. Vishnevskia-Dai V, et al. *Ophthalmology.* 2015;122(4):866–868.e3 PMID: 25556113
77. Nassetta L, et al. *J Antimicrob Chemother.* 2009;63(5):862–867 PMID: 19287011
78. Kimberlin DW, et al. *J Pediatr.* 2003;143(1):16–25 PMID: 12915819
79. Groth A, et al. *Int J Pediatr Otorhinolaryngol.* 2012;76(10):1494–1500 PMID: 22832239
80. Stahelin-Massik J, et al. *Eur J Pediatr.* 2008;167(5):541–548 PMID: 17668240
81. Ongkasuwan J, et al. *Pediatrics.* 2008;122(1):34–39 PMID: 18595984
82. Rosenfeld RM, et al. *Otolaryngol Head Neck Surg.* 2014;150(1Suppl):S1–S24 PMID: 24491310
83. Dohar JE. *Pediatr Infect Dis J.* 2003;22(4):299–308 PMID: 12690268
84. Carfrae MJ, et al. *Otolaryngol Clin North Am.* 2008;41(3):537–549 PMID: 18435997
85. Kaushik V, et al. *Cochrane Database Syst Rev.* 2010;(1):CD004740 PMID: 20091565
86. Hoberman A, et al. *N Engl J Med.* 2011;364(2):105–115 PMID: 21226576
87. Tähtinen PA, et al. *N Engl J Med.* 2011;364(2):116–126 PMID: 21226577
88. Lieberthal AS, et al. *Pediatrics.* 2013;131(3):e964–e999 PMID: 23439909
89. Rovers MM, et al. *Lancet.* 2006;368(9545):1429–1435 PMID: 17055944
90. Venekamp RP, et al. *Cochrane Database Syst Rev.* 2013;1:CD000219 PMID: 23440776
91. Hoberman A, et al. *Clin Pediatr (Phila).* 2011;50(2):114–120 PMID: 21098526

92. Pichichero ME. *Pediatr Clin North Am.* 2013;60(2):391–407 PMID: 23481107
93. Macfadyen CA, et al. *Cochrane Database Syst Rev.* 2006;(1):CD005608 PMID: 16437533
94. Kutz JW Jr, et al. *Expert Opin Pharmacother.* 2013;14(17):2399–2405 PMID: 24093464
95. Haynes DS, et al. *Otolaryngol Clin North Am.* 2007;40(3):669–683 PMID: 17544701
96. Wald ER, et al. *Pediatrics.* 2009;124(1):9–15 PMID: 19564277
97. Wald ER, et al. *Pediatrics.* 2013;132(1):e262–e280 PMID: 23796742
98. Sharma S, et al. *JAMA Otolaryngol Head Neck Surg.* 2014;140(11):1070–1073 PMID: 25317572
99. Chow AW, et al. *Clin Infect Dis.* 2012;54(8):e72–e112 PMID: 22438350
100. Brook I. *Int J Pediatr Otorhinolaryngol,* 2016;84:21–26 PMID: 27063747
101. Ellison SJ. *Br Dent J.* 2009;206(7):357–362 PMID: 19357666
102. Robertson DP, et al. *BMJ.* 2015;350:h1300 PMID: 25804417
103. American Academy of Pediatrics. Diphtheria. In: Kimberlin DW, et al, eds. *Red Book: 2015 Report of the Committee on Infectious Diseases.* 2015:325–329
104. Wheeler DS, et al. *Pediatr Emerg Care.* 2008;24(1):46–49 PMID: 18212612
105. Sobol SE, et al. *Otolaryngol Clin North Am.* 2008;41(3):551–566 PMID: 18435998
106. Nasser M, et al. *Cochrane Database Syst Rev.* 2008;(4):CD006700 PMID: 18843726
107. Amir J, et al. *BMJ.* 1997;314(7097):1800–1803 PMID: 9224082
108. Kimberlin DW, et al. *Clin Infect Dis.* 2010;50(2):221–228 PMID: 20014952
109. Riordan T. *Clin Microbiol Rev.* 2007;20(4):622–659 PMID: 17934077
110. Kizhner V, et al. *J Laryngol Otol.* 2013;127(7):721–723 PMID: 23701713
111. Ridgway JM, et al. *Am J Otolaryngol.* 2010;31(1):38–45 PMID: 19944898
112. Goldenberg NA, et al. *Pediatrics.* 2005;116(4):e543–e548 PMID: 16147971
113. Agrafiotis M, et al. *Am J Emerg Med.* 2015;33(5):733.e3–733.e4 PMID: 25455045
114. Baldassari CM, et al. *Otolaryngol Head Neck Surg.* 2011;144(4):592–595 PMID: 21493241
115. Shulman ST, et al. *Clin Infect Dis.* 2012;55(10):e86–e102 PMID: 22965026
116. Lennon DR, et al. *Arch Dis Child.* 2008;93(6):474–478 PMID: 18337284
117. American Academy of Pediatrics. Group A streptococcal infections. In: Kimberlin DW, et al, eds. *Red Book: 2015 Report of the Committee on Infectious Diseases.* 2015:732–744
118. Casey JR, et al. *Diagn Microbiol Infect Dis.* 2007;57(3Suppl):39S–45S PMID: 17292576
119. Altamimi S, et al. *Cochrane Database Syst Rev.* 2012;8:CD004872 PMID: 22895944
120. Abdel-Haq N, et al. *Pediatr Infect Dis J.* 2012;31(7):696–699 PMID: 22481424
121. Cheng J, et al. *Otolaryngol Head Neck Surg.* 2013;148(6):1037–1042 PMID: 23520072
122. Brown NK, et al. *Pediatr Infect Dis J.* 2015;34(4):454–456 PMID: 25760568
123. Shargorodsky J, et al. *Laryngoscope.* 2010;120(12):2498–2501 PMID: 21108480
124. Tebruegge M, et al. *Scand J Infect Dis.* 2009;41(8):548–557 PMID: 19401934
125. Lemaître C, et al. *Pediatr Infect Dis J.* 2013;32(10):1146–1149 PMID: 23722529
126. Bender JM, et al. *Clin Infect Dis.* 2008;46(9):1346–1352 PMID: 18419434
127. Blumer JL, et al. *Pediatr Infect Dis J.* 2016;35(7):760–766 PMID: 27078119
128. Brook I. *Adv Exp Med Biol.* 2011;697:117–152 PMID: 21120724
129. Agarwal R, et al. *Future Microbiol.* 2013;8(11):1463–1474 PMID: 24199804
130. Schuh S. *Curr Opin Pediatr.* 2011;23(1):110–114 PMID: 21157348
131. Zobell JT, et al. *Pediatr Pulmonol.* 2013;48(6):525–537 PMID: 23359557
132. Chmiel JF, et al. *Ann Am Thorac Soc.* 2014;11(7):1120–1129 PMID: 25102221
133. Flume PA, et al. *Am J Respir Crit Care Med.* 2009;180(9):802–808 PMID: 19729669
134. Bhatt JM. *Eur Respir Rev.* 2013;22(129):205–216 PMID: 23997047
135. Mayer-Hamblett N, et al. *Pediatr Pulmonol.* 2013;48(10):943–953 PMID: 23818295
136. Chmiel JF, et al. *Ann Am Thorac Soc.* 2014;11(8):1298–1306 PMID: 25167882
137. Ryan G, et al. *Cochrane Database Syst Rev.* 2012;12:CD008319 PMID: 23235659139
138. Saiman L. *Paediatr Respir Rev.* 2007;8(3):249–255 PMID: 17868923
139. Waters V, et al. *Cochrane Database Syst Rev.* 2008;(3):CD006961 PMID: 18646176
140. Langton Hewer SC, et al. *Cochrane Database Syst Rev.* 2014;(11):CD004197 PMID: 25383937
141. Cheer SM, et al. *Drugs.* 2003;63(22):2501–2520 PMID: 14609360
142. Hutchinson D, et al. *Expert Opin Pharmacother.* 2013;14(15):2115–2124 PMID: 23992352

143. Mogayzel PJ Jr, et al. *Am J Respir Crit Care Med.* 2013;187(7):680–689 PMID: 23540878

144. Southern KW, et al. *Cochrane Database Syst Rev.* 2012;11:CD002203 PMID: 23152214

145. Moskowitz SM, et al. *Pediatr Pulmonol.* 2008;43(9):874–881 PMID: 18668689

146. American Academy of Pediatrics. Pertussis (whooping cough). In: Kimberlin DW, et al, eds. *Red Book: 2015 Report of the Committee on Infectious Diseases.* 2015:608–621

147. Altunaiji S, et al. *Cochrane Database Syst Rev.* 2007;(3):CD004404 PMID: 17636756

148. Kilgore PE, et al. *Clin Microbiol Rev.* 2016;29(3):449–486 PMID: 27029594

149. Wang K, et al. *Cochrane Database Syst Rev.* 2014;(9):CD003257 PMID: 25243777

150. Jain S, et al. *N Engl J Med.* 2015;372(9):835–845 PMID: 25714161

151. Bradley JS, et al. *Clin Infect Dis.* 2011;53(7):e25–e76 PMID: 21880587

152. Esposito S, et al. *Pediatr Infect Dis J.* 2012;31(6):e78–e85 PMID: 22466326

153. Queen MA, et al. *Pediatrics.* 2014;133(1):e23–e29 PMID: 24324001

154. Ambroggio L, et al. *J Pediatr.* 2012;161(6):1097–1103 PMID: 22901738

155. Leyenaar JK, et al. *Pediatr Infect Dis J.* 2014;33(4):387–392 PMID: 24168982

156. Bradley JS, et al. *Pediatr Infect Dis J.* 2007;26(10):868–878 PMID: 17901791

157. Hidron AI, et al. *Lancet Infect Dis.* 2009;9(6):384–392 PMID: 19467478

158. Wunderink RG, et al. *Clin Infect Dis.* 2012;54(5):621–629 PMID: 22247123

159. Freifeld AG, et al. *Clin Infect Dis.* 2011;52(4):e56–e93 PMID: 21258094

160. American Thoracic Society, et al. *Am J Respir Crit Care Med.* 2005;171(4):388–416 PMID: 15699079

161. Foglia E, et al. *Clin Microbiol Rev.* 2007;20(3):409–425 PMID: 17630332

162. Srinivasan R, et al. *Pediatrics.* 2009;123(4):1108–1115 PMID: 19336369

163. Boselli E, et al. *Intensive Care Med.* 2007;33(9):1519–1523 PMID: 17530217

164. Kollef MH, et al. *Curr Opin Infect Dis.* 2013;26(6):538–544 PMID: 24126716

165. St Peter SD, et al. *J Pediatr Surg.* 2009;44(1):106–111 PMID: 19159726

166. Islam S, et al. *J Pediatr Surg.* 2012;47(11):2101–2110 PMID: 23164006

167. Aziz A, et al. *Surg Infect (Larchmt).* 2008;9(3):317–323 PMID: 18570573

168. Marhuenda C, et al. *Pediatrics.* 2014;134(5):e1301–e1307 PMID: 25349313

169. American Academy of Pediatrics. Chlamydial infections. In: Kimberlin DW, et al, eds. *Red Book: 2015 Report of the Committee on Infectious Diseases.* 2015:284–294

170. American Academy of Pediatrics. Cytomegalovirus infection. In: Kimberlin DW, et al, eds. *Red Book: 2015 Report of the Committee on Infectious Diseases.* 2015:317–322

171. Kotton CN, et al. *Transplantation.* 2013;96(4):333–360 PMID: 23896556

172. Erard V, et al. *Clin Infect Dis.* 2015;61(1):31–39 PMID: 25778751

173. American Academy of Pediatrics. Tularemia. In: Kimberlin DW, et al, eds. *Red Book: 2015 Report of the Committee on Infectious Diseases.* 2015:839–841

174. Levy ER, et al. *Clin Infect Dis.* 2013;56(11):1573–1578 PMID: 23463636

175. American Academy of Pediatrics. Coccidioidomycosis. In: Kimberlin DW, et al, eds. *Red Book: 2015 Report of the Committee on Infectious Diseases.* 2015:302–305

176. American Academy of Pediatrics. Histoplasmosis. In: Kimberlin DW, et al, eds. *Red Book: 2015 Report of the Committee on Infectious Diseases.* 2015:445–448

177. Wheat LJ, et al. *Clin Infect Dis.* 2007;45(7):807–825 PMID: 17806045

178. D'Mello T, et al. *MMWR Morb Mortal Wkly Rep.* 2015;64(8):206–212 PMID: 25742380

179. American Academy Pediatrics Committee on Infectious Diseases. *Pediatrics.* 2015;136(4):792–808 PMID: 26347430

180. Kimberlin DW, et al. *J Infect Dis.* 2013;207(5):709–720 PMID: 23230059

181. Yang K, et al. *Ann Pharmacother.* 2007;41(9):1427–1435 PMID: 17666573

182. Badal RE, et al. *Pediatr Infect Dis J.* 2013;32(6):636–640 PMID: 23838732

183. Johnson MM, et al. *J Thorac Dis.* 2014;6(3):210–220 PMID: 24624285

184. Biondi E, et al. *Pediatrics.* 2014;133(6):1081–1090 PMID: 24864174

185. Cardinale F, et al. *J Clin Microbiol.* 2013;51(2):723–724 PMID: 23224091

186. Aidsinfo.gov. https://aidsinfo.nih.gov/contentfiles/lvguidelines/oi_guidelines_pediatrics.pdf. Accessed September 19, 2016

187. Caselli D, et al. *J Pediatr.* 2014;164(2):389–392.e1 PMID: 24252793

188. Michalopoulos A, et al. *Crit Care Clin.* 2008;24(2):377–391 PMID: 18361952
189. Micek ST, et al. *Medicine (Baltimore).* 2011;90(6):390–395 PMID: 22033455
190. Micek ST, et al. *Crit Care.* 2015;19:219 PMID: 25944081
191. American Academy of Pediatrics. Respiratory syncytial virus. In: Kimberlin DW, et al, eds. *Red Book: 2015 Report of the Committee on Infectious Diseases.* 2015:667–676
192. Villarino ME, et al. *JAMA Pediatr.* 2015;169(3):247–255 PMID: 25580725
193. Meehan WP III, et al. *Pediatr Emerg Care.* 2010;26(12):875–880 PMID: 21088637
194. Biondi E, et al. *Pediatrics.* 2013;132(6):990–996 PMID: 24218461
195. Byington CL, et al. *Pediatrics.* 2003;111(5pt1):964–968 PMID: 12728072
196. Mischler M, et al. *Hosp Pediatr.* 2015;5(6):293–300 PMID: 26034160
197. Ishimine P. *Emerg Med Clin North Am.* 2013;31(3):601–626 PMID: 23915596
198. Greenhow TL, et al. *Pediatr Infect Dis J.* 2014;33(6):595–599 PMID: 24326416
199. Hakim H, et al. *Am J Infect Control.* 2007;35(2):102–105 PMID: 17327189
200. Luthander J, et al. *Acta Paediatr.* 2013;102(2):182–186 PMID: 23121094
201. Russell CD, et al. *J Med Microbiol.* 2014;63(Pt6):841–848 PMID: 24623637
202. Ligon J, et al. *Pediatr Infect Dis J.* 2014;33(5):e132–e134 PMID: 24732394
203. Baddour LM, et al. *Circulation.* 2005;111(23):e394–e434 PMID: 15956145
204. Johnson JA, et al. *Mayo Clin Proc.* 2012;87(7):629–635 PMID: 22766082
205. Russell HM, et al. *Ann Thorac Surg.* 2013;96(1):171–174 PMID: 23602067
206. Baddour LM, et al. *Circulation.* 2015;132(15):1435–1486 PMID: 26373316
207. Tacke D, et al. *Curr Opin Infect Dis.* 2013;26(6):501–507 PMID:24126720
208. Wilson W, et al. *Circulation.* 2007;116(15):1736–1754 PMID: 17446442
209. Silberbach M. *Pediatr Rev.* 2008;29(5):169–170 PMID: 18450838211.
210. Lutmer JE, et al. *Ann Am Thorac Soc.* 2013;10(3):235–238 PMID: 23802820
211. Demmler GJ. *Pediatr Infect Dis J.* 2006;25(2):165–166 PMID: 16462296
212. Denno DM, et al. *Clin Infect Dis.* 2012;55(7):897–904 PMID: 22700832
213. Pfeiffer ML, et al. *J Infect.* 2012;64(4):374–386 PMID: 22266388
214. Butler T. *Trans R Soc Trop Med Hyg.* 2012;106(7):395–399 PMID: 22579556
215. Wong CS, et al. *Clin Infect Dis.* 2012;55(1):33–41 PMID: 22431799
216. Bennish ML, et al. *Clin Infect Dis.* 2006;42(3):356–362 PMID: 16392080
217. Smith KE, et al. *Pediatr Infect Dis J.* 2012;31(1):37–41 PMID: 21892124
218. Tribble DR, et al. *Clin Infect Dis.* 2007;44(3):338–346 PMID: 17205438
219. Steffen R, et al. *JAMA.* 2015;313(1):71–80 PMID: 25562268
220. Paredes-Paredes M, et al. *Curr Gastroenterol Rep.* 2011;13(5):402–407 PMID: 21773708
221. DuPont HL, et al. *J Travel Med.* 2009;16(3):149–160 PMID: 19538575
222. Ouyang-Latimer J, et al. *Antimicrob Agents Chemother.* 2011;55(2):874–878 PMID: 21115800
223. O'Ryan M, et al. *Expert Rev Anti Infect Ther.* 2010;8(6):671–682 PMID: 20521895
224. Koo HL, et al. *Curr Opin Gastroenterol.* 2010;26(1):17–25 PMID: 19881343
225. Advice for travelers. *Med Lett Drugs Ther.* 2015;57(1466):52–58 PMID: 25853663
226. Kantele A, et al. *Clin Infect Dis.* 2015;60(6):837–846 PMID: 25613287
227. Riddle MS, et al. *Clin Infect Dis.* 2008;47(8):1007–1014 PMID: 18781873
228. Butler T. *Clin Infect Dis.* 2008;47(8):1015–1016 PMID: 18781871
229. Janda JM, et al. *Clin Microbiol Rev.* 2010;23(1):35–73 PMID: 20065325
230. American Academy of Pediatrics. *Campylobacter* infections. In: Kimberlin DW, et al, eds. *Red Book: 2015 Report of the Committee on Infectious Diseases.* 2015:273–275
231. Fullerton KE, et al. *Pediatr Infect Dis J.* 2007;26(1):19–24 PMID: 17195700
232. Kirkpatrick BD, et al. *Curr Opin Gastroenterol.* 2011;27(1):1–7 PMID: 21124212
233. Leibovici-Weissman Y, et al. *Cochrane Database Syst Rev.* 2014;6:CD008625 PMID: 24944120
234. Pant C, et al. *Curr Med Res Opin.* 2013;29(8):967–984 PMID: 23659563
235. American Academy of Pediatrics. *Clostridium difficile.* In: Kimberlin DW, et al, eds. *Red Book: 2015 Report of the Committee on Infectious Diseases.* 2015:298–301
236. Kelly CP, et al. *N Engl J Med.* 2008;359(18):1932–1940 PMID: 18971494
237. Khanna S, et al. *Clin Infect Dis.* 2013;56(10):1401–1406 PMID: 23408679
238. Rimbara E, et al. *Nat Rev Gastroenterol Hepatol.* 2011;8(2):79–88 PMID: 21293508

239. McColl KE. *N Engl J Med.* 2010;362(17):1597–1604 PMID: 20427808

240. Bontems P, et al. *J Pediatr Gastroenterol Nutr.* 2011;53(6):646–650 PMID: 21701406

241. American Academy of Pediatrics. *Helicobacter pylori* infections. In: Kimberlin DW, et al, eds. *Red Book: 2015 Report of the Committee on Infectious Diseases.* 2015:379–381

242. Fallone CA, et al. *Gastroenterology.* 2016;151(1):51–69.e14 PMID: 27102658

243. Kalach N, et al. *Ann Gastroenterol.* 2015;28(1):10–18 PMID: 25608573

244. American Academy of Pediatrics. *Giardia intestinalis* (formerly *Giardia lamblia* and *Giardia duodenalis*) infections. In: Kimberlin DW, et al, eds. *Red Book: 2015 Report of the Committee on Infectious Diseases.* 2015:353–355

245. Bula-Rudas FJ, et al. *Adv Pediatr.* 2015;62(1):29–58 PMID: 26205108

246. Haeusler GM, et al. *Adv Exp Med Biol.* 2013;764:13–26 PMID: 23654054

247. Trivedi NA, et al. *J Postgrad Med.* 2012;58(2):112–118 PMID: 22718054

248. Frenck RW Jr, et al. *Clin Infect Dis.* 2004;38(7):951–957 PMID: 15034826

249. Effa EE, et al. *Cochrane Database Syst Rev.* 2008;(4):CD006083 PMID: 18843701

250. Effa EE, et al. *Cochrane Database Syst Rev.* 2011;(10):CD004530 PMID: 21975746

251. Begum B, et al. *Mymensingh Med J.* 2014;23(3):441–448 PMID: 25178594

252. National Antimicrobial Resistance Monitoring System, Centers for Diseases Control and Prevention. http://www.cdc.gov/narms/reports/index.html. Accessed September 19, 2016

253. Basualdo W, et al. *Pediatr Infect Dis J.* 2003;22(4):374–377 PMID: 12712971

254. American Academy of Pediatrics. *Shigella* infections. In: Kimberlin DW, et al, eds. *Red Book: 2015 Report of the Committee on Infectious Diseases.* 2015:706–709

255. Abdel-Haq NM, et al. *Pediatr Infect Dis J.* 2000;19(10):954–958 PMID: 11055595

256. Abdel-Haq NM, et al. *Int J Antimicrob Agents.* 2006;27(5):449–452 PMID: 16621458

257. El Qouqa IA, et al. *Int J Infect Dis.* 2011;15(1):e48–e53 PMID: 21131221

258. Fallon SC, et al. *J Surg Res.* 2013;185(1):273–277 PMID: 23835072

259. Lee SL, et al. *J Pediatr Surg.* 2010;45(11):2181–2185 PMID: 21034941

260. Chen CY, et al. *Surg Infect (Larchmt).* 2012;13(6):383–390 PMID: 23231389

261. Solomkin JS, et al. *Clin Infect Dis.* 2010;50(2):133–164 PMID: 20034345

262. Sawyer RG, et al. *N Engl J Med.* 2015;372(21):1996–2005 PMID: 25992746

263. Fraser JD, et al. *J Pediatr Surg.* 2010;45(6):1198–1202 PMID: 20620320

264. Bradley JS, et al. *Pediatr Infect Dis J.* 2001;20(1):19–24 PMID: 11176562

265. Cruz AT, et al. *Int J Tuberc Lung Dis.* 2013;17(2):169–174 PMID: 23317951

266. Hlavsa MC, et al. *Clin Infect Dis.* 2008;47(2):168–175 PMID: 18532886

267. Alrajhi AA, et al. *Clin Infect Dis.* 1998;27(1):52–56 PMID: 9675450

268. Arditi M, et al. *Pediatr Infect Dis J.* 1990;9(6):411–415 PMID: 2367163

269. Ballinger AE, et al. *Cochrane Database Syst Rev.* 2014;4:CD005284 PMID: 24771351

270. Warady BA, et al. *Perit Dial Int.* 2012;32(Suppl2):S32–S86 PMID: 22851742

271. Preece ER, et al. *ANZ J Surg.* 2012;82(4):283–284 PMID: 22510192

272. Workowski K. *Ann Intern Med.* 2013;158(3):ITC2-1 PMID: 23381058

273. Santillanes G, et al. *Pediatr Emerg Care.* 2011;27(3):174–178 PMID: 21346680

274. Klin B, et al. *Isr Med Assoc J.* 2001;3(11):833–835 PMID: 11729579

275. Smith JC, et al. *Adv Exp Med Biol.* 2013;764:219–239 PMID: 23654071

276. Centers for Disease Control and Prevention. *MMWR Morb Mortal Wkly Rep.* 2012;61(31):590–594 PMID: 22874837

277. Centers for Disease Control and Prevention. *MMWR Morb Mortal Wkly Rep.* 2007;56(14):332–336 PMID: 17431378

278. James SH, et al. *Clin Pharmacol Ther.* 2010;88(5):720–724 PMID: 20881952

279. Fife KH, et al. *Sex Transm Dis.* 2008;35(7):668–673 PMID: 18461016

280. Stephenson-Famy A, et al. *Obstet Gynecol Clin North Am.* 2014;41(4):601–614 PMID: 25454993

281. Mitchell C, et al. *Infect Dis Clin North Am.* 2013;27(4):793–809 PMID: 24275271

282. Cohen SE, et al. *Infect Dis Clin North Am.* 2013;27(4):705–722 PMID: 24275265

283. Manhart LE, et al. *Clin Infect Dis.* 2015;61(Suppl 8):S802–S817 PMID: 26602619

284. O'Brien G. *Pediatr Rev.* 2008;29(6):209–211 PMID: 18515339

285. das Neves J, et al. *Drugs.* 2008;68(13):1787–1802 PMID: 18729533

286. Bumbulienė Ž, et al. *Postgrad Med J.* 2014;90(1059):8–12 PMID: 24191064
287. Jasper JM, et al. *Pediatr Emerg Care.* 2006;22(8):585–586 PMID: 16912629
288. Hansen MT, et al. *J Pediatr Adolesc Gynecol.* 2007;20(5):315–317 PMID: 1786890
289. Yogev R, et al. *Pediatr Infect Dis J.* 2004;23(2):157–159 PMID: 14872183
290. Bonfield CM, et al. *J Infect.* 2015;71(Suppl1):S42–S46 PMID: 25917804
291. Tunkel AR, et al. *Clin Infect Dis.* 2008;47(3):303–327 PMID: 18582201
292. Bitnun A, et al. *Can J Infect Dis Med Microbiol.* 2015;26(2):69–72 PMID: 26015788
293. Kotton CN, et al. *Transplantation.* 2010;89(7):779–795 PMID: 20224515
294. Abzug MJ, et al. *J Pediatr Infect Dis Soc.* 2016;5(1):53–62 PMID: 26407253
295. Doja A, et al. *J Child Neurol.* 2006;21(5):384–391 PMID: 16901443
296. James SH, et al. *Clin Pharmacol Ther.* 2010;88(5):720–724 PMID: 20881952
297. Brouwer MC, et al. *Cochrane Database Syst Rev.* 2013;6:CD004405 PMID: 23733364
298. Fritz D, et al. *Neurology.* 2012;79(22):2177–2179 PMID: 23152589
299. Tunkel AR, et al. *Clin Infect Dis.* 2004;39(9):1267–1284 PMID: 15494903
300. Prasad K, et al. *Cochrane Database Syst Rev.* 2008;(1):CD002244 PMID: 18254003
301. Kandasamy J, et al. *Childs Nerv Syst.* 2011;27(4):575–581 PMID: 20953871
302. Al-Dabbagh M, et al. *Adv Exp Med Biol.* 2011;719:105–115 PMID: 22125038
303. National Institute for Health and Care Excellence. Urinary tract infection in under 16s: diagnosis and management. http://www.nice.org.uk/guidance/CG54. Reviewed July 2016. Accessed September 19, 2016
304. Montini G, et al. *N Engl J Med.* 2011;365(3):239–250 PMID: 21774712
305. Cheng CH, et al. *J Pediatr.* 2010;156(1):82–86 PMID: 19782999
306. Chen WL, et al. *Pediatr Neonatal.* 2015;56(3):176–182 PMID: 25459491
307. Perez F, et al. *Clin Infect Dis.* 2015;60(9):1326–1329 PMID: 25586684
308. Strohmeier Y, et al. *Cochrane Database Syst Rev.* 2014;7:CD003772 PMID: 25066627
309. Bocquet N, et al. *Pediatrics.* 2012;129(2):e269–e275 PMID: 22291112
310. American Academy of Pediatrics Subcommittee on Urinary Tract Infection, Steering Committee on Quality Improvement and Management. *Pediatrics.* 2011;128(3):595–610 PMID: 21873693
311. Craig JC, et al. *N Engl J Med.* 2009;361(18):1748–1759 PMID: 19864673
312. Williams GJ, et al. *Adv Exp Med Biol.* 2013;764:211–218 PMID: 23654070
313. RIVUR Trial Investigators, et al. *N Engl J Med.* 2014;370(25):2367–2376 PMID: 24795142
314. American Academy of Pediatrics. Actinomycosis. In: Kimberlin DW, et al, eds. *Red Book: 2015 Report of the Committee on Infectious Diseases.* 2015:225–226
315. Brook I. *South Med J.* 2008;101(10):1019–1023 PMID: 18791528
316. Thomas RJ, et al. *Expert Rev Anti Infect Ther.* 2009;7(6):709–722 PMID: 19681699
317. American Academy of Pediatrics. Brucellosis. In: Kimberlin DW, et al, eds. *Red Book: 2015 Report of the Committee on Infectious Diseases.* 2015:268–270
318. Shen MW. *Pediatrics.* 2008;121(5):e1178–e1183 PMID: 18450861
319. Mile B, et al. *Trop Doct.* 2012;42(1):13–17 PMID: 22290107
320. Franco MP, et al. *Lancet Infect Dis.* 2007;7(12):775–786 PMID: 18045560
321. Florin TA, et al. *Pediatrics.* 2008;121(5):e1413–e1425 PMID: 18443019
322. Zangwill KM. *Adv Exp Med Biol.* 2013;764:159–166 PMID: 23654065
323. Klassen TP, et al. *Cochrane Database Syst Rev.* 2005;(4):CD002980 PMID: 16235308
324. American Academy of Pediatrics. Varicella-zoster virus infections. In: Kimberlin DW, et al, eds. *Red Book: 2015 Report of the Committee on Infectious Diseases.* 2015:846–860
325. Kimberlin DW, et al. *Clin Infect Dis.* 2010;50(2):221–228 PMID: 20014952
326. Saez-Llorens X, et al. *Antimicrob Agents Chemother.* 2009;53(5):1912–1920 PMID: 19273678
327. Ismail N, et al. *Clin Lab Med.* 2010;30(1):261–292 PMID: 20513551
328. Schutze GE, et al. *Pediatr Infect Dis J.* 2007;26(6):475–479 PMID: 17529862
329. Wormser GP, et al. *Clin Infect Dis.* 2006;43(9):1089–1134 PMID: 17029130
330. Averbuch D, et al. *Haematologica.* 2013;98(12):1826–1835 [Erratum: *Haematologica.* 2014;99(2):400] PMID: 24323983
331. Freifeld AG, et al. *Clin Infect Dis.* 2011;52(4):e56–e93 PMID: 21258094
332. Miedema KG, et al. *Eur J Cancer.* 2016;53:16–24 PMID: 26700076
333. Arnon SS. *Pediatrics.* 2007;119(4):785–789 PMID: 17403850

334. Newburger JW, et al. *Circulation.* 2004;110(17):2747–2771 PMID: 15505111

335. Newburger JW, et al. *N Engl J Med.* 2007;356(7):663–675 PMID: 17301297

336. Kobayashi T, et al. *Lancet.* 2012;379(9826):1613–1620 PMID: 22405251

337. Son MB, et al. *J Pediatr.* 2011;158(4):644–649 PMID: 21129756

338. Son MB, et al. *Pediatr Rev.* 2013;34(4):151–162 PMID: 23547061

339. American Academy of Pediatrics. Leprosy. In: Kimberlin DW, et al, eds. *Red Book: 2015 Report of the Committee on Infectious Diseases.* 2015:506–510

340. Griffith ME, et al. *Curr Opin Infect Dis.* 2006;19(6):533–537 PMID: 17075327

341. American Academy of Pediatrics. Leptospirosis. In: Kimberlin DW, et al, eds. *Red Book: 2015 Report of the Committee on Infectious Diseases.* 2015:510–513

342. American Academy of Pediatrics. Lyme disease. In: Kimberlin DW, et al, eds. *Red Book: 2015 Report of the Committee on Infectious Diseases.* 2015:516–525

343. Shapiro ED. *N Engl J Med.* 2014;370(18):1724–1731 PMID: 24785207

344. Sood SK. *Infect Dis Clin North Am.* 2015;29(2):281–294 PMID: 25999224

345. Wiersinga WJ, et al. *N Engl J Med.* 2012;367(11):1035–1044 PMID: 22970946

346. Chetchotisakd P, et al. *Lancet.* 2014;383(9919):807–814 PMID: 24284287

347. Griffith DE, et al. *Am J Respir Crit Care Med.* 2007;175(4):367–416 [Erratum: *Am J Respir Crit Care Med.* 2007;175(7):744–745] PMID: 17277290

348. Philley JV, et al. *Semin Respir Crit Care Med.* 2013;34(1):135–142 PMID: 23460013

349. Kasperbauer SH, et al. *Clin Chest Med.* 2015;36(1):67–78 PMID: 25676520

350. Henkle E, et al. *Clin Chest Med.* 2015;36(1):91–99 PMID: 25676522

351. Wilson JW. *Mayo Clin Proc.* 2012;87(4):403–407 PMID: 22469352

352. American Academy of Pediatrics. Nocardiosis. In: Kimberlin DW, et al, eds. *Red Book: 2015 Report of the Committee on Infectious Diseases.* 2015:571–572

353. Koirala J. *Infect Dis Clin North Am.* 2006;20(2):273–287 PMID: 16762739

354. Stenseth NC, et al. *PLoS Med.* 2008;5(1):e3 PMID: 18198939

355. American Academy of Pediatrics. Plague. In: Kimberlin DW, et al, eds. *Red Book: 2015 Report of the Committee on Infectious Diseases.* 2015:624–626

356. Kersh GJ. *Expert Rev Anti Infect Ther.* 2013;11(11):1207–1214 PMID: 24073941

357. Anderson A, et al. *MMWR Recomm Rep.* 2013;62(RR-03):1–30 PMID: 23535757

358. Woods CR. *Pediatr Clin North Am.* 2013;60(2):455–470 PMID: 23481111

359. American Academy of Pediatrics. Rocky Mountain spotted fever. In: Kimberlin DW, et al, eds. *Red Book: 2015 Report of the Committee on Infectious Diseases.* 2015:682–684

360. American Academy of Pediatrics. Tetanus. In: Kimberlin DW, et al, eds. *Red Book: 2015 Report of the Committee on Infectious Diseases.* 2015:773–778

361. Brook I. *Expert Rev Anti Infect Ther.* 2008;6(3):327–336 PMID: 18588497

362. Curtis N. *Arch Dis Child.* 2014;99(12):1062–1064 PMID: 25395586

363. Dellinger RP, et al. *Crit Care Med.* 2013;41(2):580–637 PMID: 23353941

364. Harik NS. *Pediatr Ann.* 2013;42(7):288–292 PMID: 23805970

Chapter 7

1. Qureshi ZA, et al. *Clin Infect Dis.* 2015;60(9):1295–1303 PMID: 25632010

2. Fishban J, et al. *Clin Infect Dis.* 2010;51(1):79–84 PMID: 20504234

3. Hsu AJ, et al. *Clin Infect Dis.* 2014;58(10):1439–1448 PMID: 24501388

4. Bonnin RA, et al. *Expert Rev Anti Infect Ther.* 2013;11(6):571–583 PMID: 23750729

5. Brook I. *South Med J.* 2008;101(10):1019–1023 PMID: 18791528

6. Janda JM, et al. *Clin Microbiol Rev.* 2010;23(1):35–73 PMID: 20065325

7. Rahamat-Langendoen JC, et al. *J Clin Periodontol.* 2011;38(8):702–706 PMID: 21539594

8. Thomas RJ, et al. *Expert Rev Anti Infect Ther.* 2009;7(6):709–722 PMID: PMC2739015

9. Ismail N, et al. *Clin Lab Med.* 2010;30(1):261–292 PMID: 20513551

10. Therriault BL, et al. *Ann Pharmacother.* 2008;42(11):1697–1702 PMID: 18812563

11. Bradley JS, et al. *Pediatrics.* 2014;133(5):e1411–e1436 PMID: 24777226

12. American Academy of Pediatrics. *Bacillus cereus* infections. In: Kimberlin DW, et al, eds. *Red Book: 2015 Report of the Committee on Infectious Diseases.* 2015:255–256

13. Bottone EJ. *Clin Microbiol Rev.* 2010;23(2):382–398 PMID: 20357358

14. Wexler HM. *Clin Microbiol Rev.* 2007;20(4):593–621 PMID: 17934076
15. Snydman DR, et al. *Clin Infect Dis.* 2010;50(Suppl1):S26–S33 PMID: 20067390
16. Florin TA, et al. *Pediatrics.* 2008;121(5):e1413–e1425 PMID: 18443019
17. Massei F, et al. *Infect Dis Clin North Am.* 2005;19(3):691–711 PMID: 16102656
18. Foucault C, et al. *Emerg Infect Dis.* 2006;12(2):217–223 PMID: 16494745
19. Tiwari T, et al. *MMWR Recomm Rep.* 2005;54(RR-14):1–16 PMID: 16340941
20. American Academy of Pediatrics. Pertussis (whooping cough). In: Kimberlin DW, et al, eds. *Red Book: 2015 Report of the Committee on Infectious Diseases.* 2015:608–621
21. Shapiro ED. *N Engl J Med.* 2014;370(18):1724–1731 PMID: 24785207
22. American Academy of Pediatrics. Lyme disease. In: Kimberlin DW, et al, eds. *Red Book: 2015 Report of the Committee on Infectious Diseases.* 2015:516–525
23. Wormser GP, et al. *Clin Infect Dis.* 2006;43(9):1089–1134 PMID: 17029130
24. American Academy of Pediatrics. *Borrelia* infections. In: Kimberlin DW, et al, eds. *Red Book: 2015 Report of the Committee on Infectious Diseases.* 2015:265–267
25. Dworkin MS, et al. *Infect Dis Clin North Am.* 2008;22(3):449–468 PMID: 18755384
26. American Academy of Pediatrics. Brucellosis. In: Kimberlin DW, et al, eds. *Red Book: 2015 Report of the Committee on Infectious Diseases.* 2015:268–270
27. Shen MW. *Pediatrics.* 2008;121(5):e1178–e1183 PMID: 18450861
28. Mile B, et al. *Trop Doct.* 2012;42(1):13–17 PMID: 22290107
29. American Academy of Pediatrics. *Burkholderia* infections. In: Kimberlin DW, et al, eds. *Red Book: 2015 Report of the Committee on Infectious Diseases.* 2015:270–272
30. Waters V. *Curr Pharm Des.* 2012;18(5):696–725 PMID: 22229574
31. King P, et al. *Antimicrob Agents Chemother.* 2010;54(1):143–148 PMID: 19805554
32. Horsley A, et al. *Cochrane Database Syst Rev.* 2012;10:CD009529 PMID: 23076960
33. Wiersinga WJ, et al. *N Engl J Med.* 2012;367(11):1035–1044 PMID: 22970946
34. Cheng AC, et al. *Am J Trop Med Hyg.* 2008;78(2):208–209 PMID: 18256414
35. Chetchotisakd P, et al. *Lancet.* 2014;383(9919):807–814 PMID: 24284287
36. Fujihara N, et al. *J Infect.* 2006;53(5):e199–e202 PMID: 16542730
37. American Academy of Pediatrics. *Campylobacter* infections. In: Kimberlin DW, et al, eds. *Red Book: 2015 Report of the Committee on Infectious Diseases.* 2015:273–275
38. Ternhag A, et al. *Clin Infect Dis.* 2007;44(5):696–700 PMID: 17278062
39. Kirkpatrick BD, et al. *Curr Opin Gastroenterol.* 2011;27(1):1–7 PMID: 21124212
40. Oehler RL, et al. *Lancet Infect Dis.* 2009;9(7):439–447 PMID: 19555903
41. Jolivet-Gougeon A, et al. *Int J Antimicrob Agents.* 2007;29(4):367–373 PMID: 17250994
42. Wang HK, et al. *J Clin Microbiol.* 2007;45(2):645–647 PMID: 17135428
43. Blasi F, et al. *Clin Microbiol Infect.* 2009;15(1):29–35 PMID: 19220337
44. Burillo A, et al. *Infect Dis Clin North Am.* 2010;24(1):61–71 PMID: 20171546
45. Workowski KA, et al. *MMWR Recomm Rep.* 2015;64(RR-03):1–137 PMID: 26042815
46. Kohlhoff SA, et al. *Expert Opin Pharmacother.* 2015;16(2):205–212 PMID: 25579069
47. American Academy of Pediatrics. Chlamydial infections. In: Kimberlin DW, et al, eds. *Red Book: 2015 Report of the Committee on Infectious Diseases.* 2015:284–294
48. Workowski KA, et al. *MMWR Recomm Rep.* 2010;59(RR-12):1–110 PMID: 21160459
49. Campbell JI, et al. *BMC Infect Dis.* 2013;13:4 PMID: 23286235
50. Sirinavin S, et al. *Pediatr Infect Dis J.* 2005;24(6):559–561 PMID: 15933571
51. Nuñez Cuadros E, et al. *J Med Microbiol.* 2014;63(Pt1):144–147 PMID: 24243285
52. Doran TI. *Clin Infect Dis.* 1999;28(2):384–394 PMID: 10064257
53. Jacoby GA. *Clin Microbiol Rev.* 2009;22(1):161–182 PMID: 19136439
54. Sobel J. *Clin Infect Dis.* 2005;41(8):1167–1173 PMID: 16163636
55. American Academy of Pediatrics. Botulism and infant botulism. In: Kimberlin DW, et al, eds. *Red Book: 2015 Report of the Committee on Infectious Diseases.* 2015:294–297
56. Hill SE, et al. *Ann Pharmacother.* 2013;47(2):e12 PMID: 23362041
57. Sammons JS, et al. *JAMA Pediatr.* 2013;167(6):567–573 PMID: 23460123
58. American Academy of Pediatrics. *Clostridium difficile.* In: Kimberlin DW, et al, eds. *Red Book: 2015 Report of the Committee on Infectious Diseases.* 2015:298–301

59. American Academy of Pediatrics. Clostridial myonecrosis. In: Kimberlin DW, et al, eds. *Red Book: 2015 Report of the Committee on Infectious Diseases.* 2015:297–298

60. American Academy of Pediatrics. *Clostridium perfringens* food poisoning. In: Kimberlin DW, et al, eds. *Red Book: 2015 Report of the Committee on Infectious Diseases.* 2015:301–302

61. American Academy of Pediatrics. Tetanus. In: Kimberlin DW, et al, eds. *Red Book: 2015 Report of the Committee on Infectious Diseases.* 2015:773–778

62. Brook I. *Expert Rev Anti Infect Ther.* 2008;6(3):327–336 PMID: 18588497

63. American Academy of Pediatrics. Diphtheria. In: Kimberlin DW, et al, eds. *Red Book: 2015 Report of the Committee on Infectious Diseases.* 2015:325–329

64. Fernandez-Roblas R, et al. *Int J Antimicrob Agents.* 2009;33(5):453–455 PMID: 19153032

65. Holdiness MR. *Drugs.* 2002;62(8):1131–1141 PMID: 12010076

66. Dalal A, et al. *J Infect.* 2008;56(1):77–79 PMID: 18036665

67. Anderson A, et al. *MMWR Recomm Rep.* 2013;62(RR-03):1–30 PMID: 23535757

68. Kersh GJ. *Expert Rev Anti Infect Ther.* 2013;11(11):1207–1214 PMID: 24073941

69. Pritt BS, et al. *N Engl J Med.* 2011;365(5):422–429 PMID: 21812671

70. Paul K, et al. *Clin Infect Dis.* 2001;33(1):54–61 PMID: 11389495

71. Ceyhan M, et al. *Int J Pediatr.* 2011;2011:215–237 PMID: 22046191

72. Hsu MS, et al. *Eur J Clin Microbiol Infect Dis.* 2011;30(10):1271–1278 PMID: 21461847

73. Siedner MJ, et al. *Clin Infect Dis.* 2014;58(11):1554–1563 PMID: 24647022

74. Harris PN, et al. *Int J Antimicrob Agents.* 2012;40(4):297–305 PMID: 22824371

75. Livermore DM, et al. *Int J Antimicrob Agents.* 2011;37(5):415–419 PMID: 21429716

76. Arias CA, et al. *Nat Rev Microbiol.* 2012;10(4):266–278 PMID: 22421879

77. American Academy of Pediatrics. Non-group A or B streptococcal and enterococcal infections. In: Kimberlin DW, et al, eds. *Red Book: 2015 Report of the Committee on Infectious Diseases.* 2015:750–573

78. Hollenbeck BL, et al. *Virulence.* 2012;3(5):421–433 PMID: 23076243

79. Veraldi S, et al. *Clin Exp Dermatol.* 2009;34(8):859–862 PMID: 19663854

80. American Academy of Pediatrics. Tularemia. In: Kimberlin DW, et al, eds. *Red Book: 2015 Report of the Committee on Infectious Diseases.* 2015:839–841

81. Hepburn MJ, et al. *Expert Rev Anti Infect Ther.* 2008;6(2):231–240 PMID: 18380605

82. Huggan PJ, et al. *J Infect.* 2008;57(4):283–239 PMID: 18805588

83. Riordan T. *Clin Microbiol Rev.* 2007;20(4):622–659 PMID: 17934077

84. Donders G. *Obstet Gynecol Surv.* 2010;65(7):462–473 PMID: 20723268

85. Ahamed SP, et al. *Neurosciences (Riyadh).* 2010;15(1):40–42 PMID: 20677591

86. Agrawal A, et al. *J Clin Microbiol.* 2011;49(11):3728–3732 PMID: 21900515

87. American Academy of Pediatrics. *Helicobacter pylori* infections. In: Kimberlin DW, et al, eds. *Red Book: 2015 Report of the Committee on Infectious Diseases.* 2015:379–381

88. McColl KE. *N Engl J Med.* 2010;362(17):1597–1604 PMID: 20427808

89. Georgopoulos SD, et al. *Expert Opin Pharmacother.* 2013;14(2):211–223 PMID: 23331077

90. Yagupsky P, et al. *Pediatrics.* 2011;127(3):557–565 PMID: 21321033

91. Weiss-Salz I, et al. *Adv Exp Med Biol.* 2011;719:67–80 PMID: 22125036

92. Petrosillo N, et al. *Expert Rev Anti Infect Ther.* 2013;11(2):159–177 PMID: 23409822

93. Nordmann P, et al. *Lancet Infect Dis.* 2009;9(4):228–236 PMID: 19324295

94. Bergen PJ, et al. *Curr Opin Infect Dis.* 2012;25(6):626–633 PMID: 23041772

95. Viasus D, et al. *Medicine (Baltimore).* 2013;92(1):51–60 PMID: 23266795

96. American Academy of Pediatrics. Leptospirosis. In: Kimberlin DW, et al, eds. *Red Book: 2015 Report of the Committee on Infectious Diseases.* 2015:510–513

97. Florescu D, et al. *Pediatr Infect Dis J.* 2008;27(11):1013–1019 PMID: 18833028

98. Bortolussi R. *CMAJ.* 2008;179(8):795–797 PMID: 18787096

99. Murphy TF, et al. *Clin Infect Dis.* 2009;49(1):124–131 PMID: 19480579

100. Chang HY, et al. *Pediatr Int.* 2011;53(1):121–123 PMID: 21342342

101. Milligan KL, et al. *Clin Pediatr (Phila).* 2013;52(5):462–464 PMID: 22267858

102. American Academy of Pediatrics. Diseases caused by nontuberculous mycobacteria. In: Kimberlin DW, et al, eds. *Red Book: 2015 Report of the Committee on Infectious Diseases.* 2015:831–841

103. Nessar R, et al. *J Antimicrob Chemother.* 2012;67(4):810–818 PMID: 22290346
104. Griffith DE, et al. *Am J Respir Crit Care Med.* 2007;175(4):367–416 PMID: 17277290
105. American Academy of Pediatrics. Tuberculosis. In: Kimberlin DW, et al, eds. *Red Book: 2015 Report of the Committee on Infectious Diseases.* 2015:805–831
106. Hlavsa MC, et al. *Clin Infect Dis.* 2008;47(2):168–175 PMID: 18532886
107. Hay RJ. *Curr Opin Infect Dis.* 2009;22(2):99–101 PMID: 19276876
108. Uslan DZ, et al. *Arch Dermatol.* 2006;142(10):1287–1292 PMID: 17043183
109. American Academy of Pediatrics. Leprosy. In: Kimberlin DW, eds. *Red Book: 2015 Report of the Committee on Infectious Diseases.* 2015:506–510
110. Doedens RA, et al. *Pediatr Infect Dis J.* 2008;27(1):81–83 PMID: 18162949
111. American Thoracic Society, et al. *MMWR Recomm Rep.* 2003;52(RR-11):1–77 PMID: 12836625
112. Waites KB, et al. *Semin Fetal Neonatal Med.* 2009;14(4):190–199 PMID: 19109084
113. Watt KM, et al. *Pediatr Infect Dis J.* 2012;31(2):197–199 PMID: 22016080
114. Bradley JS, et al. *Clin Infect Dis.* 2011;53(7):e25–e76 PMID: 21880587
115. Akaike H, et al. *Jpn J Infect Dis.* 2012;65(6):535–538 PMID: 23183207
116. Centers for Disease Control and Prevention. *MMWR Morb Mortal Wkly Rep.* 2012;61(31):590–594 PMID: 22874837
117. Wu HM, et al. *N Engl J Med.* 2009;360(9):886–892 PMID: 19246360
118. American Academy of Pediatrics. Meningococcal infections. In: Kimberlin DW, et al, eds. *Red Book: 2015 Report of the Committee on Infectious Diseases.* 2015:547–558
119. Wilson JW. *Mayo Clin Proc.* 2012;87(4):403–407 PMID: 22469352
120. American Academy of Pediatrics. Nocardiosis. In: Kimberlin DW, et al, eds. *Red Book: 2015 Report of the Committee on Infectious Diseases.* 2015:571–572
121. Casanova-Román M, et al. *Infection.* 2010;38(4):321–323 PMID: 20376528
122. Goldstein EJ. *Antimicrob Agents Chemother.* 2012;56(12):6319–6323 PMID: 23027193
123. Murphy EC, et al. *FEMS Microbiol Rev.* 2013;37(4):520–553 PMID: 23030831
124. Ozdemir O, et al. *J Microbiol Immunol Infect.* 2010;43(4):344–346 PMID: 20688296
125. Stock I, Wiedemann B. *J Antimicrob Chemother.* 2001;48(6):803–811 PMID: 11733464
126. Brook I, et al. *Clin Microbiol Rev.* 2013;26(3):526–546 PMID: 23824372
127. Nisbet M, et al. *J Antimicrob Chemother.* 2007;60(5):1097–1103 PMID: 17875606
128. Perry A, et al. *Expert Rev Anti Infect Ther.* 2011;9(12):1149–1156 PMID: 22114965
129. Saperston KN, et al. *J Urol.* 2014;191(5Suppl):1608–1613 PMID: 24679887
130. Tumbarello M, et al. *J Antimicrob Chemother.* 2004;53(2):277–282 PMID: 14688041
131. Sun HY, et al. *Chest.* 2011;139(5):1172–1185 PMID: 21540216
132. Grgurich PE, et al. *Expert Rev Respir Med.* 2012;6(5):533–555 PMID: 23134248
133. Tam VH, et al. *Antimicrob Agents Chemother.* 2010;54(3):1160–1164 PMID: 20086165
134. Freifeld AG, et al. *Clin Infect Dis.* 2011;52(4):e56–e93 PMID: 21258094
135. Velkov T, et al. *Future Microbiol.* 2013;8(6):711–724 PMID: 23701329
136. Döring G, et al. *J Cyst Fibros.* 2012;11(6):461–479 PMID: 23137712
137. Mogayzel PJ Jr, et al. *Am J Respir Crit Care Med.* 2013;187(7):680–689 PMID: 23540878
138. Saiman L. *Paediatr Respir Rev.* 2007;8(3):249–255 PMID: 17868923
139. Yamshchikov AV, et al. *Lancet Infect Dis.* 2010;10(5):350–359 PMID: 20417417
140. American Academy of Pediatrics. Rickettsial diseases. In: Kimberlin DW, et al, eds. *Red Book: 2015 Report of the Committee on Infectious Diseases.* 2015:677–680
141. Woods CR. *Pediatr Clin North Am.* 2013;60(2):455–470 PMID: 23481111
142. American Academy of Pediatrics. *Salmonella* infections. In: Kimberlin DW, et al, eds. *Red Book: 2015 Report of the Committee on Infectious Diseases.* 2015:695–702
143. Haeusler GM, et al. *Adv Exp Med Biol.* 2013;764:13–26 PMID: 23654054
144. Onwuezobe IA, et al. *Cochrane Database Syst Rev.* 2012;11:CD001167 PMID: 23152205
145. Effa EE, et al. *Cochrane Database Syst Rev.* 2008;(4):CD006083 PMID: 18843701
146. To KK, et al. *Scand J Infect Dis.* 2010;42(10):757–762 PMID: 20524786
147. Shiferaw B, et al. *Clin Infect Dis.* 2012;54(Suppl5):S458–S463 PMID: 22572670
148. American Academy of Pediatrics. *Shigella* infections. In: Kimberlin DW, et al, eds. *Red Book: 2015 Report of the Committee on Infectious Diseases.* 2015:706–709

149. Sjölund Karlsson M, et al. *Antimicrob Agents Chemother.* 2013;57(3):1559–1560 PMID: 23274665
150. Vinh H, et al. *PLoS Negl Trop Dis.* 2011;5(8):e1264 PMID: 21829747
151. Gaastra W, et al. *Vet Microbiol.* 2009;133(3):211–228 PMID: 19008054
152. American Academy of Pediatrics. Rat-bite fever. In: Kimberlin DW, et al, eds. *Red Book: 2015 Report of the Committee on Infectious Diseases.* 2015:666–667
153. Liu C, et al. *Clin Infect Dis.* 2011;52(3):e18–e55 PMID: 21208910
154. Long CB, et al. *Expert Rev Anti Infect Ther.* 2010;8(2):183–195 PMID: 20109048
155. Cheung GY, et al. *Curr Opin Infect Dis.* 2010;23(3):208–216 PMID: 20179594
156. Marchant EA, et al. *Clin Dev Immunol.* 2013;2013:586076 PMID: 23762094
157. Falagas ME, et al. *J Antimicrob Chemother.* 2008;62(5):889–894 PMID: 1866294
158. Church D, et al. *Scand J Infect Dis.* 2013;45(4):265–270 PMID: 23113657
159. American Academy of Pediatrics. Group A streptococcal infections. In: Kimberlin DW, et al, eds. *Red Book: 2015 Report of the Committee on Infectious Diseases.* 2015:732–744
160. American Academy of Pediatrics. Group B streptococcal infections. In: Kimberlin DW, et al, eds. *Red Book: 2015 Report of the Committee on Infectious Diseases.* 2015:745–750
161. Belko J, et al. *Pediatr Infect Dis J.* 2002;21(8):715–723 PMID: 12192158
162. Broyles LN, et al. *Clin Infect Dis.* 2009;48(6):706–712 PMID: 19187026
163. Stelzmueller I, et al. *Eur J Pediatr Surg.* 2009;19(1):21–24 PMID: 19221948
164. Deutschmann MW, et al. *JAMA Otolaryngol Head Neck Surg.* 2013;139(2):157–160 PMID: 23429946
165. Pichichero ME. *Pediatr Clin North Am.* 2013;60(2):391–407 PMID: 23481107
166. American Academy of Pediatrics. Pneumococcal infections. In: Kimberlin DW, et al, eds. *Red Book: 2015 Report of the Committee on Infectious Diseases.* 2015:626–638
167. Jones RN, et al. *Int J Antimicrob Agents.* 2010;36(3):197–204 PMID: 20558045
168. Kaplan SL, et al. *Pediatr Infect Dis J.* 2013;32(3):203–207 PMID: 23558320
169. Baddour LM, et al. *Circulation.* 2005;111(23):e394–e434 PMID: 15956145
170. American Academy of Pediatrics. Syphilis. In: Kimberlin DW, et al, eds. *Red Book: 2015 Report of the Committee on Infectious Diseases.* 2015:755–768
171. Turner MA, et al. *Arch Dis Child.* 2012;97(6):573–577 PMID: 21697219
172. American Academy of Pediatrics. Cholera. In: Kimberlin DW, et al, eds. *Red Book: 2015 Report of the Committee on Infectious Diseases.* 2015:860–863
173. Charles RC, et al. *Curr Opin Infect Dis.* 2011;24(5):472–477 PMID: 21799407
174. Dechet AM, et al. *Clin Infect Dis.* 2008;46(7):970–976 PMID: 18444811
175. Daniels NA. *Clin Infect Dis.* 2011;52(6):788–792 PMID: 21367733
176. Fàbrega A, et al. *Enferm Infecc Microbiol Clin.* 2012;30(1):24–32 PMID: 22019131
177. American Academy of Pediatrics. *Yersinia enterocolitica* and *Yersinia pseudotuberculosis* infections. In: Kimberlin DW, et al, eds. *Red Book: 2015 Report of the Committee on Infectious Diseases.* 2015:868–870
178. American Academy of Pediatrics. Plague. In: Kimberlin DW, et al, eds. *Red Book: 2015 Report of the Committee on Infectious Diseases.* 2015:624–626
179. Butler T. *Clin Infect Dis.* 2009;49(5):736–742 PMID: 19606935
180. Kaasch AJ, et al. *Infection.* 2012;40(2):185–190 PMID: 21789525

Chapter 8

1. Groll AH, et al. *Lancet Oncol.* 2014;15(8):e327–e340 PMID: 24988936
2. Wingard JR, et al. *Blood.* 2010;116(24):5111–5118 PMID: 20826719
3. Van Burik JA, et al. *Clin Infect Dis.* 2004;39(10):1407–1416 PMID: 15546073
4. Cornely OA, et al. *N Engl J Med.* 2007;356(4):348–359 PMID: 17251531
5. Kung HC, et al. *Cancer Med.* 2014;3(3):667–673 PMID: 24644249
6. Science M, et al. *Pediatr Blood Cancer.* 2014;61(3):393–400 PMID: 24424789
7. Bow EJ, et al. *BMC Infect Dis.* 2015;15:128 PMID: 25887385
8. Tacke D, et al. *Ann Hematol.* 2014;93(9):1449–1456 PMID: 24951122
9. Almyroudis NG, et al. *Curr Opin Infect Dis.* 2009;22(4):385–393 PMID: 19506476
10. Maschmeyer G. *J Antimicrob Chemother.* 2009;63(Suppl1):i27–i30 PMID: 19372178
11. Freifeld AG, et al. *Clin Infect Dis.* 2011;52(4):e56–e93 PMID: 21258094

12. De Pauw BE, et al. *N Engl J Med*. 2007;356(4):409–411 PMID: 17251538
13. Salavert M. *Int J Antimicrob Agents*. 2008;32(Suppl2):S149–S153 PMID: 19013340
14. Eschenauer GA, et al. *Liver Transpl*. 2009;15(8):842–858 PMID: 19642130
15. Winston DJ, et al. *Am J Transplant*. 2014;14(12):2758–2764 PMID: 25376267
16. Sun HY, et al. *Transplantation*. 2013;96(6):573–578 PMID: 23842191
17. Radack KP, et al. *Curr Infect Dis Rep*. 2009;11(6):427–434 PMID: 19857381
18. Walsh TJ, et al. *Clin Infect Dis*. 2008;46(3):327–360 PMID: 18177225
19. Thomas L, et al. *Expert Rev Anti Infect Ther*. 2009;7(4):461–472 PMID: 19400765
20. Friberg LE, et al. *Antimicrob Agents Chemother*. 2012;56(6):3032–3042 PMID: 22430956
21. Burgos A, et al. *Pediatrics*. 2008;121(5):e1286–e1294 PMID: 18450871
22. Herbrecht R, et al. *N Engl J Med*. 2002;347(6):408–415 PMID: 12167683
23. Mousset S, et al. *Ann Hematol*. 2014;93(1):13–32 PMID: 24026426
24. Blyth CC, et al. *Intern Med J*. 2014;44(12b):1333–1349 PMID: 25482744
25. Denning DW, et al. *Eur Respir J*. 2016;47(1):45–68 PMID: 26699723
26. Cornely OA, et al. *Clin Infect Dis*. 2007;44(10):1289–1297 PMID: 17443465
27. Walsh TJ, et al. *Antimicrob Agents Chemother*. 2010;54(10):4116–4123 PMID: 20660687
28. Bartelink IH, et al. *Antimicrob Agents Chemother*. 2013;57(1):235–240 PMID: 23114771
29. Marr KA, et al. *Ann Intern Med*. 2015;162(2):81–89 PMID: 25599346
30. Verweij PE, et al. *Drug Resist Updat*. 2015;21–22:30–40 PMID: 26282594
31. Kohno S, et al. *Eur J Clin Microbiol Infect Dis*. 2013;32(3):387–397 PMID: 23052987
32. Naggie S, et al. *Clin Chest Med*. 2009;30(2):337–353 PMID: 19375639
33. Revankar SG, et al. *Clin Microbiol Rev*. 2010;23(4):884–928 PMID: 20930077
34. Wong EH, et al. *Infect Dis Clin North Am*. 2016;30(1):165–178 PMID: 26897066
35. Revankar SG, et al. *Clin Infect Dis*. 2004;38(2):206–216 PMID: 14699452
36. Li DM, et al. *Lancet Infect Dis*. 2009;9(6):376–383 PMID: 19467477
37. Chowdhary A, et al. *Clin Microbiol Infect*. 2014;20(Suppl3):47–75 PMID: 24483780
38. McCarty TP, et al. *Med Mycol*. 2015;53(5):440–446 PMID: 25908651
39. Schieffelin JS, et al. *Transplant Infect Dis*. 2014;16(2):270–278 PMID: 24628809
40. Chapman SW, et al. *Clin Infect Dis*. 2008;46(12):1801–1812 PMID: 18462100
41. McKinnell JA, et al. *Clin Chest Med*. 2009;30(2):227–239 PMID: 19375630
42. Walsh CM, et al. *Pediatr Infect Dis J*. 2006;25(7):656–658 PMID: 16804444
43. Fanella S, et al. *Med Mycol*. 2011;49(6):627–632 PMID: 21208027
44. Smith JA, et al. *Proc Am Thorac Soc*. 2010;7(3):173–180 PMID: 20463245
45. Bariola JR, et al. *Clin Infect Dis*. 2010;50(6):797–804 PMID: 20166817
46. Limper AH, et al. *Am J Respir Crit Care Med*. 2011;183(1):96–128 PMID: 21193785
47. Pappas PG, et al. *Clin Infect Dis*. 2009;48(5):503–535 PMID: 19191635
48. Lortholary O, et al. *Clin Microbiol Infect*. 2012;18(Suppl7):68–77 PMID: 23137138
49. Ullman AJ, et al. *Clin Microbiol Infect*. 2012;18(Suppl7):53–67 PMID: 23137137
50. Hope WW, et al. *Clin Microbiol Infect*. 2012;18(Suppl7):38–52 PMID: 23137136
51. Cornely OA, et al. *Clin Microbiol Infect*. 2012;18(Suppl7):19–37 PMID: 23137135
52. Hope WW, et al. *Antimicrob Agents Chemother*. 2015;59(2):905–913 PMID: 25421470
53. Piper L, et al. *Pediatr Infect Dis J*. 2011;30(5):375–378 PMID: 21085048
54. Watt KM, et al. *Antimicrob Agents Chemother*. 2015;59(7):3935–3943 PMID: 25896706
55. Sobel JD. *Lancet*. 2007;369(9577):1961–1971 PMID: 17560449
56. Lopez Martinez R, et al. *Clin Dermatol*. 2007;25(2):188–194 PMID: 17350498
57. Ameen M. *Clin Exp Dermatol*. 2009;34(8):849–854 PMID: 19575535
58. Chowdhary A, et al. *Clin Microbiol Infect*. 2014;20(Suppl3):47–75 PMID: 24483780
59. Queiroz-Telles F. *Rev Inst Med Trop Sao Paulo*. 2015;57(Suppl19):46–50 PMID: 26465369
60. Galgiani JN, et al. *Clin Infect Dis*. 2005;41(9):1217–1223 PMID: 16206093
61. Anstead GM, et al. *Infect Dis Clin North Am*. 2006;20(3):621–643 PMID: 16984872
62. Williams PL. *Ann N Y Acad Sci*. 2007;1111:377–384 PMID: 17363442
63. Homans JD, et al. *Pediatr Infect Dis J*. 2010;29(1):65–67 PMID: 19884875
64. Kauffman CA, et al. *Transplant Infectious Diseases*. 2014;16(2):213–224 PMID: 24589027
65. McCarty JM, et al. *Clin Infect Dis*. 2013;56(11):1579–1585 PMID: 23463637

66. Bravo R, et al. *J Pediatr Hematol Oncol.* 2012;34(5):389–394 PMID: 22510771
67. Catanzaro A, et al. *Clin Infect Dis.* 2007;45(5):562–568 PMID: 17682989
68. Thompson GR, et al. *Clin Infect Dis.* 2016;63(3):356–362 PMID: 27169478
69. Chayakulkeeree M, et al. *Infect Dis Clin North Am.* 2006;20(3):507–544 PMID: 16984867
70. Jarvis JN, et al. *Semin Respir Crit Care Med.* 2008;29(2):141–150 PMID: 18365996
71. Perfect JR, et al. *Clin Infect Dis.* 2010;50(3):291–322 PMID: 20047480
72. Joshi NS, et al. *Pediatr Infect Dis J.* 2010;29(12):e91–e95 PMID: 20935
73. Day JN, et al. *N Engl J Med.* 2013;368(14):1291–1302 PMID: 23550668
74. Cortez KJ, et al. *Clin Microbiol Rev.* 2008;21(1):157–197 PMID: 18202441
75. Tortorano AM, et al. *Clin Microbiol Infect.* 2014;20(Suppl3):27–46 PMID: 24548001
76. Horn DL, et al. *Mycoses.* 2014;57(11):652–658 PMID: 24943384
77. Muhammed M, et al. *Medicine (Baltimore).* 2013;92(6):305–316 PMID: 24145697
78. Rodriguez-Tudela JL, et al. *Med Mycol.* 2009;47(4):359–370 PMID: 19031336
79. Wheat LJ, et al. *Clin Infect Dis.* 2007;45(7):807–825 PMID: 17806045
80. Myint T, et al. *Medicine (Baltimore).* 2014;93(1):11–18 PMID: 24378739
81. Assi M, et al. *Clin Infect Dis.* 2013;57(11):1542–1549 PMID: 24046304
82. Chayakulkeeree M, et al. *Eur J Clin Microbiol Infect Dis.* 2006;25(4):215–229 PMID: 16568297
83. Spellberg B, et al. *Clin Infect Dis.* 2009;48(12):1743–1751 PMID: 19435437
84. Reed C, et al. *Clin Infect Dis.* 2008;47(3):364–371 PMID: 18558882
85. Cornely OA, et al. *Clin Microbiol Infect.* 2014;20(Suppl3):5–26 PMID: 24479848
86. Spellberg B, et al. *Clin Infect Dis.* 2012;54(Suppl1):S73–S78 PMID: 22247449
87. Queiroz-Telles F, et al. *Clin Infect Dis.* 2007;45(11):1462–1469 PMID: 17990229
88. Menezes VM, et al. *Cochrane Database Syst Rev.* 2006;(2):CD004967 PMID: 16625617
89. Marques SA. *An Bras Dermatol.* 2013;88(5):700–711 PMID: 24173174
90. Borges SR, et al. *Med Mycol.* 2014;52(3):303–310 PMID: 24577007
91. Panel on Opportunistic Infections in HIV-Exposed and HIV-Infected Children. Guidelines for the prevention and treatment of opportunistic infections in HIV-exposed and HIV-infected children. http://aidsinfo.nih.gov/contentfiles/lvguidelines/oi_guidelines_pediatrics.pdf. Updated November 6, 2013. Accessed September 19, 2016
92. Siberry GK, et al. *Pediatr Infect Dis J.* 2013;32(Suppl2):i–KK4 PMID: 24569199
93. Kauffman CA, et al. *Clin Infect Dis.* 2007;45(10):1255–1265 PMID: 17968818
94. Aung AK, et al. *Med Mycol.* 2013;51(5):534–544 PMID: 23286352
95. Ali S, et al. *Pediatr Emerg Care.* 2007;23(9):662–668 PMID: 17876261
96. Shy R. *Pediatr Rev.* 2007;28(5):164–174 PMID: 17473121
97. Andrews MD, et al. *Am Fam Physician.* 2008;77(10):1415–1420 PMID: 18533375
98. Kakourou T, et al. *Pediatr Dermatol.* 2010;27(3):226–228 PMID: 20609140
99. Gupta AK, et al. *Pediatr Dermatol.* 2013;30(1):1–6 PMID: 22994156
100. de Berker D. *N Engl J Med.* 2009;360(20):2108–2116 PMID: 19439745
101. Ameen M, et al. *Br J Dermatol.* 2014;171(5):937–958 PMID: 25409999
102. Pantazidou A, et al. *Arch Dis Child.* 2007;92(11):1040–1042 PMID: 17954488
103. Gupta AK, et al. *J Cutan Med Surg.* 2014;18(2):79–90 PMID: 24636433

Chapter 9

1. Terrault NA, et al. *Hepatology.* 2016;63(1):261–283 PMID: 26566064
2. Lenaerts L, et al. *Rev Med Virol.* 2008;18(6):357–374 PMID: 18655013
3. Michaels MG. *Expert Rev Anti Infect Ther.* 2007;5(3):441–448 PMID: 17547508
4. Biron KK. *Antiviral Res.* 2006;71(2–3):154–163 PMID: 16765457
5. Boeckh M, et al. *Blood.* 2009;113(23):5711–5719 PMID: 19299333
6. Vaudry W, et al. *Am J Transplant.* 2009;9(3):636–643 PMID: 19260840
7. Emanuel D, et al. *Ann Intern Med.* 1988;109(10):777–782 PMID: 2847609
8. Reed EC, et al. *Ann Intern Med.* 1988;109(10):783–788 PMID: 2847610
9. *Ophthalmology.* 1994;101(7):1250–1261 PMID: 8035989
10. Musch DC, et al. *N Engl J Med.* 1997;337(2):83–90 PMID: 9211677
11. Martin DF, et al. *N Engl J Med.* 2002;346(15):1119–1126 PMID: 11948271

12. Kempen JH, et al. *Arch Ophthalmol.* 2003;121(4):466–476 PMID: 12695243
13. Studies of Ocular Complications of AIDS Research Group. The AIDS Clinical Trials Group. *Am J Ophthalmol.* 2001;131(4):457–467 PMID: 11292409
14. Dieterich DT, et al. *J Infect Dis.* 1993;167(2):278–282 PMID: 8380610
15. Gerna G, et al. *Antiviral Res.* 1997;34(1):39–50 PMID: 9107384
16. Markham A, et al. *Drugs.* 1994;48(3):455–484 PMID: 7527763
17. Kimberlin DW, et al. *J Infect Dis.* 2008;197(6):836–845 PMID: 18279073
18. Kimberlin DW, et al. *N Engl J Med.* 2015;372(10):933–943 PMID: 25738669
19. Griffiths P, et al. *Herpes.* 2008;15(1):4–12 PMID: 18983762
20. Panel on Opportunistic Infections in HIV-Exposed and HIV-Infected Children. Guidelines for the prevention and treatment of opportunistic infections in HIV-exposed and HIV-infected children. http://aidsinfo.nih.gov/contentfiles/lvguidelines/oi_guidelines_pediatrics.pdf. Updated November 6, 2013. Accessed September 19, 2016
21. Abzug MJ, et al. *J Pediatr Infect Dis Soc.* 2016;5(1):53–62 PMID: 26407253
22. Biebl A, et al. *Nat Clin Pract Neurol.* 2009;5(3):171–174 PMID: 19262593
23. Chadaide Z, et al. *J Med Virol.* 2008;80(11):1930–1932 PMID: 18814244
24. American Academy of Pediatrics. Epstein-Barr virus infections. In: Kimberlin DW, et al, eds. *Red Book: 2015 Report of the Committee on Infectious Diseases.* 2015:336–340
25. Gross TG. *Herpes.* 2009;15(3):64–67 PMID: 19306606
26. Styczynski J, et al. *Bone Marrow Transplant.* 2009;43(10):757–770 PMID: 19043458
27. Jonas MM, et al. *Hepatology.* 2016;63(2):377–387 PMID: 26223345
28. Marcellin P, et al. *Gastroenterology.* 2016;150(1):134–144.e10 PMID: 26453773
29. Chen HL, et al. *Hepatology.* 2015;62(2):375–386 PMID: 25851052
30. Wu Q, et al. *Clin Gastroenterol Hepatol.* 2015;13(6):1170–1176 PMID: 25251571
31. Hou JL, et al. *J Viral Hepat.* 2015;22(2):85–93 PMID: 25243325
32. Kurbegov AC, et al. *Expert Rev Gastroenterol Hepatol.* 2009;3(1):39–49 PMID: 19210112
33. Jonas MM, et al. *Hepatology.* 2008;47(6):1863–1871 PMID: 18433023
34. Lai CL, et al. *Gastroenterology.* 2002;123(6):1831–1838 PMID: 12454840
35. Honkoop P, et al. *Expert Opin Investig Drugs.* 2003;12(4):683–688 PMID: 12665423
36. Shaw T, et al. *Expert Rev Anti Infect Ther.* 2004;2(6):853–871 PMID: 15566330
37. Elisofon SA, et al. *Clin Liver Dis.* 2006;10(1):133–148 PMID: 16376798
38. Jonas MM, et al. *Hepatology.* 2010;52(6):2192–2205 PMID: 20890947
39. Haber BA, et al. *Pediatrics.* 2009;124(5):e1007–e1013 PMID: 19805457
40. Shneider BL, et al. *Hepatology.* 2006;44(5):1344–1354 PMID: 17058223
41. Jain MK, et al. *J Viral Hepat.* 2007;14(3):176–182 PMID: 17305883
42. Sokal EM, et al. *Gastroenterology.* 1998;114(5):988–995 PMID: 9558288
43. Jonas MM, et al. *N Engl J Med.* 2002;346(22):1706–1713 PMID: 12037150
44. Chang TT, et al. *N Engl J Med.* 2006;354(10):1001–1010 PMID: 16525137
45. Liaw YF, et al. *Gastroenterology.* 2009;136(2):486–495 PMID: 19027013
46. Keam SJ, et al. *Drugs.* 2008;68(9):1273–1317 PMID: 18547135
47. Marcellin P, et al. *Gastroenterology.* 2011;140(2):459–468 PMID: 21034744
48. Poordad F, et al. *N Engl J Med.* 2011;364(13):1195–1206 PMID: 21449783
49. Schwarz KB, et al. *Gastroenterology.* 2011;140(2):450–458 PMID: 21036173
50. Nelson DR. *Liver Int.* 2011;31(Suppl1):53–57 PMID: 21205138
51. Strader DB, et al. *Hepatology.* 2004;39(4):1147–1171 PMID: 15057920
52. Soriano V, et al. *AIDS.* 2007;21(9):1073–1089 PMID: 17502718
53. Feld JJ, et al. *N Engl J Med.* 2014;370:1594–1603 PMID: 24720703
54. Zeuzem S, et al. *N Engl J Med.* 2014;370:1604–1614 PMID: 24720679
55. Andreone P, et al. *Gastroenterology.* 2014;147:359–365.e1 PMID: 24818763
56. Ferenci P, et al. *N Engl J Med.* 2014;370:1983–1992 PMID: 24795200
57. Poordad F, et al. *N Engl J Med.* 2014;370:1973–1982 PMID: 24725237
58. Jacobson IM, et al. *Lancet.* 2014;384:403–413 PMID: 24907225
59. Manns M, et al. *Lancet.* 2014;384(9941):414–426 PMID: 24907224
60. Forns X, et al. *Gastroenterology.* 2014;146:1669–1679.e3 PMID: 24602923

61. Zeuzem S, et al. *Gastroenterology.* 2014;146:430–441.e6 PMID: 24184810

62. Lawitz E, et al. *Lancet.* 2014;384:1756–1765 PMID: 25078309

63. Afdhal N, et al. *N Engl J Med.* 2014;370:1889–1898 PMID: 24725239

64. Afdhal N, et al. *N Engl J Med.* 2014;370:1483–1493 PMID: 24725238

65. Kowdley KV, et al. *N Engl J Med.* 2014;370:1879–1888 PMID: 24720702

66. Lawitz E, et al. *N Engl J Med.* 2013;368:1878–1887 PMID: 23607594

67. Jacobson IM, et al. *N Engl J Med.* 2013;368:1867–1877 PMID: 23607593

68. Zeuzem S, et al. *N Engl J Med.* 2014;370:1993–2001 PMID: 24795201

69. Hollier LM, et al. *Cochrane Database Syst Rev.* 2008;(1):CD004946 PMID: 18254066

70. Pinninti SG, et al. Neonatal herpes disease despite maternal antenatal antiviral suppressive therapy: a multicenter case series of the first such infants reported. Paper presented at: 48th Annual Meeting of The Infectious Diseases Society of America; October 22, 2010; Vancouver, British Columbia

71. Pinninti SG, et al. *J Pediatr.* 2012;161(1):134–138 PMID: 22336576

72. Kimberlin DW, et al. *Clin Infect Dis.* 2010;50(2):221–228 PMID: 20014952

73. Abdel Massih RC, et al. *World J Gastroenterol.* 2009;15(21):2561–2569 PMID: 19496184

74. Mofenson LM, et al. *MMWR Recomm Rep.* 2009;58(RR-11):1–166 PMID: 19730409

75. Kuhar DT, et al. *Infect Control Hosp Epidemiol.* 2013;34(9):875–892 PMID: 23917901

76. Acosta EP, et al. *J Infect Dis.* 2010;202(4):563–566 PMID: 20594104

77. Kimberlin DW, et al. *J Infect Dis.* 2013;207(5):709–720 PMID: 23230059

78. McPherson C, et al. *J Infect Dis.* 2012;206(6):847–850 PMID: 22807525

79. Blumer J, et al. Safety, tolerability and pharmacokinetics (PK) of intravenous zanamivir (IVZ) treatment in hospitalized pediatric and adolescent patients with influenza: a phase II open-label, multicenter, single-arm study. Presented at: IDWeek 2016; October 26–30, 2016; New Orleans, LA

80. American Academy of Pediatrics. Measles. In: Kimberlin DW, et al, eds. *Red Book: 2015 Report of the Committee on Infectious Diseases.* 2015:535–547

81. American Academy of Pediatrics Committee on Infectious Diseases and Bronchiolitis Guidelines Committee. *Pediatrics.* 2014;134(2):415–420 PMID: 25070315

82. American Academy of Pediatrics Committee on Infectious Diseases and Bronchiolitis Guidelines Committee. *Pediatrics.* 2014;134(2):e620–e638 PMID: 25070304

83. Whitley RJ. *Adv Exp Med Biol.* 2008;609:216–232 PMID: 18193668

Chapter 10

1. Blessmann J, et al. *J Clin Microbiol.* 2003;41(10):4745–4750 PMID: 14532214

2. Haque R, et al. *N Engl J Med.* 2003;348(16):1565–1573 PMID: 1270037

3. Rossignol JF, et al. *Trans R Soc Trop Med Hyg.* 2007;101(10):1025–1031 PMID: 17658567

4. Mackey-Lawrence NM, et al. *BMJ Clin Evid.* 2011;pii:0918 PMID: 21477391

5. Fox LM, et al. *Clin Infect Dis.* 2005;40(8):1173–1180 PMID: 15791519

6. Barnett ND, et al. *Pediatr Neurol.* 1996;15(3):230–234 PMID: 8916161

7. Vargas-Zepeda J, et al. *Arch Med Res.* 2005;36(1):83–86 PMID: 15900627

8. Visvesvara GS, et al. *FEMS Immunol Med Microbiol.* 2007;50:1–26 PMID: 17428307

9. Linam WM, et al. *Pediatrics.* 2015;135(3):e744–e748 PMID: 25667249

10. Deetz TR, et al. *Clin Infect Dis.* 2003;37(10):1304–1312 PMID: 14583863

11. Chotmongkol V, et al. *Am J Trop Med Hyg.* 2009;81(3):443–445 PMID: 19706911

12. Lo Re V III, et al. *Am J Med.* 2003;114(3):217–223 PMID: 12637136

13. Jitpimolmard S, et al. *Parasitol Res.* 2007;100(6):1293–1296 PMID: 17177056

14. Checkley AM, et al. *J Infect.* 2010;60(1):1–20 PMID: 19931548

15. Bethony J, et al. *Lancet.* 2006;367(9521):1521–1532 PMID: 16679166

16. Krause PJ, et al. *N Engl J Med.* 2000;343(20):1454–1458 PMID: 11078770

17. Vannier E, et al. *Infect Dis Clin North Am.* 2008;22(3):469–488 PMID: 18755385

18. Wormser GP, et al. *Clin Infect Dis.* 2006;43(9):1089–1134 PMID: 17029180

19. Fisk T, et al. *Cyclospora cayetanensis, Isospora belli, Sarcocystis species, Balantidium coli,* and *Blastocystis hominis.* In: Mandell GL, et al, eds. *Principles and Practice of Infectious Diseases.* 2005:3228–3237

20. Murray WJ, et al. *Clin Infect Dis.* 2004;39(10):1484–1492 PMID: 15546085

21. Park SY, et al. *Pediatrics.* 2000;106(4):e56 PMID: 11015551
22. Shlim DR, et al. *Clin Infect Dis.* 1995;21(1):97–101 PMID: 7578767
23. Udkow MP, et al. *J Infect Dis.* 1993;168(1):242–244 PMID: 8515120
24. Bern C, et al. *JAMA.* 2007;298(18):2171–2181 PMID: 18000201
25. Maguire JH. Trypanosoma. In: Gorbach SL, Bartlett JG, Blacklow NR, eds. *Infectious Diseases.* 3rd ed. 2004:2327–2334
26. Miller DA, et al. *Clin Infect Dis.* 2015;60(8):1237–1240 PMID: 25601454
27. Smith HV, et al. *Curr Opin Infect Dis.* 2004;17(6):557–564 PMID: 15640710
28. Davies AP, et al. *BMJ.* 2009;339:b4168 PMID: 19841008
29. Bushen OY, et al. Cryptosporidiosis. In: Guerrant RL, Walker DH, Weller PF, eds. *Tropical Infectious Diseases.* 2006:1003–1014
30. Abubakar I, et al. *Cochrane Database Syst Rev.* 2007;(1):CD004932 PMID: 17253532
31. Jelinek T, et al. *Clin Infect Dis.* 1994;19(6):1062–1066 PMID: 7534125
32. Schuster A, et al. *Clin Infect Dis.* 2013;57(8):1155–1157 PMID: 23811416
33. Eberhard ML, et al. *Curr Opin Infect Dis.* 2002;15(5):519–522 PMID: 12686886
34. Ortega YR, et al. *Clin Microbiol Rev.* 2010;23(1):218–234 PMID: 20065331
35. Nash TE, et al. *Neurology.* 2006;67(7):1120–1127 PMID: 17030744
36. Garcia HH, et al. *Lancet Neurol.* 2014;13(12):1202–1215 PNID: 25453460
37. Lillie P, et al. *J Infect.* 2010;60(5):403–404 PMID: 20153773
38. Mitchell WG, et al. *Pediatrics.* 1988;82(1):76–82 PMID: 3288959
39. Stark DJ, et al. *Trends Parasitol.* 2006;22(2):92–96 PMID: 16380293
40. Johnson EH, et al. *Clin Microbiol Rev.* 2004;17(3):553–570 PMID: 15258093
41. Smego RA Jr, et al. *Clin Infect Dis.* 2003;37(8):1073–1083 PMID: 14523772
42. Brunetti E, et al. *Acta Trop.* 2010;114(1):1–16 PMID: 19931502
43. Grencis RK, et al. *Gastroenterol Clin North Am.* 1996;25(3):579–597 PMID: 8863041
44. Tisch DJ, et al. *Lancet Infect Dis.* 2005;5(8):514–523 PMID: 16048720
45. Mand S, et al. *Clin Infect Dis.* 2012;55(5):621–630 PMID: 22610930
46. Ottesen EA, et al. *Annu Rev Med.* 1992;43:417–424 PMID: 1580599
47. Jong EC, et al. *J Infect Dis.* 1985;152(3):637–640 PMID: 3897401
48. Calvopina M, et al. *Trans R Soc Trop Med Hyg.* 1998;92(5):566–569 PMID: 9861383
49. Johnson RJ, et al. *Rev Infect Dis.* 1985;7(2):200–206 PMID: 4001715
50. Graham CS, et al. *Clin Infect Dis.* 2001;33(1):1–5 PMID: 11389487
51. Gardner TB, et al. *Clin Microbiol Rev.* 2001;14(1):114–128 PMID: 11148005
52. Ross AG, et al. *N Engl J Med.* 2013;368(19):1817–1825 PMID: 23656647
53. Abboud P, et al. *Clin Infect Dis.* 2001;32(12):1792–1794 PMID: 11360222
54. Hotez PJ, et al. *N Engl J Med.* 2004;351(8):799–807 PMID: 15317893
55. Keiser J, et al. *JAMA.* 2008;299(16):1937–1948 PMID: 18430913
56. Steinmann P, et al. *PLoS One.* 2011;6(9):e25003 PMID: 21980373
57. World Health Organization, Technical Report Series 949. Control of the leishmaniases. Report of a meeting of the WHO Expert Committee on the Control of Leishmaniases, Geneva, 22–26 March 2010
58. Alrajhi AA, et al. *N Engl J Med.* 2002;346(12):891–895 PMID: 11907288
59. Bern C, et al. *Clin Infect Dis.* 2006;43(7):917–924 PMID: 16941377
60. Ritmeijer K, et al. *Clin Infect Dis.* 2006;43(3):357–364 PMID: 16804852
61. Monge-Maillo B, et al. *Clin Infect Dis.* 2015;60(9):1398–1404 PMID: 25601455
62. Sundar S, et al. *N Engl J Med.* 2002;347(22):1739–1746 PMID: 12456849
63. Sundar S, et al. *N Engl J Med.* 2007;356(25):2571–2581 PMID: 17582067
64. Foucault C, et al. *J Infect Dis.* 2006;193(3):474–476 PMID: 16388498
65. Fischer PR, et al. *Clin Infect Dis.* 2002;34(4):493–498 PMID: 11797176
66. Freedman DO. *N Engl J Med.* 2008;359(6):603–612 PMID: 18687641
67. Overbosch D, et al. *Clin Infect Dis.* 2001;33(7):1015–1021 PMID: 11528574
68. Arguin PM, et al. Malaria. In: Brunette GW, ed. *CDC Health Information for International Travel 2016: The Yellow Book.* 2016:236–254. http://wwwnc.cdc.gov/travel/yellowbook/2016/infectious-diseases-related-to-travel/malaria. Accessed September 19, 2016
69. Griffith KS, et al. *JAMA.* 2007;297(20):2264–2277 PMID: 17519416

70. Usha V, et al. *J Am Acad Dermatol.* 2000;42(2pt1):236–240 PMID: 10642678
71. Brodine SK, et al. *Am J Trop Med Hyg.* 2009;80(3):425–430 PMID: 19270293
72. Doenhoff MJ, et al. *Expert Rev Anti Infect Ther.* 2006;4(2):199–210 PMID: 16597202
73. Fenwick A, et al. *Curr Opin Infect Dis.* 2006;19(6):577–582 PMID: 17075334
74. Marti H, et al. *Am J Trop Med Hyg.* 1996;55(5):477–481 PMID: 8940976
75. Segarra-Newnham M. *Ann Pharmacother.* 2007;41(12):1992–2001 PMID: 17940124
76. Barisani-Asenbauer T, et al. *J Ocul Pharmacol Ther.* 2001;17(3):287–294 PMID: 11436948
77. McAuley JB. *Pediatr Infect Dis J.* 2008;27(2):161–162 PMID: 18227714
78. McLeod R, et al. *Clin Infect Dis.* 2006;42(10):1383–1394 PMID: 16619149
79. Petersen E. *Expert Rev Anti Infect Ther.* 2007;5(2):285–293 PMID: 17402843
80. Adachi JA, et al. *Clin Infect Dis.* 2003;37(9):1165–1171 PMID: 14557959
81. Diemert DJ. *Clin Microbiol Rev.* 2006;19(3):583–594 PMID: 16847088
82. DuPont HL. *Clin Infect Dis.* 2007;45(Suppl1):S78–S84 PMID: 17582576
83. Gottstein B, et al. *Clin Microbiol Rev.* 2009;22(1):127–145 PMID: 19136437
84. Fairlamb AH. *Trends Parasitol.* 2003;19(11):488–494 PMID: 14580959
85. Pépin J, et al. *Adv Parasitol.* 1994;33:1–47 PMID: 8122565
86. Bisser S, et al. *J Infect Dis.* 2007;195(3):322–329 PMID: 17205469
87. Sahlas DJ, et al. *N Engl J Med.* 2002;347(10):749–753 PMID: 12213947

Chapter 13

1. Tetzlaff TR, et al. *J Pediatr.* 1978;92(3):485–490 PMID: 632997
2. Ballock RT, et al. *J Pediatr Orthop.* 2009;29(6):636–642 PMID: 19700997
3. Peltola H, et al. *N Engl J Med.* 2014;370(4):352–360 PMID: 24450893
4. Bradley JS, et al. *Pediatrics.* 2011;128(4):e1034–e1045 PMID: 21949152
5. Rice HE, et al. *Arch Surg.* 2001;136(12):1391–1395 PMID: 11735866
6. Fraser JD, et al. *J Pediatr Surg.* 2010;45(6):1198–1202 PMID: 20620320
7. Strohmeier Y, et al. *Cochrane Database Syst Rev.* 2014;7:CD003772 PMID: 25066627
8. Drusano GL, et al. *J Infect Dis.* 2014;210(8):1319–1324 PMID: 24760199
9. Arnold JC, et al. *Pediatrics.* 2012;130(4):e821–e828 PMID: 22966033
10. Zaoutis T, et al. *Pediatrics.* 2009;123(2):636–642 PMID: 19171632
11. Liu C, et al. *Clin Infect Dis.* 2011;52(3):e18–e55 [Erratum: *Clin Infect Dis.* 2011;53(3):319] PMID: 21208910
12. Syrogiannopoulos GA, et al. *Lancet.* 1988;1(8575–8576):37–40 PMID: 2891899

Chapter 14

1. Oehler RL, et al. *Lancet Infect Dis.* 2009;9(7):439–447 PMID: 19555903
2. Wu PS, et al. *Pediatr Emerg Care.* 2011;27(9):801–803 PMID: 21878832
3. Stevens DL, et al. *Clin Infect Dis.* 2014;59(2):147–159 PMID: 24947530
4. Talan DA, et al. *Clin Infect Dis.* 2003;37(11):1481–1489 PMID: 14614671
5. Aziz H, et al. *J Trauma Acute Care Surg.* 2015;78(3):641–648 PMID: 25710440
6. American Academy of Pediatrics. Rabies. In: Kimberlin DW, eds. *Red Book: 2015 Report of the Committee on Infectious Diseases.* 2015:658–666
7. American Academy of Pediatrics. Tetanus. In: Kimberlin DW, eds. *Red Book: 2015 Report of the Committee on Infectious Diseases.* 2015:773–778
8. Wilson W, et al. *Circulation.* 2007;116(15):1736–1754 PMID: 17446442
9. Pasquali SK, et al. *Am Heart J.* 2012;163(5):894–899 PMID: 22607869
10. Pant S, et al. *J Am Coll Cardiol.* 2015;65(19):2070–2076 PMID: 25975469
11. Dayer MJ, et al. *Lancet.* 2015;385(9974):1219–1228 PMID: 25467569
12. Cohn AC, et al. *MMWR Recomm Rep.* 2013;62(RR-2):1–28 PMID: 23515099
13. American Academy of Pediatrics. Pertussis (whooping cough). In: Kimberlin DW, et al, eds. *Red Book: 2015 Report of the Committee on Infectious Diseases.* 2015:608–621
14. Centers for Disease Control and Prevention. Pertussis (whooping cough). Postexposure antimicrobial prophylaxis. http://www.cdc.gov/pertussis/outbreaks/PEP.html. Updated September 8, 2015. Accessed September 19, 2016

15. Brook I. *Expert Rev Anti Infect Ther*. 2008;6(3):327–336 PMID: 18588497
16. American Academy of Pediatrics. Tetanus. In: Kimberlin DW, et al, eds. *Red Book: 2015 Report of the Committee on Infectious Diseases*. 2015:773–778
17. Centers for Disease Control and Prevention. Tuberculosis (TB). Treatment for latent TB infection. http://www.cdc.gov/tb/topic/treatment/ltbi.htm. Updated March 8, 2016. Accessed September 19, 2016
18. American Academy of Pediatrics. Tuberculosis. In: Kimberlin DW, et al, eds. *Red Book: 2015 Report of the Committee on Infectious Diseases*. 2015:805–831
19. Centers for Disease Control and Prevention. *MMWR Morb Mortal Wkly Rep*. 2011;60(48):1650–1653 PMID: 22157884
20. ACOG Committee on Practice Bulletins. *Obstet Gynecol*. 2007;109(6):1489–1498 PMID: 17569194
21. Kimberlin DW, et al. *Pediatrics*. 2013;131(2):e635–e646 PMID: 23359576
22. American Academy of Academy Committee on Infectious Diseases. *Pediatrics*. 2015;136(4):792–808 PMID: 26347430
23. Kimberlin DW, et al. *J Infect Dis*. 2013;207(5):709–720 PMID: 23230059
24. American Academy of Pediatrics. Rabies. In: Kimberlin DW, et al, eds. *Red Book: 2015 Report of the Committee on Infectious Diseases*. 2015:658–666
25. American Academy of Pediatrics. *Pneumocystis jirovecii* infections. In: Kimberlin DW, et al, eds. *Red Book: 2015 Report of the Committee on Infectious Diseases*. 2015:638–644
26. Siberry GK, et al. *Pediatr Infect Dis J*. 2013;32(Suppl2):i–KK4 PMID: 24569199
27. Leach AJ, et al. *Cochrane Database Syst Rev*. 2006;(4):CD004401 PMID: 17054203
28. McDonald S, et al. *Cochrane Database Syst Rev*. 2008;(4):CD004741 PMID: 18843668
29. Williams GJ, et al. *Adv Exp Med Biol*. 2013;764:211–218 PMID: 23654070
30. Craig JC, et al. *N Engl J Med*. 2009;361(18):1748–1759 PMID: 19864673
31. RIVUR Trial Investigators, et al. *N Engl J Med*. 2014;370(25):2367–2376 PMID: 24795142
32. American Academy of Pediatrics Subcommittee on Urinary Tract Infection and Steering Committee on Quality Improvement and Management. *Pediatrics*. 2011;128(3):595–610 PMID: 21873693
33. *Treat Guidel Med Lett*. 2012;10(122):73–80 PMID: 22996382
34. Mangram AJ, et al. *Infect Control Hosp Epidemiol*. 1999;20(4):250–280 PMID: 10219875
35. Edwards FH, et al. *Ann Thorac Surg*. 2006;81(1):397–404 PMID: 16368422
36. Engelman R, et al. *Ann Thorac Surg*. 2007;83(4):1569–1576 PMID: 17383396
37. Hansen E, et al. *J Orthop Res*. 2014;32(Suppl1):S31–S59 PMID: 24464896
38. Saleh A, et al. *Ann Surg*. 2015;261(1):72–80 PMID: 25119119
39. Haley RW, et al. *Am J Epidemiol*. 1985;121(2):206–215 PMID: 4014116
40. Dellinger EP. *Ann Surg*. 2008;247(6):927–928 PMID: 18520218
41. Shaffer WO, et al. *Spine J*. 2013;13(10):1387–1392 PMID: 23988461

Chapter 15

1. Best EJ, et al. *Pediatr Infect Dis J*. 2011;30(10):827–832 PMID: 21577177
2. Zakova M, et al. *Ther Drug Monit*. 2014;36(3):288–294 PMID: 24695354
3. Smyth AR, et al. *Cochrane Database Syst Rev*. 2012;2:CD002009 PMID: 22336782
4. Workowski KA, et al. *MMWR Recomm Rep*. 2015;64(RR-3):1–137 PMID: 26042815
5. Gruchalla RS, et al. *N Engl J Med*. 2006;354(6):601–609 PMID: 16467547
6. Solensky R. *J Allergy Clin Immunol*. 2012;130(1):1442 PMID: 23195529
7. *Med Lett Drugs Ther*. 2012;54(1406):101 PMID: 23282790
8. Bradley JS, et al. *Pediatrics*. 2009;123(4):e609–e613 PMID: 19289450
9. Wong VK, et al. *Pediatr Infect Dis J*. 1991;10(2):122–125 PMID: 2062603
10. Bradley JS, et al. *Pediatrics*. 2014;134(1):e146–e153 PMID: 24918220
11. Bradley JS, et al. *Pediatrics*. 2011;128(4):e1034–e1045 PMID: 21949152
12. Jacobs RF, et al. *Pediatr Infect Dis J*. 2005;24(1):34–39 PMID: 15665708
13. American Academy of Pediatrics. Pertussis (whooping cough). In: Kimberlin DW, et al, eds. *Red Book: 2015 Report of the Committee on Infectious Diseases*. 2015:608–621
14. Nambiar S, et al. *Pediatrics*. 2011;127(6):1528–1532 PMID: 21555496
15. Williams K, et al. *Clin Infect Dis*. 2014;58(7):997–1002 PMID: 24363331
16. Sheu J, et al. *J Am Acad Dermatol*. 2015;72(2):314–320 PMID: 25481710

Index

Index